Dyslipidemia
A CLINICAL APPROACH

Dyslipidemia

A CLINICAL APPROACH

Merle Myerson, MD, EdD, FACC, FNLA

Director
Preventive Cardiology Program & Lipid Clinic
Pre-Exercise Heart Screening Program
Medical Director
Bassett Research Institute, Clinical Research Division
Attending Cardiologist
Bassett Medical Center
Division of Cardiology
Bassett Research Institute
Cooperstown, New York

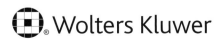 Wolters Kluwer

Philadelphia • Baltimore • New York • London
Buenos Aires • Hong Kong • Sydney • Tokyo

Senior Acquisitions Editor: Sharon Zinner
Development Editor: Ashley Fischer
Editorial Coordinators: Emily Buccieri and Kerry McShane
Marketing Manager: Dan Dressler
Production Project Manager: Barton Dudlick
Design Coordinator: Holly McLaughlin
Manufacturing Coordinator: Beth Welsh
Prepress Vendor: SPi Global

Copyright © 2019 by Wolters Kluwer

9 8 7 6 5 4 3 2 1

Printed in China

Library of Congress Cataloging-in-Publication Data
Names: Myerson, Merle, editor.
Title: Dyslipidemia : a clinical approach / [edited by] Merle Myerson.
Other titles: Dyslipidemia (Myerson)
Description: Philadelphia : Wolters Kluwer, [2019] | Includes bibliographical references and index.
Identifiers: LCCN 2017054294 | ISBN 9781496347442 (paperback)
Subjects: | MESH: Dyslipidemias—diagnosis | Dyslipidemias—therapy | Handbooks
Classification: LCC RC632.L5 | NLM WD 101 | DDC 616.3/997—dc23 LC record available at https://lccn.loc.gov/2017054294

LWW.com

This book is dedicated to my parents, Natalie and Samuel, for helping me to become a physician.

To the individuals who inspired and helped me become a cardiologist and specialist in the prevention of cardiovascular disease: Bernard Gutin, Thomas Pearson, Peter Arquin, and Henry Ginsberg and those who helped in so many other ways: Heejung Bang, Patrick McNulty, Anne Gadomski, Maria Tripp, Bo, and Cam Myerson.

To Bassett Medical Center and all my dear friends and family in Cooperstown, New York.

To the students and medical trainees for whom I hope I have imparted knowledge and inspiration to prevent the pain, suffering, and premature death due to cardiovascular disease.

To the authors, many from the national lipid association, who gave of their time and energy contributing to this text. Thank you for working with me and all the "back and forth" to make chapters better. I sincerely appreciate your help.

To Wolters Kluwer for giving me the opportunity to edit this book.

To my friends and colleagues in the National Lipid Association for helping to bring me and our field to new levels of excellence.

And, to my patients. After all, you are the reason why.

Contributors

Seth J. Baum, MD
Clinical Affiliate Professor
Charles E. Schmidt College of Medicine
Florida Atlantic University

Chief Medical Officer & President
Preventive Cardiology

Principal Investigator & Chief Medical Officer
Excel Medical Clinical Trials LLC
Boca Raton, Florida

President
The American Society for Preventive
 Cardiology (ASPC)
Jacksonville, Florida

Maria A. Bella, MS, RD, CDN
Founder
Top Balance Nutrition
New York City, New York

Piers R. Blackett, MB, ChB, FAAP, FNLA
Clinical Professor of Pediatrics
Endocrinology and Diabetes Section
Department of Pediatrics
University of Oklahoma Health Sciences Center
Oklahoma City, Oklahoma

Ashley Buffomante, MD
Clinical Instructor
Department of Internal Medicine
The Ohio State University
Columbus, Ohio

Valerie Bush, PhD
Bassett Healthcare Network
Cooperstown, New York

Emanuel M. Ebin, MD
Charles E. Schmidt College of Medicine
Florida Atlantic University
Boca Raton, Florida

Vanessa Hurta, MS, RN-BC, FNP-BC, CLS
Nurse Practitioner
Bellevue Hospital Center Lipid Clinic
New York City, New York

Marina Kawaguchi-Suzuki, PharmD, PhD
Assistant Professor
Pacific University School of Pharmacy
Hillsboro, Oregon

Kenneth Kellick, PharmD, CLS, FNLA
Clinical Pharmacy Program Manager
VA Western New York Healthcare System
Buffalo, New York

Aarthi Madhana Kumar, MBBS
Resident
Department of Medicine
Allegheny Health Network
Pittsburgh, Pennsylvania

Catherine McNeal, MD, PhD
Department of Pediatrics
Department of Internal Medicine, Division of
 Cardiology
Baylor Scott & White Health
Temple, Texas

Merle Myerson, MD, EdD, FACC, FNLA
Director
Preventive Cardiology Program & Lipid Clinic
Pre-Exercise Heart Screening Program
Medical Director
Bassett Research Institute, Clinical Research
 Division
Attending Cardiologist
Bassett Medical Center
Division of Cardiology
Bassett Research Institute
Cooperstown, New York

Madhan Nellaiyappan, MBBS
Resident
Department of Medicine
Allegheny Health Network
Pittsburgh, Pennsylvania

Connie B. Newman, MD
Adjunct Professor of Medicine
Division of Endocrinology, Diabetes and
 Metabolism
Department of Medicine
New York University School of Medicine
New York City, New York

Indu G. Poornima, MD, FACC
Associate Professor of Medicine
Division of Cardiology
Allegheny Health Network
Pittsburgh, Pennsylvania

**Joyce L. Ross, MSN, CRNP, CLS, FNLA,
FPCNA**
Immediate Past President
National Lipid Association
University of Pennsylvania (Retired)
Philadelphia, Pennsylvania

Kavita Sharma, MD, FACC
Diplomate
American Board of Clinical Lipidology
Jacksonville, Florida

Daniel Soffer, MD, FNLA, FACP
Clinical Associate Professor of Medicine
University of Pennsylvania Health System
Philadelphia, Pennsylvania

Nilay Sutaria, MD
Resident
Department of Medicine
Hospital of the University of Pennsylvania
Philadelphia, Pennsylvania

Sara Talken, MD
Department of Obstetrics and Gynecology
The University of Oklahoma Health Science
 Center
Oklahoma City, Oklahoma

Jonathan A. Tobert, MD, PhD
Academic Visitor
Nuffield Department of Population Health
University of Oxford
Oxford, United Kingdom

Ryan Turner, CSSD, CDN, RD
Senior Dietitian
Top Balance Nutrition
Sports Dietitian
New York University
New York City, New York

Michelle L. Warren, PharmD
Pharmacist
CVS Health
East Haven, Connecticut

Wayne S. Warren, MD
Assistant Clinical Professor
Yale University School of Medicine
New Haven, Connecticut

Matthew C. Weiss, MD
Fellow of Preventive Cardiology
Cardiology
New York University
New York City, New York

Robert A. Wild, MD, MPH, PhD
Presidential Professor
Chief of Gynecology
VA Med Center
Oklahoma University Health Sciences Center
Oklahoma City, Oklahoma

Don P. Wilson, MD, FNLA
Diplomate
American Board of Clinical Lipidology
Endowed Chair
Cardiovascular Health and Risk Prevention
 Program
Pediatric Endocrinology and Diabetes
Cook Children's Medical Center
Fort Worth, Texas

Preface

This book was written for practitioners and health care trainees at all levels and from all backgrounds who take care of patients with abnormal lipids. The goal was to provide clinically relevant information in a "user friendly" format along with some background information, evidence from the literature, and comment when there is conflicting or debated recommendations and, at times, author opinion.

The diagnosis and management of dyslipidemia continues to be a rapidly evolving field with new drugs, new guidelines, new markers, targets, and goals, and new risk stratification schemes. However, the basic tenet of the field of lipidology remains—that lowering the burden of atherosclerotic lipid particles is associated with reduction of risk for cardiovascular disease.

Chapters are written in an outline format to allow the reader to easily identify information that is needed at any one time but to also provide more in-depth discussion that can also be accessed as needed. Chapters start with "Key Points" to highlight areas that the authors felt

were of primary importance. Tables and algorithms are embedded to summarize information and for easy reference. Each chapter is intended to be used on its own so that some duplication of information exists along with cross references to other chapters.

For those who would like to continue to learn about lipids and prevention of cardiovascular disease, consider joining The National Lipid Association (NLA) (www.lipid.org). The NLA is a premier United States organization dedicated to enhance the practice of lipid management in clinical medicine. They are a multi-disciplinary organization including health care professionals from a wide variety of backgrounds.

The association holds many national and regional conferences, issues recommendations and expert statements, and offers numerous educational resources.

This is the first edition of this text and comments and suggestions on how to improve the content are welcome (merle.myerson@bassett.org).

Acronym List

3-Hydroxy-methylglutaryl-CoA (HMG Co-A)

Angiopoietin-like proteins (AngPTL)

Apolipoprotein A-I (apoA-I)

Apolipoprotein A-II (apoA-II)

Apolipoprotein A-V (apoA-V)

Apolipoprotein B (apoB)

Apolipoprotein B (apoB)

Atherosclerotic cardiovascular disease (ASCVD)

ATP-Binding Cassette luminal transporter type G5 and/or G8 (ABCG5/8)

ATP-Binding Cassette transporter subtype 1 (ABCA1)

Autosomal recessive hypercholesterolemia (ARH)

Cardiovascular (CV)

Cholesterol esters (CE)

Cholesteryl ester transfer protein (CETP)

Chylomicrons (CM)

Cytochrome p450 7 α-hydroxylase (aka CYP7A1)

Familial Chylomicronemia Syndrome (FCS)

Fatty acids (FA)

Free cholesterol (FC)

Free Fatty Acid (FFA)

Glycosylphosphatidylinositol-anchored HDL-binding protein 1 (GPI-HBP1)

Hepatic lipase (HL)

High-density lipoprotein cholesterol (HDL-C)

Hormone sensitive lipase (HSL)

Intermediate density lipoprotein (IDL)

LDL-cholesterol (LDL-C)

LDL-particle (LDL-P)

LDL-receptor (LDL-R)

LDL-receptor–related protein (LRP)

Lecithin cholesterol acyltransferase (LCAT)

Lipase maturation factor (LMF1)

Lipoprotein (a) [Lp(a)]

Lipoprotein lipase (LPL)

Lipoprotein X [LpX]

Lipoproteins (LP)

Liver X receptor (LXR)

Low-density lipoprotein (LDL)

Microsomal triglycerides transfer protein (MTTP)

National Lipid Association (NLA)

Niemann Pick C1-like 1 (NPC1L1)

Peroxisome-proliferating activator receptor (PPAR)

Proprotein convertase subtilisin kexin-9 (PCSK9)

Proprotein convertase subtilisin kexin-9 inhibitor (PCSK9-I)

Randomized placebo-controlled trial (RCT)

Reverse cholesterol transport (RCT)

Scavenger receptor type B1 (SR-B1)

Small dense LDL (sdLDL)

Sterol regulatory element-binding protein 2 (SREBP-2)

TG-rich lipoproteins (TRL)

Triglycerides (TG)

US Food and Drug Administration (FDA)

Very–low-density lipoprotein (VLDL)

Contents

CHAPTER 1

A Historical Perspective on Lipids and Cardiovascular Disease

Merle Myerson

Key Points

- The association of lipids with CVD became evident in the mid-19th century.
- The Framingham Heart Study was initiated in 1948 and helped to establish that blood cholesterol was a risk factor for coronary heart disease. Other observational studies followed that confirmed the association between lipids and CVD.
- The first lipid-lowering medication was developed in the late 1950s.
- Lovastatin, the first statin drug, was approved by the FDA in 1987.
- Later epidemiologic studies provided evidence that reducing cholesterol could lower mortality due to CVD.
- The National Cholesterol Education Program, Adult Treatment Panel of the NIH first published guidelines in 1988. There have since been many national guidelines for the diagnosis and management of dyslipidemia.

I.   Discovery of Blood Lipids

The history of lipids is relatively short when compared to that of other medical fields. Cholesterol was isolated from gallstones in 1784. In 1928, Michael Macheboeuf of the Pasteur Institute first described plasma lipoproteins. In 1949, John Gofman at University of California Berkeley used the newly developed ultracentrifuge to separate plasma lipoproteins by flotation.

A key advancement in the field was the work of Michael S. Brown and Joseph L. Goldstein who in 1973 showed that the defect in familial hypercholesterolemia was a deficiency in the specific receptor that recognizes LDL apolipoprotein B. This established the framework for subsequent work on cholesterol and lipoprotein metabolism.

II.   Drug Development

The 3-hydroxy-3-methylglutaryl-coenzyme A (HMG-CoA) was discovered in the early 1950s by a team led by Joseph L. Rabinowitz; however, the first FDA-approved lipid drug was cholestyramine, a bile acid sequestrant that was developed at Merck in the late 1950s. Niacin was shown to reduce lipid accumulation in the rabbit aorta in 1955. It was not until the 1970s that an inhibitor to HMG-CoA reductase was discovered, and the first statin drug, lovastatin, was approved by the FDA in 1987.

III.   Association of Lipids with Cardiovascular Disease

A. The association between risk factors and cardiovascular disease became evident by mid-19th century. Jeremy Morris' landmark study of the London transport workers initiated the modern epidemiology studies of cardiovascular risk. He found that there were more fatal myocardial infarction and more episodes of sudden death in the sedentary bus drivers when compared to the conductors who climbed up and down the steps of the double-decker buses.[1]

B. Many studies followed, and there became interest in the United States to set up a large cohort in which to study CVD risk factors. In 1948, the U.S. Public Health Service chose Framingham, Massachusetts, a town of 10 000 people, 21 miles west of Boston for a major epidemiologic study. For the first time, a large group of healthy men and women were studied prospectively. The study began in 1952, enrolled 5209 men and women aged 30-59, free of clinical CVD, and followed them with periodic interviews and extensive medical exams and blood testing. Subsequent generations have been followed, and the study has been supported by the National Heart, Lung, and Blood Institute of the NIH. The Framingham Heart Study established that blood cholesterol was a risk factor for coronary heart disease.[2]

C. Another large observational study was that led by Ancel Keys, the Seven Countries Study during the 1950s and 1960s that demonstrated the association between dietary fat, dyslipidemia, and coronary heart disease.[3]

D. The Stanford Three Community Project in the early to mid-1970s was another key project. A multimedia campaign was conducted for 2 years in two California communities. A third community was used as a control. Campaigns were designed to increase knowledge of the risk factors for CVD, to change risk-producing behaviors (smoking), and to decrease intake of calories, salt, saturated fat, and cholesterol. A composite total mortality risk score decreased by 15% in the intervention communities.[4]

E. The Lipid Research Clinics Coronary Primary Prevention Trial was the first large-scale, double-blind, placebo-controlled trial to address the lipid hypothesis and was conducted between 1973 and 1983 by the NHLBI. The trial involved 3600 men aged 39-59 years with high total cholesterol (>265 mg/dL) but no clinically evident CAD. The study showed that by lowering blood cholesterol levels by 9% with cholestyramine caused a significant (19%) reduction in CAD events.[5]

IV. Evidence Linking Treatment to Reduction in Mortality

A. Definitive proof that treatment to reduce cholesterol could lower cardiovascular *mortality* came in the mid-1990s with studies in both primary and secondary prevention. The trials used the relatively new class of drugs, the statins. Unlike the drugs used in earlier studies, cholestyramine and gemfibrozil, the statins had a stronger and more wide-ranging impact on lipids.

B. The Scandinavian Simvastatin Survival Study (4S) enrolled 4444 men and women aged 35-70 years with a history of angina or MI and total cholesterol of 212-309 mg/dL and randomized them to simvastatin or placebo and followed them for an average of 5.4 years. There were significantly more coronary deaths in the placebo group, 189 than in the simvastatin group, 111.[6]

C. Perhaps more remarkable was the West of Scotland Coronary Primary Prevention Study that randomly assigned 6595 men, aged 45-64 with a mean total cholesterol of 272 mg/dL but no known CAD to 40 mg of pravastatin or placebo and followed them for 4.9 years. The pravastatin group lowered their total cholesterol by 20% and LDL-C by 26% with no change in the placebo group. There were 248 definite coronary events in the placebo group and 174 in the pravastatin group. Relative risk reduction was 31%. There was a 32% reduction in death from all cardiovascular causes in the simvastatin group.[7]

D. Since this time, there have been countless randomized clinical trials, observational studies, and basic science work that has allowed for development of new drugs, treatment strategies, and guidelines for diagnosis and management of dyslipidemia. Studies have also established the efficacy and safety of the statin drugs such that these drugs have become first-line therapy and standard of care for the reduction of cholesterol.

V.   Development of Guidelines

A. In the United States, the NIH issued the first National Heart, Lung, and Blood Institute's National Cholesterol Education Program, Adult Treatment Panel Guidelines in 1988. Subsequent revisions were published in 1993 and 2001.

B. The planned 4th revision never materialized as the NIH determined that they should be turned over to the American Heart Association and American College of Cardiology who in 2013 issued the "ACC/AHA Guideline on the Treatment of Blood Cholesterol to Reduce Atherosclerotic Cardiovascular Risk in Adults."[8]

C. In 2015, the National Lipid Association published "Recommendations for Patient-Centered Management of Dyslipidemia."[9]

The establishment of guidelines and recommendations is a complex undertaking. Guidelines influence who will receive medication, who is labeled as "sick," and how our health care dollars are spent as well as insurance coverage. The most recent statements have provided new—and debated—algorithms, lipid goals and targets. Chapter 3 provides discussion of current guidelines and offers suggestions for clinicians.

VI.   Conclusion

Research and advancements in the field of lipidology and the prevention of ASCVD have been remarkable. It is important to continue these efforts to reduce the burden of this disease and better care for our patients.

References

1. Morris JN, Heady JA, Raffle PA, Roberts CG, Parks JW. Coronary heart-disease and physical activity of work. *Lancet*. 1953;265(6795):1053-1057.
2. Chen G, Levy D. Contributions of the Framingham heart study to the epidemiology of coronary heart disease. *JAMA Cardiol*. 2016;1(7):825-830.
3. Keys A, Menotti A, Aravanis C, et al. The seven countries study: 2,289 deaths in 15 years. *Prev Med*. 1984;13(2):141-154.
4. Farquhar JW, Fortmann SP, Flora JA, et al. Effects of communitywide education on cardiovascular disease risk factors. The Stanford Five-City Project. *JAMA*. 1990;264(3):359-365.
5. The lipid research clinics coronary primary prevention trial. Results of 6 years of post-trial follow-up. The lipid research clinics investigators. *Arch Intern Med* 1992;152(7):1399-1410.
6. Pedersen TR, Kjekshus J, Berg K, et al. Randomised trial of cholesterol lowering in 4444 patients with coronary heart disease: the Scandinavian Simvastatin Survival Study (4S). 1994. *Atheroscler Suppl*. 2004;5(3):81-87.
7. Shepherd J, Cobbe SM, Ford I, et al. Prevention of coronary heart disease with pravastatin in men with hypercholesterolemia. West of Scotland Coronary Prevention Study Group. *N Engl J Med*. 1995;333(20):1301-1307.
8. Stone NJ, Robinson J, Lichtenstein AH, et al. 2013 ACC/AHA guideline on the treatment of blood cholesterol to reduce atherosclerotic cardiovascular risk in adults: a report of the American College of Cardiology/American Heart Association Task Force on Practice Guidelines. *J Am Coll Cardiol* 2013;63:2889-2934.
9. Jacobson TA, Ito MK, Maki KC, et al. National Lipid Association recommendations for patient-centered management of dyslipidemia: Part 1— executive summary. *J Clin Lipidol*. 2014;8(5):473-488.

CHAPTER 2

Basic Lipid and Lipoprotein Biochemistry for Clinical Lipidologists

Daniel Soffer and Nilay Sutaria

Key Points

- Lipid physiology and metabolism are complex. It is helpful to be familiar with the biochemistry in order to understand lipid abnormalities.
- Cholesterol is found in all cells and tissues in humans and is needed for structure (cell membranes) and as the building blocks for steroid hormones.
- Plasma lipids are transported by molecules called lipoproteins.
- Apolipoproteins regulate the activity and function of the lipoprotein.
- The hepatic LDL receptor is the key component for removal of cholesterol from the body.
- The function of the HDL particle (to perform reverse cholesterol transport) is felt to be more clinically relevant than the cholesterol content of the HDL particle.
- Regulatory enzymes play an important role in lipid metabolism.

I.   Introduction

Atherosclerotic cardiovascular disease (ASCVD) is the most significant clinical manifestations of excess lipid and lipoprotein levels in humans.[1] Atherosclerosis is a complicated process that requires the deposition of apolipoprotein B (apoB)–containing lipoproteins, in particular low density lipoprotein (LDL) in the subendothelial space of the arterial circulation and the subsequent inflammatory reaction, ultimately resulting in either gradual or stepwise narrowing of the arterial lumen, or to an abrupt blood flow occlusion from superimposed thrombosis.

The plaque can form in any portion of the arterial tree, but there is a distinct predisposition for this to occur at arterial branch points where arterial flow currents are nonlinear and turbulent, putting higher stress on the endothelium at those sites.[2] Other systemic conditions make the endothelium more susceptible to the initiation of atheroma formation, including high systemic blood pressure, hyperglycemia/insulin resistance, smoking (related circulating toxins), hormonal, noradrenergic, and genetic factors.

Apolipoprotein A containing lipoproteins (high density lipoprotein [HDL]) serve as a brake on atherosclerosis. These lipoproteins contain multiple anti-atherogenic proteins that turn off the process and simultaneously siphon cholesterol from peripheral cells enabling a stabilization of plaque and remodeling process.

This chapter is meant to be a summary of the major concepts of lipid and lipoprotein physiology, so the practicing clinician can have a more informed shared treatment discussion with the patient.

I hope you enjoy reading about the details of lipids and lipoprotein metabolism as much as I have enjoyed writing this chapter. The huge clinical impact of cardiometabolic disorders on our society is what captured my interest in the field originally, but it is the elegance of the physiology that really drew me in. This chapter is not meant to be an exhaustive review of every physiologic factor but the highlights from our field and especially those expected to have clinical implications.

II.   Lipids

Lipids are organic molecules defined by their physical-chemical characteristic of poor solubility in organic solvents and in an alcohol or aqueous environment (like blood).

They come in many different varieties and can serve different biological functions. The solubility quality enables lipids to be the primary interface between cells and tissues and ultimately to create a regulatory barrier too. The rich carbon bonds in fatty acids render them efficient energy-carrying molecules and prone to functional restructuring by stepwise catalyzed reactions.

It is also the solubility characteristic that compels lipids to be transported in the aqueous bloodstream of animals in carrier particles called **lipoproteins (LP)**. There is also complex interaction among LP particles and between LP and cells that results in the variety of lipid and lipoprotein patterns that emerge in health and disease.

The major lipids include **sterols, fatty acids (and associated carrier macromolecules [eg, triglycerides, phospholipids]), phospholipids, eicosanoids, and sphingolipids**. It is beyond the scope of this chapter to review the role of eicosanoids and sphingolipids in detail, but key features of the others are addressed.

A. Sterols Sterols include both **cholesterol** (animal derived) and **phytosterols** (plant derived), which are similar in structure and function and are metabolized differently by humans.

1. **Cholesterol**
    a. **Cholesterol** is ubiquitous in human physiology. It is found in all cells and tissues and can be synthesized by all living cells. It is found in its most abundant state as **free cholesterol (FC)**, which is its amphipathic form (primarily nonpolar molecule, with small polar hydroxyl moiety), and as **cholesterol esters (CE)**, which are the result of esterification of the hydroxyl group with a fatty acid moiety (Fig. 2.1).
    b. Cholesterol is a complex polycyclic hydrocarbon derived from acetyl-CoA, a simpler 2-carbon molecule that undergoes transformation and combination in the cholesterol synthetic pathway (Fig. 2.2). Acetyl-CoA is modified to form

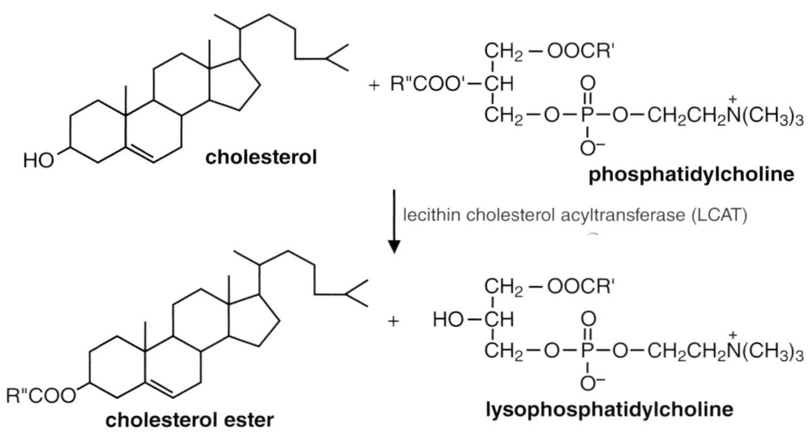

FIGURE 2.1: Chemical structure of free cholesterol and cholesterol ester. (Redrawn with permission from Christie W. Cholesterol and Cholesterol Esters. The American Oil Chemists' Society Lipid Library website. http://lipidlibrary.aocs.org/index.cgm. Updated January 6, 2014. Accessed May 26, 2017.)

Cholesterol Biosynthesis

Acetyl-CoA
↓
HMG-CoA Reductase
HMG-CoA ─────────────→ Mevalonate

| Statins |

Mevalonate-PP ────→ Isopentenyl-Adenin

Isopentenyl-PP ────→ Isoprenylation of Proteins

geranylgeranyl transferase

Geranyl-PP

Geranylgeranyl-PP

Cholesterol ◄── Squalene ◄── Farnesyl-PP + Isopentenyl-PP

farnesyl transferase ────→ Isoprenylation of Proteins

FIGURE 2.2: Cholesterol synthetic pathway.

acetoacetyl-CoA and then again to form **3-hydroxymethylglutaryl-CoA (HMG-CoA),** which is then reduced to **mevalonate** by *HMG-CoA reductase,* the rate-limiting catalytic step in cholesterol synthesis.

c. HMG-CoA reductase is inhibited by **statin drugs**. It is postulated that some of the side effects attributed to statins are the result of cellular deficiencies of the noncholesterol products of this metabolic pathway. **Coenzyme Q10 (ubiquinol)** has been used to offset muscle-associated symptoms though this approach has not been consistently validated in randomized placebo-controlled clinical trials.[3]

d. FC is found in cellular and organelle/nuclear membranes where its rigid hydro-carbon backbone can insert into the phospholipid sheets providing form to otherwise amorphous membranes (Fig. 2.3). The polycyclic structure also serves as the building block for **steroid hormones** (including estrogen, testosterone, aldosterone, cortisol, vitamin D, and others) and **bile salts**. While every cell can synthesize its own cholesterol, only specialized cells have the necessary enzymatic capacity to transform cholesterol into hormones and bile salts.

e. Circulating **high-density lipoprotein (HDL)** particles participate in the process of removing cholesterol from peripheral cells and ultimately delivering cholesterol to hepatocytes and conversion to bile for fecal excretion; this is known as **reverse cholesterol transport (RCT).** Specific mechanisms of HDL-mediated RCT and bile salt synthesis are described later.

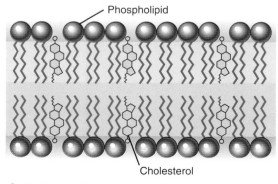

Phospholipid

Cholesterol

A. Cholesterol in plasma membrane

FIGURE 2.3: FC embedded in phospholipid membranes.

2. **Phytosterols/stanols** Phytosterols are noncholesterol sterols and part of a regular human diet and can be added to processed foods and supplements. Humans lack the enzymes necessary to effectively absorb and catabolize phytosterols; however, a rare autosomal recessive disorder (sitosterolemia or phytosterolemia) results in increased absorption of phytosterols with toxic accumulation in tissues and coronary artery disease.

B. **Fatty acids** Fatty acids **(FA)** are the basic building block of lipids. They are characterized as a carboxylic acid with short, medium, and long chains. The chemical formula structure is that of a hydrocarbon chain and a terminal carboxyl (–COOH) group. FA can be saturated (no double bonds), monounsaturated (single double bond), or polyunsaturated (multiple double bonds). They have both common and scientific names. FA nomenclature is determined by the number of carbons and the presence and location of double bonds.

1. Humans are able to hydrolyze the carbon bonds in FA, breaking off two carbon moieties for beta-oxidation, resulting in significant energy harvest. Compared to the oxidation of carbohydrate, fatty acid oxidation yields more than twice as much energy (yield of 9 cal/g FA compared to 4 cal/g carbohydrate or protein).

2. Double bonds put a "kink" in the chain preventing simple stacking of FA, which affects the melting point of the fat. Double bonds can be in the *cis*-configuration, which flattens out the FA chain, resulting in physical characteristics that have more in common with saturated compared to other unsaturated FA.

3. FA are dietary components and may be synthesized by humans as well. The most abundant saturated fatty acid in nature is hexadecanoic (aka palmitic) acid. All of the even-numbered saturated fatty acids from C_2 to C_{30} have been found in nature, but only the C_{14} to C_{18} homologues are likely to be encountered in appreciable concentrations in glycerolipids, other than in a restricted range of commercial fats and oils.[4] FA are considered essential FA if they cannot be synthesized by humans (eg, linoleic acid). They may be carried in the circulation in **triglycerides (TG)** and on phospholipids, may be esterified to other molecules (eg, cholesterol esters [CE]), or may be in their free fatty acid (FFA) form bound to albumin.

C. **Triglycerides** Triglycerides (TG) are the main dietary source of FA. They are composed of **glycerol** (a 3-carbon backbone) with FA moieties esterified to each carbon. Triglycerides, which are nonpolar molecules, are carried in the core of lipoproteins, alongside of cholesterol ester, oriented away from the aqueous environment of blood.

D. **Phospholipids** Phospholipids also have a glycerol backbone with FA moieties esterified at two of the carbons, but instead of a third FA, they have a phosphate head (providing small polar region) resulting in an amphipathic molecule. Phospholipids aggregate with each other in mono- and bilayer sheets, spheres, or micelles (Fig. 2.4). They are drawn together by the van der Waals (strong short-range electrostatic attraction between large nonpolar molecules) force from the long hydrocarbon chains, orienting polar heads to an aqueous environment. The amphipathic structure makes PL ideal emulsifiers and membrane constituents.

III.   Lipoproteins

Lipoproteins (LP) are large carrier macroparticles for lipids. They all share the same basic structure with a phospholipid outer shell interspersed with FC, exchangeable enzymes, and the principle structural **apolipoprotein(s)** that can span the outer shell and the core. Nonpolar lipids (CE, TG, fat-soluble vitamins) are found in the core.

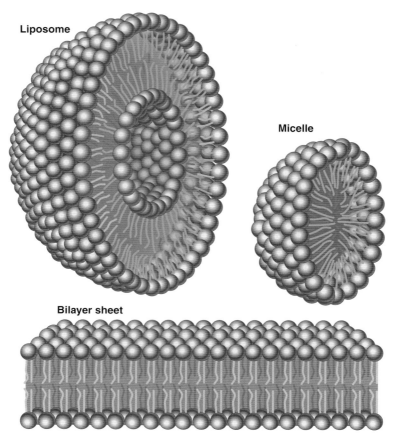

FIGURE 2.4: Phospholipids.

Lipoproteins are named according to the protein-to-lipid density after separation by ultracentrifugation, but the families of LP have other identifying features as well, including electrophoresis pattern, apolipoprotein content, lipid content, derivation, and function.

Regardless of methodology, measurement of the cholesterol content of the various LPs (eg, the cholesterol content of the LDL particle, known as "LDL-C") has been the traditional tool for estimating quantity and potential physiologic impact in an individual and remains a useful tool for assessing CVD risk. However, the lipoprotein-cholesterol content does not always tell the whole story since particles can vary in size/volume/density not only within an individual but between individuals, and particles may have variable function that is not necessarily reflected by the cholesterol content. LDL particle number or apoB predicts risk for ASCVD and several guidelines include apoB as a target for treatment.[5] Table 2.1 summarizes the characteristics of the lipoproteins.

A. Chylomicrons Chylomicrons (CM) are the largest and lowest density LP, ranging from the size of other apoB-containing LP to as large as ~1000 nm (approximately the size of some viruses). The main structural protein is apolipoprotein B-48 (apoB-48) and is intestinally derived. It is synthesized with apoA-I, apoA-II, and apoA-IV, and it will acquire apoC-I, apoC-II, apoC-III, and apoE in circulation. The lipid content is roughly

Table 2.1. Lipoproteins

Class (Origin)	Primary Apolipoproteins	Diameter (nm)	Density (g/mL)	Molecular Weight (kDa)	Electrophoresis Mobility	Composition (%) Core TG	CE	Surface FC	PL	Pro	Major Apos
Chylomicrons (intestine)	ApoB-48 ApoA-I, apoA-V ApoC-II, apoC-III ApoE	80-500	<0.93	50 000-1 000 000	α_2	86	3	2	7	2	B-48, E, A-I, A-II, A-IV, C
VLDL (liver)	ApoB-100 ApoA-I, apoA-V ApoC-II, apoC-III ApoE	30-80	0.95-1.006	10 000-80 000	Pre-β	55	12	7	18	8	B-100, C-I, C-II, C-III, E
IDL (lipoprotein)	ApoB-100 ApoE	25-35	1.006-1.019	5000-10 000	Slow pre-β	23	29	9	19	19	B-100, E
LDL (lipoprotein)	ApoB-100	21.6	1.019-1.063	2300	β	6	42	8	22	22	B-100
HDL₂ (liver, intestine, lipoprotein)	ApoA-I, apoA-II	10	1.063-1.125	400	α	5	17	5	33	40	A-I, A-II
HDL₃ (liver, intestine, lipoprotein)	ApoA-I, apoA-II	7.5	1.125-1.210	200	α	3	13	4	25	55	A-I, A-II
Lp(a) (liver, serum)	ApoB-100, apo(a)	30	1.055-1.085	LDL + apo(a)	Slow pre-β	3	33	9	22	33	B-100, apo(a)

TG, triglyceride; CE, cholesterol ester; FC, free cholesterol; PL, phospholipid; Pro, protein.
(Reprinted with permission from Durrington P. Hyperlipidaemia, Diagnosis and Management. 3rd ed. London: Hodder Arnold; 2007.)

>6:1 TG: cholesterol. The chylomicron delivers TG from the gut for energy or fat storage to peripheral adipose or muscle and cholesterol ester to the liver. As the chylomicron particle loses TG, it becomes a much smaller chylomicron remnant.

B. Very-low-density lipoprotein

1. **VLDL** undergoes a very similar synthesis and lifespan as the CM, but it originates in the hepatocyte. ApoB-100 is the principle structural protein, and it contains apoA-I, apoA-II, apoA-IV, apoC-I, apoC-II, apoC-III, and apoE. The lipid content is <5:1 TG: cholesterol.

C. Intermediate density lipoprotein

1. **IDL** is derived from the metabolism of VLDL. Its primary structural protein is apoB-100 and is an intermediary between VLDL and the transition to LDL. Its lipid content is intermediate between VLDL and LDL.

D. Low-density lipoprotein LDL is derived from the sequential condensation of VLDL to IDL then to LDL. Therefore, its main structural protein is also apoB-100, and since its TG content is low, it does not contain the other apolipoproteins required to modulate lipoprotein lipase (LPL) activity, the principle regulator of **TG-rich lipoproteins (TRL)** (process described later). Circulatory clearance of LDL is mediated by the interaction between apoB and the LDL receptor, which is expressed primarily on hepatocytes but also found in peripheral macrophages and other cells at lower levels.

E. High-density lipoprotein HDL are small dense LP, hepatic, intestine, and LP derived. This family of LP includes nascent (discoidal) HDL, HDL3, and HDL2 and their respective subcategorizations. Unlike the LP described above, HDL does not contain apoB. ApoA-I is the only apolipoprotein found on nascent HDL. HDL3 and HDL2 can have either apoA-I, apoA-II, or both, though apoA-II as the only apoA is rarely found. The formation of HDL is not as sequential as the apoB-containing LP.

The proteome associated with HDL is extensive and reflects its role in various functions in health and disease. HDL are known to carry over two hundred different proteins associated with various aspects of inflammation, thrombosis, and lipoprotein metabolism.[6]

F. Lipoprotein(a) Lp(a) is composed of an LDL with disulfide bond between apoB and an apolipoprotein (a). Apo(a) is synthesized by hepatocytes, and the complex of LDL-apo(a) is formed in the circulation. Apo(a) shares genetic and structural homology with plasminogen,[7] and there is evidence that high levels of Lp(a) in the circulation act as a competitive plasminogen inhibitor; thus, Lp(a) may contribute to ASCVD risk because of its ability to initiate/propagate the atheroma like LDL but also precipitate atherothrombosis because of its prothrombotic moiety.[8]

Lp(a) catabolism is not perfectly understood, but it has been suggested that at least some of its clearance is mediated by the LDL-R.[9] Medicines that result in upregulation of the LDL-R (bile acid sequestrants, cholesterol absorption inhibitor [ezetimibe], statins) do not reduce Lp(a); however, PCSK9 inhibitors, which directly result in delayed LDL-R degradation, do reduce Lp(a) levels by 20%-30%.[10] Lp(a) is found in almost all individuals, but the concentration distribution is widely skewed. 80% of the population has "normal" levels, while some individuals can have very high levels.[11] There is some controversy about whether mass measurements should be favored over molar to estimate concentration and potential pathogenicity. Regardless of measure, high levels are independently associated with higher CV risk.[12] The clinical aspects of Lp(a) are discussed in Chapter 14 and measurement issues in Chapter 5.

IV. Apolipoproteins

Apolipoproteins are proteins associated with lipoproteins. Their presence dictates the LP interactions with other LP's and with cells.

A. Apolipoprotein A

1. **Apolipoprotein A-I** (apoA-I) is the main structural protein on HDL; the gene is found on chromosome 11. In addition to providing the structural foundation for HDL, it acts as a promotor of cholesterol efflux and **lecithin cholesterol acyltransferase (LCAT)**, the HDL-associated enzyme responsible for esterification of free cholesterol on lipoproteins. Inherited deficiency in apoA-1 is one of the major causes of inherited very low HDL-C levels (typically <10 mg/dL); other causes include abnormalities in **ATP-binding cassette transporter subtype 1 (ABCA1)** and LCAT.

2. **Apolipoprotein A-II** (apoA-II) is the second most abundant protein found on HDL and only rarely would be found on HDL without apoA-I. Its gene is on chromosome 1, and deficiency states may be associated with hypercholesterolemia.

3. **Apolipoprotein A-V** (apoA-V) is also expressed on HDL and most closely associated with its role in regulating catabolism of TRL, and genetic defects have been associated with severe hypertriglyceridemia and coronary heart disease.[13] Its gene is found proximal to the apoA-I cluster on chromosome 11.

B. Apolipoprotein B

Apolipoprotein B (apoB) is the main structural protein in non-HDL and the principle LDL receptor ligand. There are two main variants, **apoB-48** (intestinal origin) and **apoB-100** (hepatic origin). The *APOB* gene resides on chromosome 2, and it encodes a protein with 4563 amino acids, >500 kDa, making it one of the largest human proteins. At least partly due to its size, only one apoB can be associated with each LP, and it will remain with that LP for its entire "life cycle" (from synthesis to clearance). ApoB spans the LP membrane with its mostly hydrophobic structure buried in the CE/TG-rich core and its quaternary structure, and thus, its affinity for the LDL-R can be affected by the size of the LP.

Inherited defects in the *APOB* gene that result in apoB with defective binding to the LDL-R are an uncommon cause of **familial hypercholesterolemia**, known as **familial defective apolipoprotein B-100**.

C. Apolipoprotein C

All of the apoC subtypes are ~8 kDa hepatically derived apolipoproteins whose main function is regulation of TRL metabolism/LPL modulation.

1. **ApoC-I** ApoC-I is an LPL inhibitor. There are no recognized cases of apoC-I genetic defects associated with clinical lipid/lipoprotein disorders.

2. **ApoC-II** At physiologic levels, **apoC-II** acts as a stimulator of LPL activity, promoting the clearance of TRL (CM, VLDL, and remnant particles). ApoC-II deficiency is a recognized cause of **familial chylomicronemia syndrome (FCS)**,[14] and unlike the more commonly recognized LPL deficiency, individuals may respond to the acute administration of plasma to transiently correct hyperchylomicronemia.

Table 2.2.   Common ApoE Polymorphisms

Protein	Apo E-2	Apo E-3	Apo E-4
Residue at position 112	Cysteine	Cysteine	Arginine
Residue at position 158	Cysteine	Arginine	Arginine
% LDL-R binding affinity	1	100	100
% allelic frequency in population	7	78	14
Clinical association	Type III HL	Normal	CVD and Alzheimer disease

(Reprinted with permission from Phillips MC. Apolipoprotein E isoforms and lipoprotein metabolism. *IUBMB Life*. 2014;66(9):616-623.)

3. **ApoC-III** ApoC-III is an LPL inhibitor, and there is a well-recognized inverse relationship between apoC-III activity and serum TG level.[15] ApoC-III is found on both apoA- and apoB-containing LP, mostly on HDL when serum TG levels are low and on TG-rich lipoproteins (TRL) when TG levels are high.[16] In addition to inhibiting LPL, it also has a role in enhancing VLDL synthesis and inhibiting hepatic receptor–mediated uptake of TRL and remnants and inhibiting hepatic lipase (HL).

D. **Apolipoprotein E** ApoE is a 34-kDa constituent of TRL and is a ligand for the LDL receptor-related protein (LRP) and LDL-R and also regulates lipid transport and cholesterol homeostasis in the brain. The LDL-R binding site spans positions 135-150 on the *APOE* gene (found on chromosome 19), and there are three common genetic polymorphisms (apoE-2, apoE-3, and apoE-4) that result from single amino acid substitutions at positions 112 and 158 (Table 2.2).

1. Allele frequency of E2, E3, E4 in the human population are 7%, 78%, 14%, respectively.[17] The pairing of apoE genes results in the following apoE phenotypes (E-2/E-2, E-2/E-3, E-2/E-4, E-3/E-4, E-3/E-3, E-4/E-4). E-3, which has optimal affinity for the LRP and LDL-R, is the most common polymorphism in the general population (Table 2.3).

2. Inheritance of the E-2/E-2 genotype, which occurs in <2% of the general population, results in inhibited TRL remnant clearance and high levels of cholesterol-enriched remnant particles. In the right clinical scenario (a "second hit"), an individual with the E-2/E-2 phenotype, who has weight gain, insulin resistance/type 2 diabetes mellitus, excessive alcohol intake, particular medications, pregnancy, and endocrinopathies, accumulation of remnant particles will occur, manifesting **type III according to the Fredrickson classification (dysbetalipoproteinemia).** Remnant particle remodeling and conversion to LDL, which does not contain apoE, result in normal LDL clearance. The diagnosis of type III HL is made in the right clinical context and should include the presence of eruptive xanthomas, often with pathognomonic orange palmar creases, and combined hyperlipidemia typically with both TC and TG levels >300 mg/dL. The hyperlipidemia will fluctuate considerably, dependent on the "second hit." The VLDL-C: TG >0.3 and relatively low apoB levels are seen. Higher CV

Table 2.3.   Common ApoE Phenotypes

Phenotype	E-2/E-2	E-2/E-3	E-3/E-3	E-3/E-4	E-4/E-4	E-2/E-4
Frequency in population (%)	<2	23	60	12	<1	<2

Reprinted with permission from Durrington P. *Hyperlipidaemia, Diagnosis and Management*. 3rd ed. London: Hodder Arnold; 2007.

risk is expected and the lipid abnormality should be treated. The apoE-2/E-2 state is necessary, but not sufficient to manifest type III hyperlipoproteinemia. Treatments are directed at correcting the second hit, but lipid-lowering medicine can help as well.[18]

3. Individuals with apoE-4 have higher LDL-C levels and also have a lifetime ~50% risk of developing Alzheimer/dementia.[19,20] Given the ethical and medicosocial complexity of identifying an early marker of dementia risk, genetic counseling is strongly encouraged before testing for apoE phenotype.

E. **Apolipoprotein (a)** Apolipoprotein (a) has genetic homology and is structurally similar to plasminogen. Apo(a) is secreted by hepatocytes and then forms a disulfide bond with the apoB on LDL to form Lp(a) (described earlier in chapter in Lp(a) section). Apo(a) has a single peptide region and many repeating amino acid sequences that fold into characteristic repeating domains (referred to as Kringle units [after the Danish pastry]) forming a "tail" with potential prothrombotic qualities, adherent to LDL. The size of the apo(a) is dictated by the number of repeating Kringle IV2 units and is inversely proportional to the serum Lp(a) concentration,[21] suggesting that large apo(a) is not efficiently synthesized or secreted, limiting its ability to compound with LDL in the circulation.

V. Intestinal Regulation

A. Fat globules

1. Fats are consumed as a macronutrient fraction of food. The act of chewing and mingling of food particles with saliva initiates the process of converting food into digestible smaller particles, allowing for interaction with and absorption by small intestine enterocytes.

2. The fat in our diet is segregated from other macronutrients in our food in large fat globules. Gastric and then pancreatic lipases act on the large globules converting them into smaller and smaller droplets. Dietary fats are also mixed in with the phospholipids and free cholesterol from enterocyte sloughing and with bile salts, so intestinal lumen fat content is not just dietary fat. The fat globule is further emulsified by bile salts, which act as a deterrent to break down fat globules into the so-called **mixed micelle**.

   a. The micelle is a spherical particle composed of a phospholipid outer shell and free cholesterol with core nonpolar fatty elements (mono- and diglycerides, fat-soluble vitamins). Intestinal lumen micelles are small enough to penetrate the unstirred water layer of the small intestine, which allows for enterocyte fat absorption.

B. Sterol absorption
Cholesterol and phytosterols are incorporated into intestinal micelles, along with other dietary and intestinal fats. Phytosterols have a higher affinity for intestinal micellar inclusion compared to cholesterol.[22] Therefore, when phytosterols intake is high, cholesterol inclusion in micelles is reduced, which reduces availability for enterocyte cholesterol absorption. When taken as dietary supplements, phytosterols/stanols can lower serum total cholesterol levels by as much as 5%-10%.[23]

The micelles penetrate the unstirred water layer allowing interaction with the luminal membrane of small intestine. Cholesterol and phytosterols are pumped into enterocytes by the **Niemann-Pick C1-like 1 (NPC1L1)** luminal membrane transporter. Under normal physiologic circumstances, however, phytosterols are pumped right back out into the lumen by the **ATP-binding cassette luminal transporter type G5 and/or G8 (ABCG5/8)**. Inherited defects in either/both ABCG5/8 are responsible for the autosomal recessive condition, **sitosterolemia, which is associated with xanthomas and premature ASCVD**. This condition may be effectively treated with the NPC1L1 inhibitor, ezetimibe.

C. **Bile salts as emulsifier bile acids** are stored in the gall bladder in the form of mixed micelles combined with phospholipids and cholesterol. Bile is released into the intestinal lumen due to gall bladder contraction in response to consumption of a meal. The bile acts as a detergent, emulsifying intestinal micelles, and ultimately, 95% of the bile is reabsorbed in the ileum. The 5% of bile lost in the feces is replaced with endogenous bile acid synthesis, keeping the total body bile acid pool stable. Interventions that interrupt recycling of bile acids (eg, bile acid sequestrant resins and ileal resection) result in upregulation of **cytochrome p450 7 α-hydroxylase (aka CYP7A1),** the rate-limiting enzyme responsible for bile salt synthesis by the hepatocyte. Since these therapies affect cholesterol absorption in the ileum, and the **cholesterol absorption inhibitor, ezetimibe,** interrupts it in the duodenum/jejunum, the therapies can be used together for a potentially additive effect.

D. **Fatty acid absorption** Nonpolar fats (mono-, di-, and triglycerides, fat-soluble vitamins) can traverse the enterocyte luminal membrane directly without the need for transport protein.

VI.   Lipoprotein Metabolism

Lipoprotein metabolism is complex. The schematic (Fig. 2.5) and following text provide a broad outline. A firm understanding of the process can best be achieved by reading an in-depth description while looking at schematics for each step and for the process as a whole. Intestinal fats are absorbed by enterocytes and then packaged into chylomicrons (CM),

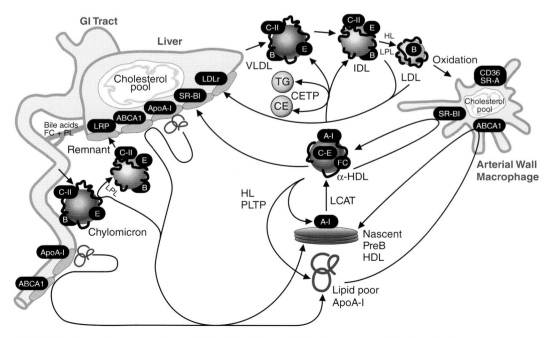

FIGURE 2.5: Lipoprotein metabolism. (Adapted with permission from Brewer HB. High-density lipoproteins: a new potential therapeutic target for the prevention of cardiovascular disease. *Arterioscler Thromb Vasc Biol.* 2004;24:387-391.)

which are secreted into the lymphatics before merging with the venous circulation. CM are metabolized in circulation to remnant particles before uptake by the liver.

The liver packages fats into VLDL, which is secreted directly into the hepatic venous circulation. These TRL then circulate distributing the energy-rich TG to peripheral tissue. The ultimate remodeling and condensation into LDL particles favor uptake by the **LDL receptor (LDL-R)**.

HDL particles are synthesized by a variety of tissues and behave like scavengers in the circulation. They facilitate removal of accumulated oxysterols in the periphery, exchange lipid with other lipoproteins in circulation, and can then deliver the oxysterol to either hepatocytes or steroidogenic tissue.

A. Lipoprotein assembly Chylomicrons (CM) and VLDL are synthesized and secreted from enterocytes and hepatocytes, respectively, utilizing almost identical cellular machinery. This is not really an unexpected phenomenon since the liver is considered by biologists as a highly specialized collection of cells with similar embryologic gut origin with increased functional capacity.

B. Exogenous pathway

1. Apolipoprotein B-48 (apoB-48), which is the truncated version of apoB, is the principle structural protein of CM. FC, phospholipid, CE, TG (formed from long chain FA [>C14]), and apolipoproteins A-I, A-II, and A-IV are packaged by **microsomal triglyceride transfer protein (MTTP)** in the endoplasmic reticulum (ER). The particle is then transported to the Golgi and then to the endosome and released into lymphatic channels at the basolateral membrane. CM will travel in lymphatic channels converging at the thoracic duct where they can then enter the venous circulation at the superior vena cava.

2. CM metabolism requires an orchestrated interaction with other exchangeable enzymes/proteins acquired in the circulation, including apolipoproteins C-I, C-II, and C-III and apolipoprotein E. ApoC-II promotes interaction of CM with lipoprotein lipase (LPL) expressed on vascular endothelium, particularly in tissues with high-energy requirements (eg, muscle, kidney, heart). The FA can then undergo hydrolysis/oxidation in cells/tissues with high-energy requirement or for storage in adipocytes. ApoC-III inhibits LPL (and probably hepatic lipase [HL]) function. Sequential condensation of CM in circulation effectively reduces the surface area and exchangeable enzymes including apoC-II and apoC-III, and lipids can be transferred to other lipoproteins, ultimately transforming the CM into CM remnant whose hepatic uptake will be mostly mediated by the LDL receptor–related protein (LRP) interaction with its primary ligand, apoE. CM remnants appear to be atherogenic, while CM are too large to penetrate the arterial endothelium. Excess CM and CM remnants predispose to pancreatitis and dermatologic manifestations (eruptive xanthomas).

C. Endogenous pathway

1. VLDL undergo an almost identical synthetic process as CM. Apolipoprotein B-100 is the principle structural protein of VLDL. FC, phospholipid, CE, TG, apolipoproteins A-I and A-V, apoC-II and apoC-III, and apoE are packaged by microsomal triglyceride transfer protein (MTTP) in the endoplasmic reticulum (ER), released from the Golgi into an endosome for export into the hepatic sinusoids where it can join the peripheral circulation. The exact mechanisms that prevent immediate lipolysis by **hepatic lipase (HL)** and uptake by the LRP are not fully understood, but this phenomenon is integral to metabolic pathway since immediate lipolysis by newly secreted TRL would be a useless waste of precious

metabolic machinery. It has been suggested that potential explanations for delayed TRL lipolysis includes the role of apoC-III as HL inhibitor[24] and distortion of the tertiary structure of apoE and apoB in newly formed VLDL in its fully lipidated and largest state, which results in diminished affinity for the LDL-R and LRP.

2. VLDL will circulate where it can interact with LPL in the periphery, resulting in the hydrolysis of FA and stepwise condensation to IDL and then to LDL. Along with delipidation, enzymes and apolipoproteins can be exchanged in the circulation. It is the stepwise gradual change that results in the characteristic "family" of LP with ranges of size and lipid content, while the exchange of proteins results in the transition from one family to the next. VLDL remnant particles and LDL are atherogenic.

D. Hepatic receptor–mediated clearance

1. **LDL receptor**

   a. Under normal physiologic circumstances, FA hydrolysis results in the condensation of TRL to relatively TG-poor LDL. LDL is then cleared from the circulation by way of its interaction with the hepatic **LDL-R**. The LDL-R is expressed on hepatic and nonhepatic cells; however, it does not seem to play a critical role outside of the liver. The LDL-R is not a necessary regulator of extrahepatic cholesterol, and nonliver cells can keep up with demand by synthesizing cholesterol on their own or by uptake by other means.[25] The LDL-R does play a critical role in hepatic uptake and in serum LDL-C regulation however.

   b. Accumulation of LDL in the circulation is known to promote atherosclerosis proportional to the time-averaged exposure to high concentrations[26] and the inverse relation between LDL-R and LDL-C activity has been clearly demonstrated.[27]

   c. **The LDL-R** family describes a family of endocytic cell surface proteins that bind and internalize lipoprotein and other lipid carrier complexes. The general structure of all of the LDL-R family is the same with the following elements: ligand binding domain, epidermal growth factor–like domain, transmembrane anchor, and cytosolic domain.

   d. The LDL receptor (*LDLR*) gene is located on chromosome 19 in humans and is composed of 18 exons. Its expression results in a complex protein with >800 amino acids in sequence. The extracellular component extends into the space of Disse where the LDL-binding domain can interact with apoB-100 (and/or apoE) on circulating LP.

   e. *LDLR* gene expression is regulated by the **sterol regulatory element-binding protein (SREBP-2)**, which is the same nuclear protein that regulates expression of the genes that code for HMG-CoA reductase and **proprotein convertase subtilisin kexin-9 (PCSK9)**.

   f. The LDL-R is expressed on the luminal membrane in **clathrin**-coated pits. It forms a trimer complex with the LP and hepatically derived **PCSK9**. The complex is taken up into the clathrin-coated endosome where it can merge with lysosomes promoting degradation of the LP to its constituent elements. The LDL-R may be recycled >150×,[28] limited by the presence of PCSK9, which signals the degradation of the LDL-R (Fig. 2.6).

   g. Both loss of function and gain of function PCSK9 gene mutations have been identified and are associated with low LDL-C/low CV risk and high LDL-C/high CV risk, respectively.[29] The latter is inherited in an autosomal dominant manner and represents an uncommon cause of **familial hypercholesterolemia (FH)**. The *PCSK9* gene is located on chromosome 1 at position 32.3.[30] Fully humanized monoclonal antibody is now available as pharmacologic therapy for PCSK9 inhibition.[31]

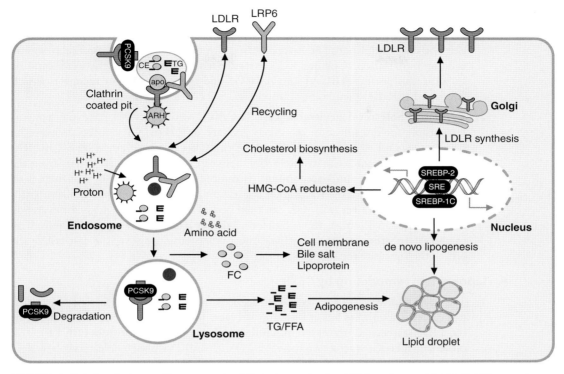

FIGURE 2.6: Cellular cholesterol homeostasis. (CE cholesteryl ester; FFA free fatty acid; LDL-R, LDL-receptor; LRP, LDL receptor-related protein; PCSK9, proprotein convertase subtilisin kexin 9; SREBP sterol regulatory element binding protein; TG triglyceride.) (Adapted from Go GW, Mani A. Low density lipoprotein receptor (LDLR) family orchestrates cholesterol homeostasis. *Yale J Biol Med.* 2012;85(1):19-28.)

    h. There are >1100 allelic variants in the *LDLR* gene known to be associated with familial hypercholesterolemia (FH), resulting in reduced or no LDL binding.[32] Most of the pharmacotherapy for treating FH results in upregulation of the LDL-R (statins, BAS, CAI, PCSK9i), which explains some of the blunted response to these therapies in FH patients who have so-called null receptor mutations or absent response in the most severe cases of homozygous FH with extremely limited receptor activity.

    i. The cytosolic domain of the LDL-R interacts with the **LDL-R adaptor protein 1** to facilitate membrane anchoring. Defects in the *LDLRAP* gene (found on chromosome 1) are known to be associated with the autosomal recessive rare cause of familial hypercholesterolemia (aka **autosomal recessive hypercholesterolemia [ARH]**).

  2. **VLDL receptor (VLDL-R)** The VLDL-R is widely expressed in adipocytes, skeletal muscle, and the heart and endothelium, but not by hepatocytes.[33] In addition to facilitated uptake of TRL in peripheral tissues, the VLDL-R also has a role in modulating LPL expression.

  3. **LDL receptor–related protein (LRP)** The **LDL receptor–related protein (LRP)** is a family of related cell surface receptors with multiple known functions associated with the modulation of inflammation and lipoprotein transport. Chylomicron remnants and other triglyceride-rich lipoproteins are hepatically cleared from the circulation by apoE-mediated interaction with the LRP.[34–36] Similar to the LDL-R, LRP-1 has been shown in experimental models to be upregulated in response to treatment with statin drugs.[37]

E. High-density lipoprotein metabolism

1. HDL is multifunctional, but its best known role is as peripheral scavenger. It mediates the disposal of peripheral oxysterols, as a protection against accumulation and cellular intoxication. Cellular FC is transferred onto HDL by the ATP-binding cassette transporters **ABCA1** and **ABCG1** and by the **scavenger receptor class B subtype 1 (SR-B1)** membrane transporter.

2. **Lecithin cholesterol acyltransferase (LCAT),** which is the principle enzyme responsible for esterification of FC, is resident on HDL. CE can be delivered to hepatocytes and steroidogenic cells where the CE can be siphoned by SR-B1. The hepatic/steroidogenic cellular interaction between HDL and SR-B1 differs from the interaction between apoB-containing LP and the LDL-R or LRP in that there is no holoparticle uptake of the LP. Rather the receptor acts as a membrane transporter for the lipid alone. In liver cells, CE can then be metabolized to bile acids for excretion into the intestinal lumen, thus completing **direct RCT** (referring to the movement of cholesterol from periphery to liver/intestine). Steroidogenic tissue can utilize the CE as the substrate for steroid hormones.

F. Lipoprotein remodeling by CETP

1. The transition from VLDL to IDL to LDL is not a simple or perfectly linear transformation. The process has at least another layer of complexity mediated primarily by the HDL-associated glycoprotein, **cholesteryl ester transfer protein (CETP)**. This protein enables the interaction between TG-rich and TG-poor (cholesteryl ester–rich) lipoproteins and the one-to-one exchange of TG for CE. In this way, lipoproteins undergo lipid remodeling as well as the protein exchange as previously described.

2. The mechanism of lipid exchange mediated by CETP allows for a diversity of LP particles, high capacitance for cholesterol esterification since CE does not have be carried only by HDL (the site of the principle cholesterol-esterifying enzyme, LCAT), and for an alternative pathway for RCT.

3. RCT can follow the direct route, from peripheral cell (foam cell) to HDL, to liver, and ultimately to excretion in the feces, described above or by an indirect route. CETP enables CE to be transferred from HDL to TRL in exchange for TG, allowing the CE to take an alternative pathway for disposal by the liver. This pathway of cholesterol ester from periphery to HDL to apoB-containing LP to hepatocytes is described as **indirect RCT**.

4. CETP activity is increased in individuals with the highest TG levels and in the insulin-resistant state. These individuals tend to have the so-called atherogenic dyslipidemia characterized by high TG, low HDL-C, and **small dense LDL (sdLDL)** with discordance between levels of LDL-C and non–HDL-C/apoB/LDL-particle count (LDL-P).[38,39]

5. CETP-mediated lipid exchange between TRL and HDL results in HDL particles that are cholesterol poor/TG enriched, which interact with peripheral lipases. Sequential interaction of these HDL particles with LPL and HL results in lipid-poor HDL. The delipidated very small protein dense HDL is susceptible to cubilin-mediated renal elimination and subsequent low HDL-C and HDL-particle count (HDL-P) levels typically seen in the insulin-resistant hypertriglyceridemic state.

6. TRL are transformed by CETP activity into cholesterol-enriched, denser particles, with increased atherogenic properties.[40] LDL particles, in particular, are condensed and have less cholesterol per particle, often referred to as pattern B.[41]

7. Since LDL-C underperforms as a CV risk marker compared to non–HDL-C, apoB, and LDL-P in individuals with atherogenic lipid triad,[42] several organizations including the 2015 National Lipid Association call for using non–HDL-C as the primary target of therapy rather than LDL-C.[43,44]

G. Major regulatory enzymes

1. **Lipoprotein lipase (LPL)**

   a. Lipoprotein lipase (LPL) is responsible for removing TG/fatty acids from circulating TRL and ultimately delivering FA to tissues with high-energy requirements.

   b. It is expressed in adipose, heart, brain, and skeletal muscle though not found in liver. LPL is a glycoprotein, active as a dimer of two glycosylated 55-kDa subunits. After LPL is synthesized, it is chaperoned from the endoplasmic reticulum for excretion by **lipase maturation factor (LMF1)**. **Glycosylphosphatidylinositol-anchored HDL-binding protein 1 (GPIHBP1)** then transports LPL from the subendothelium and is responsible for anchoring it to the endothelium luminal membrane. Genetic defects in *LMF1* (at chromosome 16p13.3)[45] and in *GPIHBP1* (at chromosome 8q24.3) are identified and associated with severe hypertriglyceridemia and are rare variants of the **familial chylomicronemia syndrome (FCS)**.[46]

   c. LPL is anchored by its sulfated proteoglycan-binding site to luminal membrane heparan sulfate. The enzymatic portion of LPL is then available in the capillary lumen for interaction with circulating LP, with a higher affinity for larger, lower density TRL (CM and nascent VLDL). Interaction between the TRL and LPL facilitates the transfer of TG to LPL, enabling subsequent hydrolysis of fatty acid and cellular uptake mediated primarily by cell surface scavenger receptor CD36. In this way, fat calories are exchanged from TRL to cells for storage or FA oxidation.

   d. The *LPL* gene is located at chromosome 8p22 and its expression and activity is highly regulated, but most of its physiologic function is regulated by posttranslational factors including insulin (sensitivity) and other hormones (eg, prolactin in mammary tissue), noradrenergic stimulation,[47] feeding/glucose levels, transiently by heparin, apolipoprotein cofactors (apoC-II, apoC-III, apoA-V), and **angiopoietinlike proteins (AngPTL)**.[48] Adipose expresses LPL in particularly high concentration.

2. **Angiopoietinlike proteins** This class of regulatory proteins has a major role in the metabolism of TRL. AngPTL3 and AngPTL8 appear to have a mostly endocrine function, participating as LPL stimulator in circulation, while AngPTL4 acts more like a paracrine hormone, inhibiting LPL by the numerous cells that express it in response to local needs. Its transcription is regulated by **peroxisome-proliferating activator receptor (PPAR)**, stimulated by the presence of FA.[49] Loss of function genetic mutations have been identified that are associated with low TG levels.[50]

   a. AngPTL3 and AngPTL8 are also LPL inhibitors but, unlike AngPTL4, are expressed primarily by hepatocytes (and adipose tissue—AngPTL8), regulated by leptin, insulin, and the nuclear liver X receptor (LXR).[51–53] Their central (hepatic) expression and distal/peripheral activity make them behave more like endocrine than paracrine hormones.

   b. LPL has its primary purpose to facilitate energy storage and has been referred to as the "gatekeeper" for calorie storage.[54] CD36 is highly regulated by many of the same pathways as LPL, which makes sense since they work in concert to facilitate cellular uptake of long chain FA and fat-soluble vitamins.[55]

3. **Hormone-sensitive lipase (HSL)** Hormone-sensitive lipase (HSL) is an intracellular lipase expressed primarily in adipocytes, but also found in other cells including steroidogenic tissue. As its name suggests, its activity is stimulated by counterregulatory noradrenergic/hormonal activity facilitating the release of free fatty acids (FFA) from adipose tissue. The enzyme can catalyze the lipolysis of triglycerides, diglycerides, monoglycerides, and cholesteryl ester. FFA are complexed with circulating albumin, which enable FFA to be transported in circulation without lipoprotein inclusion. The *HSL* gene is found on chromosome 19q13.3. It is not clear whether genetic defects in HSL are associated with specific cardiometabolic disorders such as obesity, lipodystrophy, or lipid/lipoprotein disorders though this is clearly an important regulator of normal lipid metabolism.[56]

4. **Hepatic lipase (HL)** Hepatic lipase (HL) is a 67-kDa glycoprotein, expressed and active as a monomer by hepatocytes and similar to LPL, is released from its binding by heparin infusion. It is preferentially active on smaller, denser TRL and HDL.

VII. Putting It All Together

A. Lipids have poor solubility in blood so they must be carried in the circulation by lipoproteins. Triglyceride is an efficient energy-carrying molecule and needs to be transported from its source (gut/liver) to the periphery for storage or energy utilization in fat, muscle, etc. Cholesterol is a complex heterocyclic hydrocarbon that can be synthesized by all cells, but which can be catabolized by specialized cells (liver, steroid producing) only.

B. Fats are digested, then absorbed in the gut, and packaged together in enterocytes into chylomicrons (CM) for transport into lymphatics to the venous circulation and ultimately to the liver for processing. CM are cleared from the circulation within 12 hours of a meal in an individual under normal metabolic circumstances.

C. VLDL are secreted by the hepatocyte after a meal to deliver TG to the periphery. VLDL synthesis is regulated by hepatocyte FA availability since its other principle elements (apoB-100 and cholesterol) are constitutive and stable in the hepatocyte. VLDL circulates and condenses to IDL and then to LDL as a result of interaction with LPL, which facilitates the TG removal from TRL. Multiple proteins help regulate LPL function, and inherited defects in these helper proteins result in accumulation of CM, CM remnants, and VLDL remnants. Once the apoB-containing LP has shed its core TG content and converted to LDL, LDL-R–mediated uptake is favored.

D. Overproduction of VLDL (from overconsumption of calories, excessive hepatic return of FA in the insulin-resistant state), reduced caloric utilization (sedentary lifestyle or peripheral metabolic muscle disorders), and/or defects in the many genes responsible for modulating the apoB-containing LP condensation/clearance will result in incomplete clearance of TRL.

E. Defects in genes responsible for the normal clearance of LDL and dietary excess will result in high levels of LDL (LDL-C and LDL-P). High levels of TRL and LDL are a significant contributor to the development of atherosclerosis. The process is accelerated by concomitant CV risk factors or absent protective mechanisms and occurs as a function of the height of apoB-containing LP and time exposure to high levels.

F. High levels of circulating remnant TRL and LDL both promote the development of atherosclerosis by triggering the endothelial inflammatory reaction resulting in foam cell formation. The present standard is to direct therapy at improving clearance of apoB-containing LP and, in some cases, to inhibit synthesis of TRL precursors.

G. HDL act as scavenger particles capable of interacting with foam cells in the periphery, enabling cholesterol efflux and removal of cholesterol from the arterial wall and, because of their rich anti-inflammatory protein cargo, also turn off the atherosclerotic process directly. It is impaired HDL function, not necessarily low HDL-C levels, that results in high ASCVD risk. This further suggests that targeting improvements in HDL function and cholesterol efflux should reduce cardiovascular risk.

VIII. Conclusion

Lipid biochemistry is complex, but a basic understanding of lipid metabolism is important in understanding the various lipid abnormalities and management options. This chapter has provided an overview of lipid metabolism for the clinician and an introduction for those who wish to delve further into this area of study.

References

1. Available at: http://www.cdc.gov/heartdisease/facts.htm. Accessed October 21, 2015.
2. Warboys CM, Amini N, De luca A, Evans PC. The role of blood flow in determining the sites of atherosclerotic plaques. *F1000 Med Rep.* 2011;3:5.
3. Banach M, Serban C, Sahebkar A, et al. Effects of coenzyme Q10 on statin-induced myopathy: a meta-analysis of randomized controlled trials. *Mayo Clin Proc.* 2015;90(1):24-34.
4. Available at: http://lipidlibrary.aocs.org/Primer/content.cfm?ItemNumber=39371&navItemNumber=19200. Accessed July 23, 2016.
5. Barter PJ, Ballantyne CM, Carmena R, et al. Apo B versus cholesterol in estimating cardiovascular risk and in guiding therapy: report of the thirty-person/ten-country panel. *J Intern Med.* 2006;259(3):247-258.
6. Barter PJ, Nicholls S, Rye KA, Anantharamaiah GM, Navab M, Fogelman AM. Antiinflammatory properties of HDL. *Circ Res.* 2004;95(8):764-772.
7. Anglés-cano E, Rojas G. Apolipoprotein(a): structure-function relationship at the lysine-binding site and plasminogen activator cleavage site. *Biol Chem.* 2002;383(1):93-99.
8. Ichinose A, Suzuki K, Saito T. Apolipoprotein(a) and thrombosis: molecular and genetic bases of hyper-lipoprotein(a)-emia. *Semin Thromb Hemost.* 1998;24(3):237-243.
9. Raal FJ, Giugliano RP, Sabatine MS, et al. PCSK9 inhibition-mediated reduction in Lp(a) with evolocumab: an analysis of 10 clinical trials and the LDL receptor's role. *J Lipid Res.* 2016;57:1086-1096.
10. Raal FJ, Giugliano RP, Sabatine MS, et al. Reduction in lipoprotein(a) with PCSK9 monoclonal antibody evolocumab (AMG 145): a pooled analysis of more than 1,300 patients in 4 phase II trials. *J Am Coll Cardiol.* 2014;63(13):1278-1288.
11. Nordestgaard BG, Chapman MJ, Ray K, et al. Lipoprotein(a) as a cardiovascular risk factor: current status. *Eur Heart J.* 2010;31:2844-2853.
12. The CARDIoGRAMplusC4D Consortium. Large-scale association analysis identifies new risk loci for coronary artery disease. *Nat Genet.* 2013;45(1):25-33.
13. Ye H, Zhou A, Hong Q, et al. Positive association between APOA5 rs662799 polymorphism and coronary heart disease: a case–control study and meta-analysis. *PLoS One.* 2015;10(8):e0135683.
14. Baggio G, Manzato E, Gabelli C, et al. Apolipoprotein C-II deficiency syndrome. Clinical features, lipoprotein characterization, lipase activity, and correction of hypertriglyceridemia after apolipoprotein C-II administration in two affected patients. *J Clin Invest.* 1986;77(2):520-527.
15. Schonfeld G, George PK, Miller J, Reilly P, Witztum J. Apolipoprotein C-II and C-III levels in hyperlipoproteinemia. *Metabolism.* 1979;28(10):1001-1010.
16. Sacks FM, Zheng C, Cohn JS. Complexities of apolipoprotein C-III metabolism. *J Lipid Res.* 2011;52(6):1067-1070.
17. Phillips MC. Apolipoprotein E isoforms and lipoprotein metabolism. *IUBMB Life.* 2014;66(9):616-623.
18. Hopkins PN, Brinton EA, Nanjee MN. Hyperlipoproteinemia type 3: the forgotten phenotype. *Curr Atheroscler Rep.* 2014;16(9):440.
19. Bu G. Apolipoprotein E and its receptors in Alzheimer's disease: pathways, pathogenesis and therapy. *Nat Rev Neurosci.* 2009;10:333-344.

20. Liu CC, Kanekiyo T, Xu H, Bu G. Apolipoprotein E and Alzheimer disease: risk, mechanisms and therapy. *Nat Rev Neurol*. 2013;9:106-118.
21. Kronenberg F, Utermann G. Lipoprotein(a): resurrected by genetics. *J Intern Med*. 2013;273(1):6-30.
22. Gleize B, Nowicki M, Daval C, Koutnikova H, Borel P. Form of phytosterols and food matrix in which they are incorporated modulate their incorporation into mixed micelles and impact cholesterol micellarization. *Mol Nutr Food Res*. 2016;60(4):749-759.
23. Eating you way to lower cholesterol. Foods fortified with plant sterols or stanols can help nudge down high cholesterol. *Harv Heart Lett*. 2006;16(7):3.
24. Brown WV, Ference BA, Kathiresan S. JCL roundtable: lessons from genetic variants altering lipoprotein metabolism. *J Clin Lipidol*. 2016;10:448-457.
25. Osono Y, Woollett LA, Herz J, Dietschy JM. Role of the low density lipoprotein receptor in the flux of cholesterol through the plasma and across the tissues of the mouse. *J Clin Invest*. 1995;95:1124.
26. Tsimikas S, Brilakis ES, Miller ER, et al. Oxidized phospholipids, Lp(a) lipoprotein, and coronary artery disease. *N Engl J Med*. 2005;353(1):46-57.
27. Bilheimer DW. Metabolic studies in familial hypercholesterolemia: evidence for a gene-dosage effect in vivo. *J Clin Invest*. 1979;64(2):524-533.
28. Goldstein JL, Brown MS. The LDL receptor. *Arterioscler Thromb Vasc Biol*. 2009;29(4):431-438.
29. Horton JD, Cohen JC, Hobbs HH. Molecular biology of PCSK9: its role in LDL metabolism. *Trends Biochem Sci*. 2007;32(2):71-77.
30. Available at: http://www.ncbi.nlm.nih.gov/gene/255738. Accessed July 23, 2016.
31. Fitzgerald K, Frank-kamenetsky M, Shulga-morskaya S, et al. Effect of an RNA interference drug on the synthesis of proprotein convertase subtilisin/kexin type 9 (PCSK9) and the concentration of serum LDL cholesterol in healthy volunteers: a randomised, single-blind, placebo-controlled, phase 1 trial. *Lancet*. 2014;383(9911):60-68.
32. Soutar AK, Naoumova RP. Mechanisms of disease: genetic causes of familial hypercholesterolemia. *Nat Clin Pract Cardiovasc Med*. 2007;4(4):214-225.
33. Takahashi S, Kawarabayasi Y, Nakai T, Sakai J, Yamamoto T. Rabbit very-low-density lipoprotein receptor: a low-density lipoprotein receptor-like protein with distinct ligand specificity. *Proc Natl Acad Sci U S A*. 1992;89(19):9252-9256.
34. Beisiegel U, Weber W, Ihrke G, Herz J, Stanley KK. The LDL-receptor-related protein, LRP, is an apolipoprotein E-binding protein. *Nature*. 1989;341(6238):162-164.
35. de Faria E, Fong LG, Komaromy M, Cooper AD. Relative roles of the LDL receptor, the LDL receptor-like protein, and hepatic lipase in chylomicron remnant removal by the liver. *J Lipid Res*. 1996;37(1):197-209.
36. May P. The low-density lipoprotein receptor-related protein 1 in inflammation. *Curr Opin Lipidol*. 2013;24(2):134-137.
37. Moon JH, Kang SB, Park JS, et al. Up-regulation of hepatic low-density lipoprotein receptor-related protein 1: a possible novel mechanism of antiatherogenic activity of hydroxymethylglutaryl-coenzyme A reductase inhibitor Atorvastatin and hepatic LRP1 expression. *Metabolism*. 2011;60(7):930-940.
38. Clarenbach JJ, Grundy SM, Palacio N, Vega GL. Relationship of apolipoprotein B levels to the number of risk factors for metabolic syndrome. *J Investig Med*. 2007;55(5):237-247.
39. Kathiresan S, Otvos JD, Sullivan LM, et al. Increased small low-density lipoprotein particle number: a prominent feature of the metabolic syndrome in the Framingham Heart Study. *Circulation*. 2006;113(1):20-29.
40. Patsch JR. Triglyceride-rich lipoproteins and atherosclerosis. *Atherosclerosis*. 1994;110(suppl):S23-S26.
41. Chait A, Brazg RL, Tribble DL, Krauss RM. Susceptibility of small, dense, low-density lipoproteins to oxidative modification in subjects with the atherogenic lipoprotein phenotype, pattern B. *Am J Med*. 1993;94(4):350-356.
42. Dallmeier D, Koenig W. Strategies for vascular disease prevention: the role of lipids and related markers including apolipoproteins, low-density lipoproteins (LDL)-particle size, high sensitivity C-reactive protein (hs-CRP), lipoprotein-associated phospholipase A2 (Lp-PLA$_2$) and lipoprotein(a) (Lp(a)). *Best Pract Res Clin Endocrinol Metab*. 2014;28(3):281-294.
43. Jacobson TA, Ito MK, Maki KC, et al. National lipid association recommendations for patient-centered management of dyslipidemia: part 1—full report. *J Clin Lipidol*. 2015;9(2):129-169.
44. Jacobson TA, Maki KC, Orringer CE, et al. National lipid association recommendations for patient-centered management of dyslipidemia: part 2. *J Clin Lipidol*. 2015;9(6 suppl):S1-S122.e1.
45. Cefalù AB, Noto D, Arpi ML, et al. Novel LMF1 nonsense mutation in a patient with severe hypertriglyceridemia. *J Clin Endocrinol Metab*. 2009;94(11):4584-4590.
46. Buonuomo PS, Bartuli A, Rabacchi C, Bertolini S, Calandra S. A 3-day-old neonate with severe hypertriglyceridemia from novel mutations of the GPIHBP1 gene. *J Clin Lipidol*. 2015;9(2):265-270.
47. Ricart-jané D, Cejudo-martín P, Peinado-onsurbe J, López-tejero MD, Llobera M. Changes in lipoprotein lipase modulate tissue energy supply during stress. *J Appl Physiol*. 2005;99(4):1343-1351.
48. Kersten S. Physiological regulation of lipoprotein lipase. *Biochim Biophys Acta*. 2014;1841(7):919-933.

49. Georgiadi A, Lichtenstein L, Degenhardt T, et al. Induction of cardiac Angptl4 by dietary fatty acids is mediated by peroxisome proliferator-activated receptor beta/delta and protects against fatty acid-induced oxidative stress. *Circ Res.* 2010;106(11):1712-1721.

50. Romeo S, Pennacchio LA, Fu Y, Boerwinkle E, et al. Population-based resequencing of ANGPTL4 uncovers variations that reduce triglycerides and increase HDL. *Nat Genet* 2007;39:513-516.

51. Inukai K, Nakashima Y, Watanabe M, et al. ANGPTL3 is increased in both insulin-deficient and -resistant diabetic states. *Biochem Biophys Res Commun.* 2004;317:1075-1079.

52. Shimamura M, Matsuda M, Ando Y, et al. Leptin and insulin down-regulate angiopoietin-like protein 3, a plasma triglyceride-increasing factor. *Biochem Biophys Res Commun.* 2004;322:1080-1085.

53. Kaplan R, Zhang T, Hernandez M, et al. Regulation of the angiopoietin-like protein 3 gene by LXR. *J Lipid Res.* 2003;44:136-143.

54. Greenwood MR. The relationship of enzyme activity to feeding behavior in rats: lipoprotein lipase as the metabolic gatekeeper. *Int J Obes.* 1985;9(suppl 1):67-70.

55. Goldberg IJ, Eckel RH, Abumrad NA. Regulation of fatty acid uptake into tissues: lipoprotein lipase- and CD36-mediated pathways. *J Lipid Res.* 2009;50(suppl):S86-S90.

56. Kraemer FB, Shen WJ. Hormone-sensitive lipase: control of intracellular tri-(di-)acylglycerol and cholesteryl ester hydrolysis. *J Lipid Res.* 2002;43(10):1585-1594.

Guidelines and Risk Scores

Merle Myerson

Key Points

■ Guidelines have been established for the diagnosis and management of dyslipidemia; however, there are varying approaches taken by different issuing organizations.

■ Risk scores and algorithms help determine the intensity of lipid-lowering therapy.

■ The American College of Cardiology and American Heart Association 2013 Guideline eliminated lipid targets and goals; however, many US and international organizations continued to endorse their use.

I. Introduction

A. Guidelines have been established for diagnosis and management of dyslipidemia within the United States by various professional organizations as well as internationally. The establishment of a guideline is a complex undertaking. Guidelines influence who will receive medication, who is labeled as "sick," and how our health care dollars are spent as well as insurance coverage.

B. Risk scores and algorithms have also been developed to help determine the intensity of lipid-lowering therapy. These scores are, in some part, an evolving science because potential drivers of risk and disease development continue to emerge.

C. This chapter focuses on the two current statements in the United States, that of the "2013 American College of Cardiology/American Heart Association (ACC/AHA) Guideline on the Treatment of Blood cholesterol to Reduce Atherosclerotic Cardiovascular Risk in Adults"[1] and the "2014 National Lipid Association Recommendations for Patient-Centered Management of Dyslipidemia."[2]

II. Evolution of Guidelines in the United States

The National Heart, Lung, and Blood Institute's (NHLBI) National Cholesterol Education Program, Adult Treatment Panel (NCEP ATP) issued their first guidelines in 1988 with updates in 1993 and 2001. A fourth revision was planned, and in 2007, the NHLBI convened an expert panel to update the guidelines. In 2008, the ATP IV panel was appointed; however, in 2013 the NHLBI asked the ACC and AHA to take on the task of developing updated guidelines on treatment of cholesterol.

III. United States Guidelines

A. American College of Cardiology/American Heart Association Guideline and Risk Calculator

1. The ACC/AHA determined that statin therapy should be used for those in one of four groups (Box 3.1) with either moderate- or high-dose statin (Box 3.2).

2. The ACC/AHA committee considered only evidence from randomized clinical trials (RCT) and did not include post-hoc analyses or RCTs, observational studies, or genetic studies. They felt that "Only one approach has been evaluated in multiple

---

BOX 3.1 | 2013 ACC/AHA Guidelines: 4 Groups to Treat With Statins

- 4 groups treated with moderate- to high-dose statins
  - Those with history atherosclerotic CV events
  - Those with LDL-C ≥ 190
  - Those with diabetes 1 or 2 age 40-75
  - Those with 10 y risk ASCVD with pooled cohort equations ≥ 7.5% age 40-74

- Depending on risk, add moderate- or high-dose statins
- No evidence for using the LDL-C and non-HDL-C goals of ATP III

RCTS—the use of fixed doses of cholesterol-lowering drugs to reduce atherosclerotic cardiovascular disease (ASCVD) risk." And that "Because the overwhelming body of evidence came from statin RCTs, the Expert Panel appropriately focused on these statin RCTs to develop evidence-based guidelines."

3. Treatment for older persons was not addressed as "Fewer people > 75 years of age were included in the statin RCTS reviewed" and "RCT evidence does not support/ exist for initiation of high-intensity statin therapy for secondary prevention or for any therapy for primary prevention."

4. The committee acknowledged that their process did not provide for a comprehensive approach to the detection, evaluation, and treatment of lipid disorders.

5. Most important, the committee eliminated targets and goals for treatment. If a person was in one of the four treatment groups, the person would be treated with a statin; however, LDL-C was not a target and neither were there goals for treatment.

6. The committee developed a new risk calculator, the "Pooled Cohort Equations," to estimate 10-year ASCVD risk for the identification of candidates for statin therapy.

BOX 3.2 | 2013 ACC/AHA Statin Levels

Statins Levels
- High dose
  - Rosuvastatin (Crestor)   20-40 mg
  - Atorvastatin   40-80 mg
- Moderate dose
  - Rosuvastatin (Crestor)   5-10 mg
  - Atorvastatin   10-20 mg
  - Simvastatin   20-40 mg
  - Pitavastatin (Livalo)   2-4 mg
  - Pravastatin   40-80 mg
  - Lovastatin   40 mg
  - Fluvastatin (Lescol) XL   40 bid or XL 80
- Low dose   Any lower dose than moderate
  - Simavastatin 10 mg
  - Pravastatin 10-20 mg
  - Lovastatin 20 mg
  - Fluvastatin 20-40 mg
  - Pitavastatin 1 mg

7. Information from population-based cohort studies funded by NHLBI was used to develop this scoring system and includes sex, age, race (White or African American), total cholesterol, HDL cholesterol, systolic blood pressure, treatment for high blood pressure (if systolic blood pressure is >120 mm Hg), diabetes, and smoking.

B. National Lipid Association recommendations for patient-centered management of dyslipidemia

1. Committee used evidence from RCT (including primary, subgroup, and pooled analyses), epidemiological, mechanistic, and genetic studies.

2. Maintained targets for therapy: LDL-C and Non-HDL-C with apolipoprotein B as a secondary, optional target of treatment and goals

3. Statins were first-line therapy unless triglycerides were >500 mg/dL although the role of nonstatins was endorsed

4. Used risk scoring based on NCEP ATP III, Framingham, and ACC/AHA Pooled Cohort Equations (see Chapter 5 for the NLA risk scoring plan). Table 3.1 compares the Framingham and Pooled Cohort Equations risk schemes.

5. Targets and goals listed in Table 3.2

C. Lipid targets and goals

1. The ACC/AHA Guideline was both criticized and applauded for their new approach; however, many did not agree with the elimination of targets and goals.

2. Existing Canadian,[3] European,[4] and International Atherosclerosis Society[5] have all continued to endorse targets and goals.

Table 3.1. Risk Scores: Framingham, Pooled Cohort Equations		
	Framingham Risk Score	**Pooled Cohort Equations (ACC/AHA)**
Population	General population from one area. Framingham MA (USA)	Population-based cohort studies funded by NHLBI
Age	30-74 y	
Data collection	1968-1971 original Framingham cohort, 1971-1975 and 1984-1987 Offspring Studies	Varied
Years risk prediction	10-y risk of CHD events 30-y risk of CHD and stroke	10-y risk of ASCVD
Variables	Sex, age, total cholesterol, HDL-C, smoking status, systolic blood pressure (treated/not treated), diabetes	Sex, age, race (white or black), total cholesterol, HDL-C, systolic blood pressure, treatment for high blood pressure (if systolic > 120 mm Hg), diabetes, smoking status
Guidelines using score	NCEP ATP III Canadian Cardiovascular Society International Atherosclerosis Society National Lipid Association Recommendations	2013 ACC/AHA Guideline on the Treatment of Blood Cholesterol to Reduce Atherosclerotic Cardiovascular Risk in Adults National Lipid Association Recommendations
Discrimination and calibration in HIV+	e-statistics: 0.65, 0.71, 0.77 O/E: 1.18, 1.51	e-statistics: 0.65, 0.71 O/E: 1.20; may be better than FRS at higher categories of predicted risk
Notes		Risk scores account for white and black race Eliminated targets for LDL-C

Data from DeFilippis AP, Young R, Carrubba CJ, et al. An analysis of calibration and discrimination among multiple cardiovascular risk scores in a modern multiethnic cohort. *Ann Intern Med* 2015;162:266-275.

Table 3.2. National Lipid Association Targets and Goals for Therapy			
		Treatment Goal	
Risk Category	Non-HDL-C	LDL-C	Apo B[a]
Low	<130	<100	<90
Moderate	<130	<100	<90
High	<130	<100	<90
Very High	<100	<70	<80

[a]Apo B is an optional target of treatment.
All values are in mg/dL.

3. Research supports use of goals, in particular lower LDL-C goals to lower risk for ASCVD.[6,7]

4. The National Lipid Association Recommendations continue to endorse lipid targets and goals.

D. Role of biomarkers and noninvasive tests

1. Other markers and testing have been shown to predict risk for ASCVD but are not part of risk stratification schemes or guidelines.

2. Both the NLA Recommendations and the ACC/AHA Guideline discuss where use of additional risk indicators may be considered for risk refinement. In general, these indicators are helpful in intermediate-risk persons. The ACC/AHA Guidelines state that they are useful "In selected individuals who are not in 1 of the 4 statin benefit groups, and for whom a decision to initiate statin therapy is otherwise unclear."[1]

3. Factors to consider include the following:
   a. Coronary Artery Calcium is an indicator of subclinical disease and a score ≥ 300 Agatston units or ≥75 percentile for age, sex, and ethnicity is considered high risk.
   b. C-reactive protein ≥ 2.0 mg/L.
   c. Lp(a) ≥ 50 mg/dL (protein) using an isoform-insensitive assay.

IV. Summary

Guidelines and risk scoring systems are important and helpful in determining how we treat patients with dyslipidemia or at risk for ASCVD. In the United States, we currently have two approaches, that of the ACC/AHA and that of the NLA. Both groups advocate risk stratification and management reflecting the level of risk; however, the two approaches differ in terms of cutoffs and qualifications for treatment, use of lipid targets and goals, and endorsement of nonstatin therapy. As always, the clinician should use these documents to help guide clinical judgment for his or her individual patients.

References

1. Stone NJ, Robinson J, Lichtenstein AH, et al. 2013 ACC/AHA Guideline on the Treatment of Blood Cholesterol to Reduce Atherosclerotic Cardiovascular Risk in Adults: A Report of the American College of Cardiology/American Heart Association Task Force on Practice Guidelines. *J Am Coll Cardiol*. 2014 Jul 1;63(25 Pt B):2889–2934.
2. Jacobson TA, Ito MK, Maki KC, et al. National Lipid Association recommendations for patient-centered management of dyslipidemia: part 1–executive summary. *J Clin Lipidol*. 2014;8(5):473-488.
3. Anderson TJ, Gregoire J, Hegele RA, et al. 2012 update of the Canadian Cardiovascular Society guidelines for the diagnosis and treatment of dyslipidemia for the prevention of cardiovascular disease in the adult. *Can J Cardiol*. 2013;29(2):151-167.

4. Catapano AL, Chapman J, Wiklund O, Taskinen MR. The new joint EAS/ESC guidelines for the management of dyslipidaemias. *Atherosclerosis.* 2011;217(1):1.
5. Expert Dyslipidemia Panel of the International Atherosclerosis Society Panel members. An International Atherosclerosis Society position paper: global recommendations for the management of dyslipidemia—full report. *J Clin Lipidol.* 2014;8(1):29-60.
6. Cannon CP, Blazing MA, Giugliano RP, et al. Ezetimibe added to statin therapy after acute coronary syndromes. *N Engl J Med.* 2015;372(25):2387-2397.
7. Boekholdt SM, Hovingh GK, Mora S, et al. Very low levels of atherogenic lipoproteins and the risk for cardiovascular events: a meta-analysis of statin trials. *J Am Coll Cardiol.* 2014;64(5):485-494.

Lipid Measurement

Valerie Bush and Merle Myerson

Key Points

- Reliable and valid measurement of lipid levels is important to the diagnosis and management of dyslipidemia.
- There are many sources of analytic variation. The reliability of an analytical method is dependent upon the accuracy (bias) and precision (reproducibility).
- Lipid testing has traditionally been performed in the fasting state primarily because of the effect of food on triglycerides and the calculation of LDL-C using the Friedewald formula.
- Calculation of the LDL-C using the Friedewald formula has been used for clinical management, guidelines, and research.
- The Friedewald formula is optimal for calculation of LDL-C when triglycerides are <150. The accuracy is reduced as triglyceride level increases, and the formula should not be used when triglycerides are >400 mg/dL.
- Direct measurement of LDL-C and calculation by the Friedewald formula are not the same, and the determinations can vary significantly.

I. Introduction

A. The diagnosis of dyslipidemia and assessment of risk for cardiovascular disease are made by measuring plasma concentration of lipids and lipoproteins. Guidelines and standards for clinical chemistry laboratories that perform these measurements have been established to help assure the measurements are both reliable and valid.

B. Accurate determination of serum lipids, lipoproteins, and apolipoproteins is dependent on controlling analytical and preanalytical factors. However, the heterogeneity and complexity of lipid particles present challenges for their analysis.

C. Traditionally, lipid measurements have been expressed in terms of their cholesterol content of the particle, for example, "LDL cholesterol" is the measurement of the cholesterol content of the LDL particle.

D. Analytically, cholesterol has a known molecular structure that can be accurately and precisely measured. Conversely, triglycerides and lipoproteins vary in biochemical composition and structure. Primary considerations are summarized below.

E. This chapter is intended to provide background information on measurement of lipids and lipoproteins so the clinician may understand how measurement issues are relevant for management of lipids in their patients.

II. Laboratory Performance and Certification

A. Standardization programs The Centers for Disease Control (CDC) and World Health Organization (WHO) provide accuracy-based programs for standardizing and ensuring quality of lipid measurements. These programs monitor the precision and accuracy of methods by using independent internal and external quality controls, international reference standards, and protocols to identify and reduce errors due to preanalytical factors. These standards exist for total cholesterol, triglycerides, high density lipoprotein cholesterol (HDL), apolipoprotein A-I (apoA-I), and apolipoprotein B (apoB). Measurement standardization ensures the credibility of results and valid comparability among different laboratories, population studies, and clinical trials. The CDC-Laboratory Standardization Program is not a proficiency testing (PT) program, in which performance assessment often is based on peer group means, not on traceability to accuracy standards.[1]

B. **Reference methods** Reference methods provide accuracy targets that are fully validated and credentialed through the Joint Committee for Traceability in Laboratory Medicine. Other methods, although not formally credentialed, have been accepted by consensus. Various methods should be capable of similar accuracy and precision such that lipid measurements among laboratories are as if they had been made in a single laboratory, regardless of the method used. Laboratory standardization programs facilitate achieving this goal. Regardless of improving analytical measurements, there are still sources of variation that can occur in the testing process (preanalytical, analytical, and postanalytical).

C. **Laboratory certification** In 1995, the National Cholesterol Education Program (NCEP) (NCEP Recommendations on Lipoprotein Measurement NIH publication 95-3044 Bethesda, 1995) issued recommendations for acceptable lipid and lipoprotein measurements. These have formed the basis for national laboratory lipid certification.

III. Sources of Test Variation

Interpreting test results requires an association with a reference range among other factors. The diagnostic usefulness of an abnormal result will vary with the sensitivity and specificity of the test and with the prevalence of the disease in the population tested.[2] For cholesterol and other lipids, criteria from evidence-based medical and laboratory principles for reference ranges and interpretation of those ranges are used.[3] These ranges are fixed and have accounted for some sources of variation. Common sources of variability are described below.

A. **Analytical variation** Every analytical method has some intrinsic sources of variability. Although these cannot be completely eliminated, they can be minimized with good laboratory quality practices.

1. **Accuracy and precision** The reliability of an analytical method is dependent upon the accuracy (bias) and precision (reproducibility). Accuracy is subject to systematic variation, which is the difference between the result obtained and the true value of measured component. Bias can be constant or proportional to the value of the analyte measured. For example, bias can be affected by changes in instrumentation, methodologies for the same analyte or reagent, and calibrator lots. Precision is measured by replicate analysis of the same sample and is influenced by random error. An example of random error is temperature fluctuations during the analytical reaction. Random variation exhibits a Gaussian distribution with a symmetrical bell-shaped curve.

2. **Standard deviation and coefficient of variation and total analytical error of a measurement** The width of dispersion of the distribution can be calculated as the standard deviation. The standard deviation relative to the mean is the coefficient of variation (CV).[4] Errors associated with accuracy and precision are combined as total analytical error. The NCEP guidelines state that the total error of a test should be within the criteria from the reference test as shown in Table 4.1.

3. **Proficiency testing** Proficiency testing programs provide a mechanism for laboratories to assess the accuracy of laboratory tests. These have been required in the

Table 4.1. **Analytical Performance Criteria for Assays Used to Assess CVD Risk**

Analyte	Maximum Allowable Bias[a]	Maximum Allowable Imprecision
TC[b]	≤3.0%	≤3.0% CV
HDL-C[b]	≤5.0%	≤4% CV at ≥ 42 mg/dL ≤1.7 mg/dL SD at <42 mg/dL
LDL-C[b]	≤4%	CV ≤ 4%
TG[c]	≤5%	CV ≤ 5%

Source: CDC CRMLN. Procedures for Certification of Clinical Laboratories. https://www.cdc.gov/labstandards/crmln_clinical.html

[a]Bias to the reference method

CV, coefficient of variation; SD, standard deviation; TC, total cholesterol; HDL-C, high density lipoprotein cholesterol; LDL-C, low density lipoprotein cholesterol.

[b]https://www.cdc.gov/labstandards/crmln_clinical.html

[c]Fallest-Strobl PC, Olafsdottir E, Wiebe D, Westgard JO. Comparison of NCEP performance specifications for triglycerides, HDL-, and LDL-cholesterol with operating specifications based on NCEP clinical and analytical goals. *Clin Chem*. 1995;43(11):2164-2168.

United States since the Clinical Laboratory Improvement Act of 1988 (CLIA '88).[4,5] These regulations also specify performance standards laboratories must achieve. Laboratory accreditation programs survey laboratories against these regulations and provide feedback for areas of improvement. Any failures require a corrective action plan.

B. **Preanalytical variation** Prior to any analytical measurement, the patient and specimen must be prepared for testing. Preanalytical variations from differences in patient lifestyle, altered lipid metabolism due to disease or genetics, source of blood specimen, and conditions of sample handling can all impact the result. Biologic variability is well understood in endocrinology where hormones change in rhythmic cycles or over the lifespan of an individual. Biologic variation may not result in clinically significant changes, but it is important to be aware of them, particularly when they can lead to misdiagnosis or mistreatment strategies. Cooper et al. provide an excellent review of preanalytical variables associated with lipid measurements.[6]

1. **Posture** Posture can influence total cholesterol, HDL-C, triglycerides, apoA-1, apoB, and Lp(a). Postural effects on cholesterol are well recognized but are thought to be related to shifts in plasma volume when changing position. Going from the standing to sitting position can lower total cholesterol by ~5%.[7] The mechanism for these shifts for triglyceride and lipoprotein values is not clear because lipids and lipoproteins do not easily diffuse between vascular and extravascular spaces. Nevertheless and for practicality, the CDC NCEP guidelines recommend patients sit quietly for 5 minutes prior to venipuncture.[8]

2. **Plasma or serum or whole blood** Either plasma or serum can be used to measure most lipids, lipoproteins, and apolipoproteins. Heparinized plasma is typically the anticoagulant of choice for lipid testing due to its convenience for testing other chemistry analytes.[9] Total cholesterol and HDL-C have shown biases from ethylenediaminetetraacetic acid (EDTA) plasma compared to serum.[10] Some older references have suggested a conversion formula for calculating an equivalent serum value from plasma. This was to accommodate the dilution from liquid additives in the blood collection tube. Most blood collection tubes today contain a dry additive without any dilutional effects. Long-term refrigerated or frozen storage of plasma lipids and lipoproteins has been demonstrated to have little impact on recovery for up to 1 month.[11]

3. **Fingerstick whole blood sample** Whole blood samples from a fingerstick used with "desktop analyzers" or other "point-of-care" whole blood measurements exhibited

greater analytical variation than serum laboratory-based analysis.[12] These are often used at health fairs and screenings as well as in clinician offices, but it is best to confirm point-of-care results with standard laboratory testing for diagnosis and management.[13]

4. **Fasting vs nonfasting**
   a. Historically, lipid profile testing has required a fasting specimen. The rationale being that postprandial changes to triglycerides and lipoprotein composition would impact calculation of LDL cholesterol when using the Friedewald equation. Cholesterol, HDL-C and lipoproteins do not clinically differ between fasting and nonfasting specimens to the extent where it would have clinical relevance.[14,15]
   b. Triglycerides are subject to clinically significant fluctuations associated with the fasting or nonfasting state[16,17] and show the greatest variation in relation to when and what food was eaten prior to blood testing. Ingested fat will reach a peak at about 3-6 hours and decline to fasting level by 10-12 hours.[14] Alcohol and other foods can also influence triglyceride levels.[18,19] NCEP guidelines recommend fasting for 9 hours prior to lipid testing.[20] Although nonfasting samples are considerably more convenient for patients, the decision points used by the current guidelines are based on fasting triglyceride measurements.
   c. Nonfasting triglyceride values
      i. Early studies linked nonfasting triglyceride values to increased cardiac risk of myocardial infarct or ischemic heart disease.[21] More recently, some European organizations[22] along with the Women's Health Study[17] have recommended the use of a nonfasting specimen for routine lipid profile testing. An American Heart Association Statement on Triglycerides states that in patients with normal baseline triglycerides, consumption of a low-fat breakfast before blood testing would not be expected to raise the triglyceride level above 200 mg/dL. Therefore, if nonfasting level is ≥200 mg/dL, a fasting lipid profile is recommended to diagnose hypertriglyderidemia.[23]

IV. Methods of Measurement

A. **Basic lipid panel** Among the first methods used was that of ultracentrifugation whereby plasma was separated and measured based on size, shape, and density. The CDC reference methods for cholesterol, HDL-C, and triglyceride by ultracentrifugation are complex and time consuming, and for these reasons, most instrument manufacturers and laboratories have adopted simpler methods for routine clinical use. These methods are traceable to a reference method and require very small amounts (microliters) of sample.

1. **Total cholesterol** Cholesterol, with its known molecular structure, can be accurately and precisely measured by well-established automated standardized methods. Cholesterol is usually measured enzymatically in a series of coupled reactions that hydrolyze cholesterol esters and produce by-products that are measured in a single photometric reagent. Manufacturers of these reagents provide calibration materials specific to their formulation that are traceable to the CDC reference method.

2. **HDL-C** HDL-C is most commonly measured after the separation of apoB-100 containing lipoproteins using one of several polyanion-divalent cation combinations. Other newer approaches measure HDL-C directly without a preliminary separation step by rendering the cholesterol in HDL more reactive than that of other lipoproteins.

3. **Triglycerides** Triglycerides are measured enzymatically directly in serum or plasma. Several types of methods have been employed, but all utilize a lipase-catalyzed hydrolysis of triglycerides to glycerol and free fatty acids as the first step. With the generation of glycerol, any glycerol that may be present in the sample contributes to the

triglyceride measured, although usually not medically significant. The rare condition of glycerokinase deficiency may demonstrate 50- to 100-fold levels of glycerol in serum.[24]

4. **LDL-C**
   a. Calculated LDL-C
      i. LDL-C has traditionally been assessed using the Friedewald formula to calculate LDL-C.[25] Calculation of LDL-C assumes that total cholesterol is the sum of HDL-C, LDL-C, IDL-C, and VLDL-C as well as lipoprotein (a).

      Friedewald Formula: LDL-C = [Total cholesterol] – [HDL-C] – [Triglyceride]/5.
      All units of measure are given in mg/dL.

      ii. The factor [TG]/5 is an estimate of VLDL-C and assumes that all triglycerides are carried by the VLDL particles and that 1/5 of VLDL is cholesterol and 4/5 is triglyceride. This formula is most accurate when triglycerides are <150 mg/dL and becomes less accurate as levels increase. The calculation remains reasonably accurate and is recommended by the NCEP for estimating LDL-C when triglycerides are <400 mg/dL.[20] When TG are >400 mg/dL, VLDL-C contains greater proportion of TG (the denominator in the TG/VLDL will be >5) thereby underestimating LDL-C. Additionally, the Friedewald formula cannot be used when chylomicrons or VLDL remnants are present with higher TG/chol ratios (LDL-C underestimated) or in type III hyperlipoproteinemia (LDL-C overestimated). Regardless, the formula has been shown to be appropriate for a majority of the population, and LCL-C calculation has been used in guidelines, in establishing goals for LDL-C, and in clinical and epidemiologic research.[26]
   b. Directly measured LDL-C
      i. Given the limitations of the Friedewald formula outlined above, it may seem that direct measurement of LDL-C would be optimal. However, the direct measurement of LDL-C is also not without limitations.[27]
      ii. The Centers for Disease Control and Prevention Lipid Standardization Program does not provide certification of direct LDL-C assays as they do for total cholesterol, HDL-C, and triglycerides. A NCEP working group published recommendations for direct measurement of LDL-C.[28]
      iii. While specific recommendations for manufacturers of LDL-C reagents are provided, results from different methods cannot be used interchangeably as biases exist.[29,30] Of the several methods available, beta-quantification is most widely used.
   c. Comparison of calculated LDL-C and directly measured LDL-C
      Studies comparing calculated and direct LDL-C measurements have shown significant differences. In a study comparing calculated LDL-C and direct LDL-C measurement, the two were correlated at $r^2 = 0.86$, but 1/3 had 15 mg/dL greater direct measurement and 25% had >20 mg/dL difference.[27] It is, therefore, important to understand that the Friedewald formula for LDL-C calculation does not report the same measure as does the direct LDL-C measurement because the calculation includes cholesterol contained in IDL and lipoprotein (a).

5. Measurement of atherosclerotic particle burden
   a. While LDL-C is still a standard measure of atherosclerotic particles, research has shown that other measures such as non–HDL-C and apolipoprotein B better reflect total particle burden and prediction of risk for cardiovascular disease. Current guidelines that recommend lipid targets provide goals for LDL-C and non–HDL-C, and some also list a goal for apoB.[31] Most patients can be assessed

using calculated LDL-C and non–HDL-C; however, in certain situations and with certain patient groups, use of apoB or LDL particle number will be helpful. These include the following:

- LDL-C calculation will not be accurate with the Friedewald formula.
- Marked discordance between LDL-C and apoB or LDL particle number has been noted (diabetes, HIV).
- High-risk patients where aggressive lipid lowering is indicated. Please see Chapter 6 for discussion on how to incorporate these two measures into clinical practice. Methods for measurement of non–HDL-C. ApoB and LDL particle number are described below.

b. Non–HDL-C

Non–HDL-C is a measure of all atherosclerotic lipid particles (VLDL-C, IDL-C, LDL-C, and lipoprotein (a)). It is calculated by subtracting the HDL-C from the total cholesterol and does not need to be measured in the fasting state.

V. Apolipoproteins and Lipoprotein (a)

As mentioned above, lipoproteins are heterogenous particles consisting of lipids and apoproteins. Common immunoassays used to measure apolipoproteins and Lp(a) utilize antibodies that recognize protein antigenic sites. The antibodies need to sufficiently recognize variable expression of the epitope (the specific part of the antigen to which an antibody binds). These epitopes are often covered by lipids and must be exposed for an optimal in vitro reaction to take place. This is typically accomplished by detergents added to the assay buffer. The CDC provides reference standards to which different assays can be calibrated against to minimize interassay variability.

A. Apolipoprotein B (ApoB)

1. Each LDL particle contains a single molecule of ApoB. As such, ApoB may be a better method of determining "total" LDL and atherogenic particles rather than LDL-C alone, which is the measurement of the cholesterol content of the LDL particle. As noted above, apolipoprotein B has been included as a target for treatment in recommendations and guidelines for diagnosis and management of dyslipidemia.

2. Two methods are commonly used, either immunonephelometry or immunoturbidimetry. Although the WHO and IFCC have facilitated standardization of ApoB methods by providing reference materials, neither method is considered definitive[32]; however, the reliability and validity of measurements by either method are considered good overall.

B. Apolipoprotein A-1
ApoA-1 is the primary protein associated with HDL-C. There are variable numbers of apoA-1 proteins on an HDL-C particle so there is no 1:1 relationship. Measurement is by either immunonephelometric or immunoturbidimetric methods. Similar to HDL-C, increased concentrations are associated with reduced risk of atherosclerotic cardiovascular disease compared to HDL-C[33]. However, apoA-1 is not often used in the general practice of lipid management.

C. Lipoprotein (a)

1. The clinical use of Lp(a) is discussed in Chapter X. Measurement of Lp(a) has been challenging due to Lp(a)'s variable isoform size. This particle, which is similar to plasminogen, is a complex structure consisting of an LDL-like particle to which an apolipoprotein (a) is covalently bound. It is very heterogeneous, in part due to a variable number of so-called "kringle" repeats in the apo(a) portion of the molecule.

2. In the past, Lp(a) has been measured by preparative ultracentrifugation, high-resolution electrophoresis or immunoprecipitation. These methods determined the amount of Lp(a) cholesterol and were time consuming.[34]

3. The existing methods are immunologic assays specific to apo(a) antigenic determinants expressed on kringle 4. Both immunoturbidimetric and ELISA methods measure Lp(a) mass. Whether to measure Lp(a) cholesterol or Lp(a) mass and their respective relationship to cardiovascular disease is controversial.

4. Standardization. An accurate standardized measurement of Lp(a), using an international reference material, has been developed by International Federation of Clinical Chemistry and Laboratory Medicine (IFCC) and approved by the National Heart, Lung, and Blood Institute (NHLBI) and the World Health Organization (WHO).[35,36]

   This IFCC reference material uses monoclonal antibody specifically directed toward an epitope present in KIV type 9; only one copy of which is present on every apo(a) molecule, regardless of size. This allows accurate measurement of Lp(a) levels irrespective of isoform size and has become the gold standard for measurement of Lp(a).[37]

VI. Advanced Measurement Methods

A. Nuclear magnetic resonance (NMR) spectroscopy

1. Nuclear magnetic resonance spectroscopy (NMR) is used to determine number of lipid particles as well as subclass particle concentration such as quantification of large and small LDL particles.

2. NMR detects lipoproteins using small amounts of serum or plasma (500 μL). This is accomplished by detecting signals emitted by terminal methyl groups on the lipid particle that are specific to each lipid entity and proportional to the particle count for a given lipoprotein class. In this way, both particle (ie, LDL or HDL) and amount are determined.[38]

3. Some limitations to NMR include the need for NMR instruments, high cost, lack of procedural standardization, and lack of universal reimbursement by insurance.

4. Clinical use

   Research has shown that LDL particle number, similar to apoB, better predicts risk for cardiovascular disease. Cole et al. reviewed the cardiovascular outcomes from 25 studies to assess the comparability of apoB and NMR lipid particle measurements to make best practice recommendations.[39] They found that both apoB and NMR particle measurements compared well with clinical outcomes and both were better than LDL-C alone. However, this working group preferred apoB measurements due to its availability, standardization, and relatively lower cost. Guidelines and statements have not recommended routine measurement of LDL particle number. Clinical utility is similar to that of apoB noted above.

B. Density gradient ultracentrifugation
This method separates lipoproteins by high-speed centrifugation into gradients based upon the density of the particle. This technique was able to identify and quantify HDL-C, subclasses of HDL-C, IDL, VLDL, and Lp(a) cholesterol. It was known commercially as the vertical auto profile (VAP) test; however, it is no longer available. Density gradient ultracentrifugation had several disadvantages, including being very time consuming, results influenced by centrifugation conditions, and medium conditions exposed to lipids in the procedure. In addition, the clinical utility of the numerous results reported was unclear.[40]

VII. Summary

Lipids and lipoproteins are important biomarkers for assessing cardiovascular disease risk and in the diagnosis and management of cardiovascular disease making measurement considerations and understanding of the measurement process important for the clinician. There are inherent sources of variability associated with lipid and lipoprotein determinations. The CDC standardization program provides accuracy-based standards for total cholesterol, HDL-C, triglycerides, apoA-1, and apoB to reduce analytical variability among laboratories. With the understanding of biochemistry, physiology, and genetic interactions of plasma lipids has come advances in analytical methods for measuring lipids, lipoproteins, and apolipoproteins.

References

1. *CDC Lipid Standardization Program.* Available at: http://www.cdc.gov/labstandards/lsp.html
2. Rottenberg RB, Simon R, Chipperfield E, et al. Efficacy of selected diagnostic tests for sexually transmitted diseases. *JAMA.* 1976;235:49-51.
3. Schetman G, Sasse E. Variability of lipid measurements: relevance for the clinician. *Clin Chem.* 1993;39(7):1495-1503.
4. Clinical Laboratory Standards Institute (CLSI). *Expression of Measurement Uncertainty in Laboratory Medicine.* CLSI document EP29-A. Wayne, PA; 2012.
5. *Standards and Certification: Laboratory Requirements.* Federal Register. 42 CFR 493. Available at: http://wwwn.cdc.gov/clia/Regulatory/default.aspx
6. Cooper GR, Myers GL, Smith SJ, et al. Blood lipid measurements. Variations and practical utility. *JAMA.* 1992;267:1652-1660.
7. Miller M, Bachorik PS, Cloey TA. Normal variation of plasma lipoproteins: postural effects on plasma concentrations of lipids, lipoproteins and apolipoproteins. *Clin Chem.* 1992;38:569-574.
8. CDC NCEP. NIH publ 90–2964; 1990.
9. Klotzsch SG, McNamara JR. Triglyceride measurements: a review of methods and interferences. *Clin Chem.* 1990;36(9):1605-1613.
10. Behesthi I, Wessels LM, Eckfeldt JH. EDTA-plasma vs serum differences cholesterol, high density lipoprotein cholesterol and triglyceride as measured by several methods. *Clin Chem.* 1994;40(11):2088-2092.
11. Kronenburg F, Lobentanz EM, König P, Utterman G, Dieplinger H. Effect of storage on the measurement of lipoprotein(a), apolipoproteins B and A-IV, total and high density lipoprotein cholesterol and triglyceride. *J Lipid Res.* 1994;35:1318-1328.
12. Kafonek SD, Donovan L, Lovejoy KL, Bachorik PS. Biological variation of lipids and lipoproteins in fingerstick blood. *Clin Chem.* 1996;42:2002-2007.
13. Lovett KM, Liang BA. Direct-to-consumer disease screening with fingerstick testing: online patient safety risks. *Clin Chem.* 2012;58(7):1091-1093.
14. Langsted A, Freiberg JJ, Borge G, Nordestgaard G. Fasting and non-fasting lipid levels. *Circulation.* 2008;118(20):2047-2056.
15. Craig SR, Amin RV, Russell DW, Paradise NF. Blood cholesterol screening. Influence of fasting state on cholesterol and management decisions. *J Gen Intern Med.* 2000;15(6):395-399.
16. Cohn JS, McNamara JR, Cohn SD, Ordovas JM, Schaefer EJ. Post-prandial plasma lipoprotein changes in human subjects of different ages. *J Lipid Res.* 1988;29:469-479.
17. White KT, Moorthy MV, Akinkoulie AO, et al. Identifying the optimal cutpoint for the diagnosis of hypertriglyceridemia in the nonfasting state. *Clin Chem.* 2015;61(9):1156-1163.
18. Crouse JR, Grundy SG. Effects of alcohol on plasma lipoproteins and cholesterol and triglyceride metabolism in man. *J Lipid Res.* 1984;25:486-496.
19. Van de Wiel A. The effect of alcohol on postprandial and fasting triglycerides. *Int J Vasc Med.* 2012.
20. NCEP. *Recommendations on Lipoprotein Measurement.* Bethesda, MD. NIH Publication No. 95-3044; 1995.
21. Nordestgaard BG, Benn M, Schnorr P, Tybjaerg-Hansen A. Nonfasting triglycerides and risk of myocardial infarction, ischemic heart disease in men and women. *JAMA.* 2007;298(3):299-308.
22. Nordestgaard BG, Langsted A, Mora S, et al. Fasting is not routinely required for determination of a lipid profile: clinical and laboratory implications including flagging at desirable concentration cutpoints-A joint consensus statement from the European atherosclerosis society and European federation of clinical chemistry and laboratory medicine. *Clin Chem.* 2016;62(7):930-946.
23. Miller M, Stone NJ, Ballantyne CM, et al. Triglycerides and cardiovascular disease: a scientific statement from the American Heart Association. *Circulation.* 2011;123:2292-2333.

24. McCabe ERB. Disorders of glycerol metabolism. In: *The Metabolic and Molecular Basis of Inherited Diseases.*
25. Friedewald WT, Levy RI, Frederickson DS. Estimation of the correlation of low-density lipoprotein cholesterol in plasma. *Clin Chem* 1972;18:499-502.
26. LaRosa JC, Chambless LE, Criqui MH, et al. Patterns of dyslipoproteinemia in selected North American populations. *Circulation.* 1986;73(suppl I):12-29.
27. Baruch L, Agarwal S, Gupta B, Haynos A, et al. Is directly measured low-density lipoprotein clinically equivalent to calculated low-density lipoprotein? *J Clin Lipidol.* 2010;4(4):259-264.
28. Bachorik PS, Ross JW. National cholesterol education program recommendations for measurement of low-density lipoprotein cholesterol. *Clin Chem.* 1995;41(10):1414-1420.
29. Korzun WJ, Nilsson G, Bachmann LM, Myers GL, et al. Difference in bias approach for commutability assessment: application to frozen pools to human serum measured by 8 direct methods for HDL and LDL. *Clin Chem.* 2015;61(8):1107-1113.
30. Stepman HCM, Tiikkainen U, Stockl D, Vesper HW, et al. Measurement for 8 common analytes in native sera identify inadequate standardization among 6 routine laboratory assays. *Clin Chem.* 2014;60(6):855-863.
31. U.S. Department of Health and Human Services. Public Health Service National Institutes of Health National Heart, Lung, and Blood Institute. NIH Publication No. 01-3305. May 2001.
32. Warnick GR, Kimberly MM, Waymack PP, Leary ET, Myers GL. Standardization of measurements for cholesterol, triglycerides, and major lipoproteins. *Lab Med.* 2008;39:481-490.
33. McQueen MJ, Hawken S, Wang X, et al. Lipids, lipoproteins, and apolipoproteins as risk markers of myocardial infarction in 52 countries (the INTERHEART study): a case control study. *Lancet.* 2008;372:224-233.
34. Baudhin LM, Hartman SJ, O'Brien JF, Meissner I, Galen RS, et al. Electrophoretic measurement of lipoprotein(a) cholesterol in plasma with and without ultracentrifugation: comparison with a immunoturbidimetric lipoprotein(a) method. *Clin Biochem.* 2004;37(6):481-488.
35. Marcovina SM, Koschinsky ML, Albers JJ, Skarlatos S. Report of the National Heart, Lung, and Blood Institute Workshop on Lipoprotein(a) and Cardiovascular Disease: recent advances and future directions. *Clin Chem.* 2003;49(11):1785-1796.
36. Dati F, Tate JR, Marcovina SM, et al. First WHO/IFCC international reference reagent for lipoprotein (a) for immunoassay, SRM 2B. *Clin Chem Lab Med.* 2004;42(6):670-676.
37. Marcovina SM, Albers JJ, Scanu AM, et al. Use of a reference material proposed by the International Federation of Clinical Chemistry and Laboratory Medicine to evaluate analytical methods for the determination of plasma lipoprotein(a). *Clin Chem.* 2000;46(12):1956-1967.
38. Cole TG, Contois JH, Csako G, McConnell JP, et al. Association of apolipoprotein B and nuclear magnetic resonance spectroscopy-derived LDL particle number with outcomes in 25 clinical studies: assessment by the AACC lipoprotein and vascular diseases division working group on best practices. *Clin Chem.* 2013;59(5):752-770.
39. Edelstein C, Pfaffinger D, Scanu AM. Advantages and limitations of density gradient ultracentrifugation in the fractionation of human serum lipoproteins: role of salts and sucrose. *J Lipid Res.* 1984;25:630-637.
40. Jeyarajah EJ, Cromwell WC, Otvos JD. Lipoprotein particle analysis by nuclear magnetic resonance spectroscopy. *Clin Lab Med.* 2006;26:847-870.

CHAPTER 5

Step-by-Step Diagnosis and Management Plan

Merle Myerson

Key Points

- Diagnosis and Management of dyslipidemia is best achieved in an ordered sequence.
- History and physical examination can provide important information for risk stratification and possible etiologies of the patient's dyslipidemia.
- Risk scoring schemes should be used along with clinical judgment, for example, deciding when additional risk indicators may change risk category.
- Lipid targets and goals were not incorporated in the 2013 ACC/AHA Guidelines but retained in the 2014 NLA Recommendations.
- Blood testing should include measures that may diagnose secondary causes of dyslipidemia and relevant comorbidities.
- Therapeutic lifestyle changes should be incorporated into all management plans.
- Assess response to therapy to determine if modification of management plan is needed.

I.   Introduction

Diagnosis and management of dyslipidemia are best achieved in an ordered sequence. As discussed in Chapter 3, there are several guidelines and recommendations for diagnosis and management of dyslipidemia in the United States. The step-by-step plan presented here is based on the NCEP ATP III,[1] the 2013 ACC/AHA Guidelines,[2] and the 2014 National Lipid Association (NLA) Recommendations.[3] The tables and boxes are meant to serve as a guide and do not constitute a defined guideline.

II.   History and Physical Examination

All patients should have a directed history and physical examination. Boxes 5.1 and 5.2 outline aspects specific for the evaluation of dyslipidemia. The metabolic syndrome is a constellation of features that both together and individually predict risk. Table 5.1 outlines the components and diagnosis of metabolic syndrome.

III.   Assessment of Risk

Chapter 4 reviewed the commonly used risk stratification schemes used in the United States. Presented here are the NLA Recommendations (see Table 5.2 and Box 5.3) that incorporate both the Framingham-based risk scoring and the ACC/AHA Pooled Cohort Equations.

Clinical judgment is also needed along with additional risk indicators that might be considered for "risk refinement" meaning that consideration of these other factors may change the risk category of a patient. These additional indicators are outlined in Box 5.5.

BOX 5.1 | History

1. Age ≥45 years in men and ≥55 years old in women
2. Personal history of cardiovascular disease: coronary artery disease, cerebrovascular disease, peripheral artery disease, abdominal aortic aneurysm
3. History of lipid abnormalities, if known
4. Family history of premature coronary heart disease: first-degree male relative <55 years old or first-degree female relative <65 years old
5. Diet history including who buys and prepares food, whether patient is institutionalized or living without a kitchen area
6. Exercise and physical activity history
7. Family history of dyslipidemia: elevated LDL-C or triglycerides
8. Cigarette smoking (personal history, living with people who smoke, exposure to secondhand smoke)
9. History of symptoms: angina, anginal equivalents
10. Hormone history: menopausal status, use of oral contraceptives, hormone replacement therapy, testosterone therapy, hormone therapy for gender reassignment
11. Determination of diabetes mellitus and metabolic syndrome (see Table 5.1)
12. Medication history, including antiretroviral therapy, psychiatric medications, hepatitis B or C medications, methadone, anabolic steroids, immunosuppression medications (cyclosporine), selective estrogen receptor modulators (SERMs)
13. Hypertension and use of blood pressure–lowering medications
14. Substance use: illicit drugs, alcohol
15. Comorbidities that can increase LDL-C: hypothyroidism, renal disease, obstructive liver disease, anorexia nervosa, Cushing syndrome, polycystic ovarian syndrome

BOX 5.2 | Physical Examination

- Height, weight, body mass index (BMI), waist circumference, blood pressure
- Evidence of hypothyroidism
- Distal pulses and auscultation for bruit over arterial beds
- Physical stigmata of elevated LDL-C: tendon xanthomas, xanthelasmas. For elevated TG: eruptive xanthomas

Table 5.1. Components of the Metabolic Syndrome[a]

Component	Defining Level
Abdominal obesity Men Women	Waist circumference ≥40 inches (35 inches in Asians) ≥35 inches (32 inches in Asians)
HDL-C Men Women	 ≤40 mg/dL ≤50 mg/dL
Triglycerides (fasting)	≥150 mg/dL
Blood pressure	≥130/≥85 mm Hg
Fasting blood glucose	≥100 mg/dL

[a]The presence of three or more components constitutes a diagnosis of metabolic syndrome.

Table 5.2.   Cardiovascular Disease Risk Classification

Risk Category	Criteria	Treatment Goal Non-HDL-C mg/dL	LDL-C mg/dL
Low	• 0–1 major ASCVD risk factors • Consider other risk indicators, if known	<130	<100
Moderate	• 2 major ASCVD risk factors • Consider quantitative risk scoring • Consider other risk indicators	<130	<100

High	• ≥3 major ASCVD risk factors
	• Diabetes mellitus (type 1 or 2)
	  ∘ 0–1 other major ASCVD risk factors and
	  ∘ No evidence of end-organ damage
	• Chronic kidney disease stage 3B or 4
	• LDL-C ≥190 mg/dL (severe hypercholesterolemia)
	• Quantitative risk score reaching the high-risk threshold[a]
		<130
		
		<100
			<100
			
			≥100

Very high	• ASCVD
	• Diabetes mellitus (type 1 or 2)
	  ∘ ≥2 other major ASCVD risk factors or
	  ∘ Evidence of end-organ damage
		<100	<70

[a]High-risk threshold is defined as ≥10% using Adult Treatment Panel III Framingham Risk Score for hard coronary heart disease (CHD; myocardial infarction or CHD death), ≥15% using the 2013 Pooled Cohort Equations for hard ASCVD (myocardial infarction, stroke, or death from CHD or stroke), or ≥45% using the Framingham long-term (to age 80) cardiovascular disease (CVD; myocardial infarction, CHD death or stroke) risk calculation. Clinicians may prefer to use other risk calculators but should be aware that quantitative risk calculators vary in the clinical outcomes predicted (eg, CHD events, ASCVD events, cardiovascular mortality); the risk factors included in their calculation; and the timeframe for their prediction (eg, 5 years, 10 years, or long-term or lifetime). Such calculators may omit certain risk indicators that can be very important in individual patients, provide only an approximate risk estimate, and require clinical judgment for interpretation.

Modified from Jacobson TA, Ito MK, Maki KC, et al. National Lipid Association recommendations for patient-centered management of dyslipidemia: Part I—executive summary. *Journal of Clinical Lipidology*, 2014:8:473-488.

BOX 5.3   Criteria for Classification of ASCVD

- Myocardial infarction or other acute coronary syndrome
- Coronary or other revascularization procedure
- Transient ischemic attack
- Ischemic stroke
- Atherosclerotic peripheral artery disease
  ∘ Includes ankle/brachial index of <0.90
- Other documented atherosclerotic diseases such as:
  ∘ Coronary atherosclerosis
  ∘ Renal atherosclerosis
  ∘ Aortic aneurysm secondary to atherosclerosis
  ∘ Carotid plaque ≥50% stenosis

BOX 5.4   Major Risk Factors for ASCVD

1. Age: male ≥45 years, female ≥55 years
2. Family history of early coronary heart disease: <55 years in male first-degree relative and <65 years in female first-degree relative
3. Current cigarette smoking
4. High blood pressure (≥140/≥90 mm Hg or on blood pressure medication)
5. Low HDL-C: male <40 mg/dL and female <50 mg/dL

BOX 5.5   Additional Risk Indicators That Might Be Considered for Risk Refinement

1. Severe disturbance in a major ASCVD risk factor (ie, multipack per day smoking, strong family history of premature coronary heart disease)
2. Indicators of subclinical disease including coronary artery calcium (≥300 Agatston units)
3. LDL-C ≥160 mg/dL and/or non–HDL-C ≥190 mg/dL
4. High-sensitivity C-reactive protein ≥2.0 mg/L
5. Lipoprotein (a) ≥50 mg/dL (protein) using an isoform-insensitive assay
6. Urine albumin-to-creatinine ratio ≥30 mg/g

IV. Establish Targets of Therapy

A. The 2013 ACC/AHA Guideline has eliminated targets for therapy, in particular LDL-C as a target and goals for LDL-C. There has been and will continue to be debate about usefulness of lipid targets and goals. The NLA Recommendations have continued to endorse targets and goals and they are included here. Table 5.3 lists goals for LDL-C as well as non–HDL-C.

B. The LDL-C should be the "first priority" for therapy unless the TG are very high (≥500 mg/dL and especially ≥1000 mg/dL) at baseline to prevent pancreatitis (see Chapter 11 for management of TG). Once TG are below 500 mg/dL, re-evaluate LDL-C for appropriate management. Note that consideration can be given to initiate therapy for both very high TG and high LDL-C simultaneously. Chapter 11 details diagnosis and management of hypertriglyceridemia.

C. For patients with TG ≥ 200 mg/dL after LDL-C goal is reached, a secondary target is to achieve a non–HDL-C 30 mg/dL higher than the LDL-C goal.

D. HDL-C is currently not a target of therapy. Goal for triglycerides is <150 mg/dL.

E. When to use measures of residual risk

1. As discussed in Chapter 4, the LDL-C may not accurately predict atherosclerotic particle burden, and that use of other measures including non–HDL-C, apolipoprotein B, and LDL particle number may better reflect total atherosclerotic particle burden and predict risk.[6–8]

2. At this time, guidelines have not endorsed measuring apoB or LDL particle number as standard practice for the general population. Suggestions for selected use include patients at high risk, known CVD, and those groups that have shown discordance between LDL-C and apoB or LDL particle number. Discordance with LDL-C lower than apoB or particle number has been shown in diabetics, metabolic syndrome, and HIV.[9,10]

3. Table 5.3 lists goals for apoB according to the NLA Recommendations and LDL particle number as noted by an NLA Expert Panel.[4] Practical considerations may limit use of these two measures as not all labs are equipped to measure these and insurance coverage is not universal. As such, use of non–HDL-C as a measure of residual risk is recommended.

Table 5.3. Targets for LDL-C, Non–HDL-C, ApoB, LDL-P				
Risk Category	**LDL-C (mg/dL)**	**Non–HDL-C (mg/dL)**	**Apolipoprotein B (mg/dL)**	**LDL-Particle Number (nmol/L)**
Very high	<70	<100	<80	<1100
High	<100	<130	<90	<1100
Moderate	<100	<130	<90	1400
Low	<100	<130	<90	*a*

*a*Measurement of LDL-P not recommended.
(Data from Third Report of the National Cholesterol Education Program (NCEP) expert panel on detection, evaluation, and treatment of high blood cholesterol in adults (adult treatment panel III) final report. *Circulation.* 2002;106(25):3143-3421; Davidson MH, Ballantyne CM, Jacobson TA, et al. Clinical utility of inflammatory markers and advanced lipoprotein testing: advice from an expert panel of lipid specialists. *J Clin Lipidol.* 2011;5(5):338-367; Jacobson T, Ito M, Bays H, et al. *NLA Recommendations for Patient-Centered Management of Dyslipidemia (Draft)*; 2014.)

V. Laboratory Evaluation

A. A basic fasting lipid panel (total cholesterol, HDL-C, TG, and calculated LDL-C and non–HDL-C) should be obtained.

B. Consideration can be given for measurement of apolipoprotein B:

1. When TG are >400 mg/dL, the calculation for LDL-C is not accurate. Direct measurement of LDL-C is not recommended as not all laboratories are able to adequately perform this test and the lab coefficient of variation is often quite large as discussed in Chapter 4. In this situation, measurement of apoB can provide information on quantity of atherosclerotic particles.

2. For those where discordance between LDL-C and non–HDL-C or apoB would be expected, see Section IV E above.

C. In addition to lipids, other blood tests are useful for the initial evaluation to rule out secondary causes of dyslipidemia and evaluate for diabetes. These are listed in Box 5.6.

VI. Clinical Intervention

A. Therapeutic lifestyle All patients should receive counseling on therapeutic lifestyle changes regardless of their risk and lipid levels. Key components are as follows:

1. Diet: Reduce intake of saturated fats to <7% of total calories and intake of cholesterol to <200 mg/d.

2. Weight reduction if indicated.

3. Increased physical activity.

4. Cessation of smoking.

5. See Chapter 10 for specific dietary recommendations for patients with hypertriglyceridemia.

BOX 5.6 | **Laboratory Evaluation**

1. Fasting lipid profile (total cholesterol, HD6-10L-C, triglycerides, calculated LDL-C).
2. Calculate non–HDL-cholesterol (apoB and LDL-P not routinely recommended).
3. Lipoprotein (a): This is a lipid particle heavily influenced by genetics, is structurally similar to plasminogen, and is independently predictive of risk. Consider measurement in patients with premature CVD, family history of premature CVD, or familial hypercholesterolemia.
4. At present, there is no clear indication for routine measurement of hs-CRP in the initial evaluation but can be considered if needed for risk refinement.

5. TSH: Evaluate for thyroid disease as this may influence lipid levels.
6. AST and ALT: Baseline testing before starting lipid medication and evaluation for obstructive liver disease.
7. Serum creatinine kinase*.
8. Serum creatinine and calculation of GFR.
9. Urinalysis.
10. Uric acid if history of gout.
11. Fasting glucose and/or HbA1c to evaluate for diabetes, prediabetes, and metabolic syndrome.

*If indicated (patient with baseline muscle soreness or muscle disease)

B. If LDL-C is mildly elevated and the patient is a low or intermediate risk, a 3-month trial of lifestyle modification can be attempted prior to initiating medical therapy. This is also the case for elevated TG (<500) as TG respond very well to diet and weight loss.

C. For those still not at goal after a trial of lifestyle or who have markedly elevated LDL-C or TG and are at higher risk, medication should be initiated in conjunction with lifestyle counseling. Chapters 8, 9, and 10 provide detail on use of the statin and nonstatin drugs and treatment of hypertriglyceridemia.

VII. Assess Response to Therapy

A. Recommendations for monitoring response to therapy are not definitive. According to the 2011 European Guidelines, recommendations "stem from consensus rather than evidence-based guidelines" and that "Response to therapy can be assessed at 6-8 weeks from initiation or dose increases for statins."[11]

B. In general, maximum LDL and TG lowering is evident by 6 weeks after starting therapy. If a patient is not at goal, titrate to higher doses or add second medication and recheck lipid levels in 6 weeks. In general, medications should be either titrated or added one at a time and rechecked prior to making additional changes.

C. Chapters 8 and 9 review statin and nonstatin drugs. While current guidelines and recommendations list statins as first-line therapy, the nonstatin drugs should be used as listed below. The 2016 ACC Expert Consensus Decision Pathway on the Role of Non-Statin Therapies for LDL-Cholesterol Lowering in the Management of Atherosclerotic Cardiovascular Disease provides specific information on the nonstatin drugs.[12] Chapter 13 reviews the new medications including PCSK9 inhibitors and mipomersen and lomitapide, both specifically for familial hypercholesterolemia.

   1. Fibrates or fish oil for markedly elevated TG (>500 mg/dL)

   2. For additional LDL-C lowering if already on maximally tolerated statin dose

VIII. Summary

The diagnosis and management of dyslipidemia is a step-by-step process using clinical judgment along with established guidelines and recommendations. Assessment of risk is important to determine the intensity of therapy. Finally, lifestyle modifications are advised for all patients, regardless of risk.

References

1. Third Report of the National Cholesterol Education Program (NCEP) expert panel on detection, evaluation, and treatment of high blood cholesterol in adults (adult treatment panel III) final report. *Circulation*. 2002;106(25):3143-3421.
2. Stone NJ, Robinson J, Lichtenstein AH, et al. 2013 ACC/AHA guideline on the treatment of blood cholesterol to reduce atherosclerotic cardiovascular risk in adults: a report of the American College of Cardiology/American Heart Association Task Force on practice guidelines. *J Am Coll Cardiol*. 2014 Jul 1;63(25 Pt B):2889-2934.
3. Jacobson TA, Ito MK, Maki KC, et al. National Lipid Association recommendations for patient-centered management of dyslipidemia: Part 1—executive summary. *J Clin Lipidol*. 2014;8(5):473-488.
4. Davidson MH, Ballantyne CM, Jacobson TA, et al. Clinical utility of inflammatory markers and advanced lipoprotein testing: advice from an expert panel of lipid specialists. *J Clin Lipidol*. 2011;5(5):338-367.
5. Jacobson T, Ito M, Bays H, et al. *NLA Recommendations for Patient-Centered Management of Dyslipidemia (Draft)*; 2014.

6. Otvos JD, Mora S, Shalaurova I, Greenland P, Mackey RH, Goff DC Jr. Clinical implications of discordance between low-density lipoprotein cholesterol and particle number. *J Clin Lipidol.* 2011;5(2):105-113.
7. Manickam P, Rathod A, Panaich S, et al. Comparative prognostic utility of conventional and novel lipid parameters for cardiovascular disease risk prediction: do novel lipid parameters offer an advantage? *J Clin Lipidol.* 2011;5(2):82-90.
8. Cromwell WC, Otvos JD, Keyes MJ, et al. LDL particle number and risk of future cardiovascular disease in the Framingham Offspring study—implications for LDL management. *J Clin Lipidol.* 2007;1(6):583-592.
9. Malave H, Castro M, Burkle J, et al. Evaluation of low-density lipoprotein particle number distribution in patients with type 2 diabetes mellitus with low-density lipoprotein cholesterol <50 mg/dl and non-high-density lipoprotein cholesterol <80 mg/dl. *Am J Cardiol.* 2012;110(5):662-665.
10. Myerson M, Lee R, Varela D, et al. Lipoprotein measurements in patients infected with HIV: is cholesterol content of HDL and LDL discordant with particle number? *J Clin Lipidol.* 2014;8(3):332-333.
11. Catapano AL, Chapman J, Wiklund O, Taskinen MR. The new joint EAS/ESC guidelines for the management of dyslipidaemias. *Atherosclerosis.* 2011;217(1):1.
12. Lloyd-Jones DM, Morris PB, Ballantyne CM, et al. 2016 ACC expert consensus decision pathway on the role of non-statin therapies for LDL-cholesterol lowering in the management of atherosclerotic cardiovascular disease risk: a report of the American College of Cardiology Task Force on clinical expert consensus documents. *J Am Coll Cardiol.* 2016;68(1):92-125.

CHAPTER 6

Lifestyle Modification in the Management of Dyslipidemia

Maria A. Bella and Ryan Turner

Key Points

- LDL cholesterol is the primary lipid target for prevention of cardiovascular disease (CVD).

- Increasing total fiber intake has been shown to improve LDL cholesterol levels.

- Metabolic syndrome is a group of risk factors associated with CVD and diabetes that can be treated with lifestyle interventions.

- High triglyceride levels are also associated with increased risk of CVD. Lifestyle modification is especially important to the treatment of hypertriglyceridemia.

- Medical nutrition therapy from a registered dietitian can help patients with dyslipidemia improve their lipid profile.

- Tobacco use is associated with an increase in TG levels and decrease in HDL cholesterol levels.

- A sedentary lifestyle is an independent risk factor for CVD. Physical activity has been shown to delay atherogenesis and increase myocardial vascularity and fibrinolysis.

Lifestyle modification is considered an essential part in the management of dyslipidemia. Both the 2015 National Lipid Association Recommendations and the 2013 ACC/AHA Guidelines state that diet, exercise, avoidance of tobacco, and maintaining a healthy weight are advised for all patients and to be used in conjunction with pharmacotherapy if needed.[1] This chapter will review the components of lifestyle therapy and outline the key information needed to counsel patients on modification.

DIET

I. Dietary Components

LDL cholesterol is the primary lipid target for prevention of cardiovascular disease (CVD). Extensive research has shown a correlation between high LDL cholesterol levels and CVD risk. A 1% decrease in LDL cholesterol levels by 1 mg/dL is associated with a 1%-2% decreased relative risk of CVD.[2] Control of triglycerides is also important and is very responsive to dietary intervention.

A. Dietary fiber

1. Increasing total fiber intake has been shown to improve LDL cholesterol levels.[3] Fiber is commonly found in fruits, vegetables, and whole grain products. Table 6.1 shows a list of foods high in total fiber. National recommendations suggest that men ages 18-50 years old require 30-38 g of total fiber per day and women between the ages of 18 and 50 years old require ~25 g of fiber per day.

2. There are two types of fiber: insoluble and soluble.
   a. Insoluble fiber is found in foods such as vegetables, wheat bran, and whole grains. It adds bulk to stool and increases transit time through the gastrointestinal tract.

Table 6.1. Fiber Content of Food Items

Fiber-Containing Food	Serving	Total Fiber	Soluble Fiber	Insoluble Fiber
Artichoke	1 medium	6.5 g	4.7 g	1.8 g
Black beans	1/2 cup	6.1 g	3.7 g	2.4 g
Blackberries	1/2 cup	3.8 g	3.1 g	0.7 g
Lentils	1/2 cup	8 g	7 g	1 g
Pear	1 small	2.9 g	1.8 g	1.1 g
Bulgur, cooked	1/2 cup	2.9 g	2.4 g	0.5 g
Raspberries	1/2 cup	4.2 g	3.8 g	0.4 g
Apple, with skin	1 medium	5.7 g	4.2 g	1.5 g
Banana	1 medium	2.8 g	2.1 g	0.7 g
Zucchini, cooked	1/2 cup	2.5 g	1.4 g	1.1 g
Spinach, cooked	1/2 cup	4.1 g	3.5 g	0.6 g
Mango	1 medium	3.7 g	2.2 g	1.5 g
Sweet potatoes	1/2 cup	3.8 g	2.4 g	1.4 g
Kiwi	1 medium	3.1 g	2.4 g	0.7 g
Apricots, fresh	4 medium	3.5 g	1.8 g	1.7 g
Cabbage, cooked	1/2 cup	1.8 g	1.0 g	0.8 g
Broccoli	1/2 cup	2.4 g	1.2 g	1.2 g

    b. Soluble fiber attracts water to form a gellike substance delaying digestion. Soluble fiber has been shown to have beneficial effects on LDL cholesterol levels.[2] Soluble fiber is found in foods such as oat bran, legumes, and nuts and seeds. It can also be found in psyllium, a common fiber supplement.

3. Increasing soluble fiber consumption to 5-10 g/d reduces LDL cholesterol levels by about 5%. The recommended intake of soluble fiber is 10-25 g/d to help lower cholesterol levels.[4]

4. Tables 6.1-6.3 list the major dietary sources and types of soluble fiber.

Table 6.2. Grams of Soluble Fiber Found in Foods

Dietary Sources of Soluble Fiber	Grams per Serving
Beans	
Black beans	4.8 g/cup
Navy beans	4.4 g/cup
Red kidney beans	4 g/cup
Oatmeal, prepared with ¾ cup dry oats	3 g/svg
Brussels sprouts, ½ cup	2 g/svg
Orange	1.8 g/svg
Flaxseeds	1.1 g/tbsp

(Adapted from Thalheimer JC. A soluble fiber primer—plus the top five foods that can lower LDL cholesterol. *Today's Dietitian.* 2013;15(12):16.)

Table 6.3. Sources of Various Types of Soluble Fiber	
Types of Soluble Fiber	**Sources**
Inulin oligofructose	Onions, sugar beets, chicory root, processed foods
Beta-glucans	Oats, oat bran, flaxseeds, beans, peas, soybeans, carrots, berries, bananas, oranges, apples
Pectin	Fruits, berries, seeds, processed foods
Psyllium	Seeds or husks of the plantago ovata plant; added to processed foods
Resistant starch	Unripe bananas, oatmeal, legumes, processed foods
Wheat dextrin	Wheat starch, processed foods

(Adapted from Zelman KM. *Types of Fiber and Their Health Benefits.* WebMD Web Site. Available at: http://www.webmd.com/diet/compare-dietary-fibers. Updated July 22, 2015. Accessed March 19, 2016.)

B. Fats: trans fatty acids and saturated fats

1. *Saturated Fat*[7] has the strongest effect on increasing your LDL levels. This fat is usually solid at room temperature. It is found mostly in foods that come from animals, such as fatty cuts of meat, poultry with skin, whole-milk dairy products, lard, and some vegetable oils, including coconut and palm oils.
   a. National recommendations for saturated fat
      i. **American Heart Association**—Recommend no more than **5%-6%** of calories should come from saturated fat in the diet. *For example, for a 2000-calorie–based diet, no more than 100-120 calories should come from saturated fat. That's about 13 g of saturated fat per day.*
      ii. **National Lipid Association**—Recommend **<7%** of total daily calories from saturated fat.
      iii. **American Diabetes Association**—Recommend people with or without diabetes to eat **<10%** of calories from saturated fat. For most people, that's about **20 g** of saturated fat per day.
      iv. **2015-2020 Dietary Guidelines for Americans**—Recommend **<10%** of total calories from saturated fat.
   b. Saturated fat adds up fast, even when consuming a healthy diet. For example, the meal plan outlined in Table 6.4 contains 2075 total calories and 34 g of saturated fat for a total of 306 calories from saturated fat, which makes up 14.7% of the day's total calories.

2. *Trans fatty acids*[7] are found mostly in foods made from hydrogenated oils and fats, such as hard margarine or shortening.

3. *Cholesterol*[7] is found only in foods that come from animals, such as liver and other organ meats, egg yolks, shrimp, whole milk, butter, cream, and cheese. Table 6.5 shows cholesterol content of various foods.

II. Examples of Diets to Lower LDL-C and Improve Cardiovascular Health

A. **The Mediterranean diet** Adherence to the Mediterranean diet is associated with reduced all-cause and cause-specific mortality (cancer and cardiovascular disease) in both men and women.[8]

The Mediterranean diet emphasizes[9]:

- Eating primarily plant-based foods, such as fruits and vegetables, whole grains, legumes, and nuts

Table 6.4.   Healthy Sample Meal Plan (15% Saturated Fat)

	Foods	Calories	Saturated Fat in grams
Breakfast	**Omelet**		
	2 eggs	144	3.2 g
	¼ cup skim milk	21	0 g
	1 ounce goat cheese	104	5.8 g
	⅛ cup onion	10	0 g
	½ cup mushrooms	22	0 g
	1 tbsp olive oil	120	2 g
Lunch	5 ounces turkey burger (lean)	234	3.4 g
	¼ avocado	81	1.2 g
	1 whole wheat bun	120	0.4 g
	10 carrot fries (with 1 tbsp olive oil)	240	2 g
Dinner	5 ounce steak	364	8.8 g
	1 cup green beans	34	0 g
	½ tbsp grass-fed butter	50	3.5 g
	1 cup brown rice	218	0.3 g
Snack	Greek yogurt 2% fat	160	2.3 g
	Walnuts (3 tbsp)	123	1.1 g
	3 tbsp blueberries	30	0 g

- Replacing butter with unsaturated fats, such as olive oil
- Using herbs and spices instead of salt to flavor foods
- Limiting red meat to no more than a few times a month
- Eating fish and poultry at least twice a week
- Drinking wine in moderation (optional)
- The importance of being physically active and enjoying meals with family and friends

B. The Portfolio Diet eating plan[10]

1. Studies have assessed the effects of a dietary portfolio for the management of hyper-lipidemia. When compared to a low-fat diet, the addition of a dietary portfolio can facilitate positive effects on lipid profiles for individuals with hyperlipidemia. The Portfolio Diet emphasizes the addition of certain food items. These recommendations

Table 6.5.   Comparison of Cholesterol Content in Foods

Food Item	Portion Size	Cholesterol (mg)
Egg, large	1 egg	186
Chicken liver	1 liver (44 g)	152
Shrimp, raw	3 oz	137
Veal, raw	4 oz	55
Sardines	1 oz	40
Butter	1 tbsp	31
Yogurt	8 oz	30
Cheddar cheese	1 oz	28
Whole milk	8 oz	24

Table 6.6. Foods to Include in the Portfolio Eating Plan		
Foods to Include	**Grams/1000 Calories**	**Suggested Daily Intake**
Plant sterols and stanols	0.94 g	2 g/d
Soluble fiber	9.8 g	20 g/d
Soy protein	22.5 g	50 g/d
Nuts	22.5 g	30 g/d

Adapted from Jenkins DJ, Jones PJ, Lamarche B, et al. Effect of a dietary portfolio of cholesterol-lowering foods given at 2 levels of intensity of dietary advice on serum lipids in hyperlipidemia: a randomized controlled trial. *JAMA*. 2011;306(8):831-839. doi:10.1001/jama.2011.1202; Heart UK The Cholesterol Charity. *The Portfolio Diet Fact Sheet*. Available at: http://heartuk.org.uk/images/uploads/healthylivingpdfs/huk_factsheet_d01_portd.pdf. Accessed April 19, 2016.

can facilitate a positive dietary change by including specific foods instead of excluding other food items. Table 6.6 outlines components of the Portfolio Diet.

2. In one study, a control group followed a heart-healthy diet that emphasized limiting intake of saturated fat while increasing intake of fruits, vegetables, beans, and whole grains.

   The intervention group that received advice from the dietary portfolio saw a 13% improvement on LDL cholesterol after 6 months. The control group that received only heart-healthy diet education saw just a 3% decrease in LDL cholesterol.

C. Diet to reduce triglyceride levels

1. Triglycerides (TG) are the lipid storage form found in adipocytes. High TG levels are associated with increased risk of CVD and very high levels associated with pancreatitis. TG are very responsive to lifestyle modification, especially diet, exercise, and weight loss.

2. If fasting TG levels are >1000 mg/dL, restricting total fat intake to 5 grams or less per day is recommended to reduce chylomicron TG input and decrease risk for pancreatitis. Within 48-72 hours of dietary fat restriction, fasting TG levels are expected to fall below 1000 mg/dL. Positive changes in TG levels are correlated with changes in very low density lipoprotein (VLDL) cholesterol levels.[12,13]

3. Table 6.7 shows lifestyle interventions and the percent lowering that can be achieved. Excessive intake of carbohydrates and alcohol are both associated with elevated TG levels. Limiting refined carbohydrates, added sugars, and fructose consumption to <100 g/d is recommended to decrease TG levels. Limit alcohol to one drink per day or completely abstain from consumption to maintain optimal TG levels.

Table 6.7. Lifestyle Interventions to Lower Triglyceride Levels	
Modification	**Alteration on TG Levels**
Lose 5%-10% body weight	↓ TG by 20% or 1.9% for every kg loss
Avoid a low-fat (10%) diet	↓ TG by 10%-15%
Add omega-3 fatty acids from oily fish or supplements	↓ TG by 5%-10%
Moderate-intensity exercise at least 150 min/wk	↓ TG by 20%-30%
Avoid trans fats/lower saturated fat	↓ TG by 1% for each gram less trans fat

(Adapted from Felando M. *Lower Your Triglycerides with Lifestyle*. Learn Your Lipids Website. Available at: http://www.learnyourlipids.com/wp-content/uploads/2014/02/TrigsTearSheet.pdf. Accessed March 20, 2016.)

Table 6.8. Body Mass Index (BMI) Classification	
Classification	**BMI (kg/m²)**
Underweight	<18.5
Normal	18.5-24.9
Overweight	25-29.9
Obese, Class I	30-34.9
Obese, Class II	34-39.9
Morbidly obese, Class III	≥40

D. Diet to raise HDL-C Replacing saturated fat intake with foods rich in monounsaturated and polyunsaturated fatty acids have a positive effect on HDL cholesterol levels. It is recommended to increase consumption of nuts, fish, and other omega-3 fatty acids containing foods. Moderate alcohol consumption has been shown to increase HDL cholesterol levels. Moderation is defined as having up to one drink per day for women and up to two drinks per day for men. While HDL-C levels are inversely associated with risk for CVD, it is not currently a target for therapy.

III.   Obesity

While dietary therapy is an important treatment for dyslipidemia, another objective is for weight reduction. According to data from the National Health and Nutrition Examination Survey (NHANES) from 2009 to 2010, about 35.7% of American adults were considered obese based on body mass index (BMI).[15] BMI is an objective calculation based on height and weight calculated as BMI = kg/m^2. Table 6.8 provides the classification of BMI. Adults with a BMI ≥ 30 are considered obese. Weight loss for overweight or obese individuals is recommended to decrease risk of CVD.

IV.   Counseling for Dietary Modification: Medical Nutrition Therapy Intervention

A. When receiving medical nutrition therapy from a trained professional, patients with dyslipidemia can have significant improvements in their lipid profile. These improvements are seen after receiving three to four individual nutrition therapy sessions of 50 minutes over a 7-week period with a registered dietitian.[16] Table 6.9 lists the improvements on lipid profile and dietary modifications after two to six visits with a registered dietitian over 6-12 weeks. While more frequent sessions with a registered dietitian are preferred,

Table 6.9. Improvements in Lipid Profile and Dietary Modifications with Medical Nutrition Therapy	
Parameter	**Improvements**
LDL cholesterol levels	7%-22% decrease
Triglyceride levels	11%-31% decrease
Saturated fat intake	2%-4% decrease
Calories per day	232-710 calories/d

Adapted from Sikand G, Kashyap ML, Yang I. Medical nutrition therapy lowers serum cholesterol and saves medication costs in men with hypercholesterolemia. *J Am Diet Assoc.* 1998;98(8):889-894; McCoin M, Sikand G, Johnson EQ, et al. The effectiveness of medical nutrition therapy delivered by registered dietitians for disorders of lipid metabolism: a call for further research. *J Am Diet Assoc.* 2008;108(2):233-239.

clinicians can supplements these visits by reinforcing nutrition education at office visits and encouraging the described interventions.

B. In one study, among men receiving medical nutrition therapy from a registered dietitian, half of those individuals no longer required antihyperlipidemic medications, with a total saving cost of $638.35 per patient.[18]

C. Medical nutrition therapy is important in maintaining adherence to nutrition advice.

    1. A registered dietitian can provide customized meal plans to fit an individual's needs. Meal plans often emphasize decreased intake of total calories and saturated fat and increased intake of fiber, plant sterols and stanols, and omega-3 fatty acids.[17]

    2. Registered dietitians utilize motivational interviewing methods to improve diet compliance. Assisting an individual identify specific goals will also facilitate behavioral changes. Maintaining a food diary or physical activity record can be an appropriate means for patient self-monitoring, which can then be discussed upon follow-up visits.

    3. Ways to gather information about a patient's diet

       a. 24-hour recall

          This tool (as shown in Box 6.1) collects retrospective data about food intake and habits. The interviewer (registered dietitian or physician) will ask questions about what food is *typically* eaten in a day. The main benefits of the 24-hour recall are that it is quick and does not require any equipment. It is a good way to gather general information about a patient's diet, but some of the downfalls include the tendency of the patient to forget what was eaten the day before, consciously or unconsciously changing reported intake to simplify recording or to impress the interviewer, or the reported day may be atypical for the patient and thus not representative of their regular diet.

       b. Food record or food diary

          This tool is a self-reported account of all foods and beverages consumed by a respondent over one or more day. It is open-ended and allows the patient to write down as much as they want. It should be done in "real time," immediately after the meal is eaten, and not retrospectively. It is helpful to have patients bring at least a 3-day food record with them to their appointment for your analysis.

BOX 6.1 | **Example of a 24-Hour Recall**

Breakfast: 2 eggs (scrambled) + 1 banana + 2 slices toast with butter
Snack: String cheese
Lunch: Turkey sandwich with lettuce and tomato, bag of chips
Snack: Chocolate
Dinner: Lasagna with green beans
Snack: Watermelon

Tips for Interviewers

- Ask additional questions to probe for more information.
- Always ask about beverage intake (including how people take their coffee).
- Remember to ask about alcohol intake.
- Ask for a "typical day."
- Ask about oils (grilled chicken can be cooked in 1-2 tbsp of olive oil).
- If the patient does not mention any sweets, ask, "What about sweets?"
- Ask about portions! How big was the bag of chips? How much chocolate?
- Food models or measuring cups can be helpful to help patients envision portion sizes.

Optional things to include:
- Calories, carbs, fat, protein, fiber
- Sodium
- Gastrointestinal symptoms (if the patient complains of stomach issues, this can help to relate any gastrointestinal symptoms to food eaten)
- Water intake
- Level of hunger before and after meal

c. Food frequency questionnaire (FFQ)

This tool is a limited checklist of foods and beverages that includes a frequency response section for subjects to report how often each item was consumed over a specified period of time. Semiquantitative FFQs collect portion size information as standardized portions or as a choice of portion sizes. Portion size information is not collected in nonquantitative FFQs. The food frequency questionnaire can be helpful because it is representative of "habitual" intake and is easy for literate subjects to complete as a self-administered form. Drawbacks include the retrospective nature, which relies upon the respondent's memory; the exclusion of foods popular to ethnic minority groups that are significant contributors of nutrients will skew the data; and it is not appropriate for low literacy populations.

CIGARETTE SMOKING, PHYSICAL ACTIVITY, PSYCHOSOCIAL FACTORS, ALCOHOL USE, HYPERTENSION, AND METABOLIC SYNDROME

I. Cigarette Smoking

A. Cigarette smoking is the primary cause of preventable morbidity and mortality worldwide. According to the 2014 Surgeon General's Report, smoking causes one of every three deaths related to CVD. Additionally, secondhand smoke increases risk of CVD by 25%-30% among nonsmokers.[19] Tobacco use is associated with an increase in TG levels and decrease in HDL cholesterol levels.[1,20]

B. Smoking cessation methods include behavior modification and pharmacological interventions, several of which have been approved by the FDA to aid in cessation.

C. Pharmaceutical interventions[21]

1. Nicotine replacement therapy (NRT) is available in the form of patches, gum, and lozenges, available over the counter and in the form of inhalers and nasal spray available by prescription. NRT uses low-dose nicotine to assist with weaning of tobacco use and limits nicotine withdrawal symptoms.

2. Varenicline (Chantix) is a partial nicotinic agonist. This medication reduces nicotine withdrawal and the urge to smoke. These work effectively when prescribed 1-2 weeks prior to smoking cessation. Common side effects include nausea, gastrointestinal issues (stomach pain, indigestion, constipation, gas, vomiting), headaches, weakness, tiredness, unusual dreams, insomnia, headache, dry mouth, or unpleasant taste in mouth.[22]

3. Other prescribed medications reduce nicotine withdrawal symptoms and the urge to smoke.[21] Bupropion (Zyban, Wellbutrin, or Aplenzin) is an antidepressant that has been associated with reducing nicotine withdrawal symptoms.

II. Physical Inactivity

A. A sedentary lifestyle is an independent risk factor for CVD. Physical activity has been shown to delay atherogenesis and increase myocardial vascularity and fibrinolysis. Coupled with weight loss among overweight and obese patients, regular exercise can improve risk factors associated with LDL cholesterol, HDL cholesterol, TG levels, blood pressure, glucose tolerance, and insulin sensitivity.[1]

B. While HDL-C is not a target for therapy, it has been shown to be inversely associated with risk for CVD. Studies have shown that physical activity can improve HDL cholesterol levels. Aerobic physical activity expenditure equivalent to about 1000-1500 calories per week (ie, about seven to 14 miles of walking per week) can produce significant changes in HDL cholesterol.[23,24] Consistent resistance exercise training 3 times per week for 6-9 weeks with 8 to 10 exercises per session has also been shown to increase HDL cholesterol.[25,26]

C. Physical activity associated with total body fat reduction has shown significant reductions in LDL cholesterol levels.[27-31] Total body fat loss can be achieved with 200-300 min/wk of moderate-intensity exercise.[28,29] The greatest reduction of total body fat percentage is seen among previously sedentary individuals when exercise energy expenditure is >2000 calories/wk, especially in individuals with higher baseline LDL cholesterol.[28,29] Exercise intensity >60% of maximum aerobic capacity is recommended than lower-intensity exercises for significant changes in lowering TG levels.[13]

D. The exercise prescription

   1. Recommended frequency, intensity, and duration
      a. The American Heart Association (AHA) recommends 150 min/wk of moderate aerobic exercise or 75 min/wk of vigorous exercise, or a combination of moderate and vigorous activity. This is equivalent to about 30 min/d 5 times per week.
      b. For individuals with hypertension or hypercholesterolemia, the AHA recommends 40 minutes of aerobic exercise of moderate to vigorous intensity 3-4 times per week to lower the risk for myocardial infarction and stroke.[32] The National Lipid Association (NLA) recommends similar goals. To improve hypercholesterolemia, physical exercise should equal 150 minutes (about 30-40 minutes of exercise 4 d/wk) or more weekly at a moderate or higher intensity. Aerobic exercise forms the core of a cardiovascular exercise program, but patients should also incorporate resistance (ie, weight lifting) and stretching exercises as well.

   2. **The exercise prescription** While formal exercise testing and prescription may not be practical in the outpatient office setting, patients can be given general counseling on an exercise program. Here are the steps:
      a. Determine the "training-sensitive zone" for heart rate during aerobic exercise. First, figure out the maximum heart rate by subtracting the patient's age in years from their age[1,2]:

---

[1]For patients <60 years old, the lower-limit target heart rate should be 60%-70% of the maximum heart rate, and the upper-limit target heart rate should be 90% of the maximum heart rate.
[2]For patients > 60 years old, the lower-limit target heart rate should be 60% of the maximum heart rate and the upper-limit maximum heart rate should be 75% of the maximum heart rate.

$$\text{Maximum Heart Rate} = 220 - \text{age (years)}$$

 i. Example: 65-year-old woman.

$$220 - 65 = 155 \ HR_{max}.$$
$$\text{Lower Limit} = 0.60 \times 155 = 93 \text{ beats/min}$$
$$\text{Upper Limit} = 0.75 \times 155 = 166 \text{ beats/min}$$

 ii. A sample "Exercise Prescription" for this 65-year-old woman:
- 5 minutes of stretching
- Walking, 5 d/wk; 2-3 miles at 3 miles/h; HR ~ 105 beats/min
- 5 minutes of strengthening exercises: sit-ups, modified push-ups, resistance bands

3. Who to screen prior to beginning an exercise program?
 a. The American College of Sports Medicine (ACSM) defines "regularly physically active" as $\geq$30 min/d of moderate-intensity exercise at least 3 d/wk for at least 3 months.
  i. Regularly physically active asymptomatic individuals without known cardiovascular disease metabolic or renal disease may continue their usual exercise and progress graduated as tolerated according to the ACMS prescription guidelines.
  ii. Physically active asymptomatic individuals with known cardiovascular disease and metabolic or renal disease whose provider has cleared them to exercise within the last 12 months do not need evaluation to continue a moderate-intensity exercise program unless they develop symptoms or change in status.
  iii. Physically inactive but asymptomatic individuals may begin light- to moderate-intensity exercise without medical clearance and in the absence of symptoms progress gradually in intensity.
  iv. Physically inactive with known cardiovascular, metabolic, or renal disease and/or those with signs or symptoms suggestive of these diseases should seek medical clearance prior to starting an exercise program regardless of intensity.[33]

III. Psychosocial Factors

CVD has been associated among individuals with type A personality.[34] The progression of atherosclerosis develops among these individuals from stress, depression, and a higher level of education. However, studies correlating CVD and psychosocial factors consistently have been inconclusive.[35]

IV. Alcohol Consumption

Moderate alcohol consumption, defined as one or two drinks per day, is associated with decreased risk of CVD.[36] A compound, called resveratrol, contained in wine has been associated with significant increases in HDL cholesterol levels and a reduction in fibrinogen.[37] However, alcohol is not a recommended intervention for disease prevention. Although alcohol consumption has been associated with increased HDL cholesterol levels, it has also been shown to increase blood pressure and total TG levels.[1]

V. Hypertension

A. Hypertension, defined as having a blood pressure higher than 140 mm Hg systolic pressure or 90 mm Hg diastolic pressure or use of antihypertensive medications, is a risk factor for CVD. The incidence of hypertension increases with age among all genders and is seen more among blacks than non-Hispanic whites.[1]

B. The Dietary Guidelines for Americans 2015-2020 recommend limiting sodium to <2300 mg/d. Restricting sodium intake even more so to <1500 mg/d is recommended for individuals who are older than 51 years, are black, or have hypertension, diabetes, or chronic renal disease.[38] A list of foods and the sodium content comparison is shown in Table 6.10.

C. **The DASH diet** The Dietary Approaches to Stop Hypertension, or simply the DASH Diet, is based on a clinical trial that examined diet modifications and its effect on combating hypertension. Funded by the National Heart, Lung, and Blood Institute (NHLBI), the DASH clinical trial emphasized increasing intake of fruits, vegetables, nuts, and low-fat dairy products and decreasing foods high in saturated fat, cholesterol, sugar, and refined carbohydrates. Eating patterns for the DASH diet are shown in Table 6.11. The DASH diet provides a balanced eating pattern rich in potassium, calcium, and magnesium to manage blood pressure.[38]

VI. Metabolic Syndrome

A. Metabolic syndrome is a constellation of risk factors associated with CVD and diabetes. It is preventable through lifestyle interventions. Metabolic syndrome is diagnosed when any of the three following criteria are present[39]:
- Waist circumference ≥35 in (88 cm) among women and >40 in (102 cm) among men
- Triglyceride levels ≥150 mg/dL

Table 6.10.	Comparison of Sodium Content in Various Food Items	
Food Item	**Portion Size**	**Sodium (mg)**
Campbell's Classic Chicken Noodle Soup	10.75 oz	2391
Iodized salt	1 tbsp	2360
Kosher Salt	1 tbsp	1920
Salami	3 oz	1920
Himalayan Salt (fine)	1 tbsp	1520
Soy sauce	1 tbsp	1029
Soy sauce (low sodium)	1 tbsp	660
Pickles	1 pickle	600
Kellogg's Raisin Bran	1 cup	350
Rao's Homemade Tomato Basil Sauce	½ cup	340
Quest Bar	1 bar	210
Popchips	100-calorie bag	160
Campbell's Low-Sodium Chicken Noodle Soup	10.75 oz	140
Creamy Peanut Butter	2 tbsp	135

Table 6.11. The DASH Diet Eating Plan Based on a 2000-Calorie Diet		
Type of Food	**Serving Size Example**	**Servings on a DASH Diet**
Grains and grain products (*include at least 3 whole grain foods each day*)	1 oz cereal, ½ cup cooked pasta	7-8/d
Vegetables	1 cup leafy, ½ cup juice	4-5/d
Low-fat or nonfat dairy foods	1 cup yogurt or milk	2-3/d
Lean meats, fish, poultry	1 oz cooked meat, poultry, or fish	2 or less per day
Nuts, seeds, and legumes	1/3 cup nuts, 1 tbsp peanut butter	4-5 times/wk
Fats and sweets	1 tbsp sugar, jam, or jellies	limited

- HDL cholesterol levels <40 mg/dL in men and <50 mg/dL in women
- Elevated blood pressure systolic ≥130 mm Hg or diastolic ≥85 mm Hg
- Elevated fasting blood glucose ≥100 mg/dL

B. Lifestyle modification is important in the treatment of metabolic syndrome as the components respond very well to lifestyle modification. As many patients with metabolic syndrome are at risk of developing manifest diabetes, it is helpful to use an intensive lifestyle modification program.

C. Among overweight adults, those with abdominal adiposity (ie, a high waist circumference) were at increased risk of type 2 diabetes and CVD, independent of BMI classification. Individuals with abdominal adiposity have an increased risk of CVD compared to overall obese individuals. This occurrence may be due to the sensitivity of the lipolytic system in the visceral adipocytes of the abdominal area. Consequently, free fatty acid (FFA) concentrations are then elevated in hepatic and portal circulation, leading to insulin resistance in peripheral tissues. Elevated portal FFA may also inhibit hepatic uptake of insulin, resulting in hyperinsulinemia.[40]

VII. Summary

Nutrition and lifestyle changes are important factors in preventing and treating cardiovascular disease. Medical nutrition therapy from a registered dietitian can help patients with dyslipidemia improve their lipid profile. Improved nutrition, increased physical activity, and tobacco smoking cessation are positive lifestyle interventions that can improve the outcomes in a patient with, or at risk for, cardiovascular disease.

References

1. Jacobson TA, Maki KC, Orringer CE, et al. National Lipid Association recommendations for patient-centered management of dyslipidemia: part 2. *J Clin Lipidol*. 2015;9(6):S1-S122.
2. Mahan LK, Escott-Stump S. *Krause's Food and the Nutrition Care Process*. 12th ed. Philadelphia, PA: Elsevier/Saunders; 2012.
3. Lembo AJ, Ullman SP. Constipation. In: Feldman M, Friedman LS, Sleisenger MH, eds. *Sleisenger & Fordtran's Gastrointestinal and Liver Disease*. 9th ed. Philadelphia, PA: Elsevier/Saunders; 2010:chap 18.
4. National Heart, Lung, and Blood Institute. *Third Report of the National Cholesterol Education Program (NCEP) Expert Panel on Detection, Evaluation, and Treatment of High Blood Cholesterol in Adults (Adult Treatment Panel III): Final Report*. NIH Publication No. 02-5215. Bethesda, MD: National Institutes of Health; 2002.
5. Thalheimer JC. A soluble fiber primer—plus the top five foods that can lower LDL cholesterol. *Today's Dietitian*. 2013;15(12):16.
6. Zelman KM. *Types of Fiber and Their Health Benefits*. Available at: http://www.webmd.com/diet/compare-dietary-fibers. Published July 22, 2015. Updated 2015. Accessed March 19, 2016.
7. National Heart, Lung, and Blood Institute. *Your Guide to Lowering Your Cholesterol with TLC (Therapeutic Lifestyle Changes)*. Bethesda, MD: National Institutes of Health, US Department of Health and Human Services; 2006.

8. Mitrou PN, Kipnis V, Thiébaut AC, et al. Mediterranean dietary pattern and prediction of all-cause mortality in a US population: results from the NIH-AARP Diet and Health Study. *Arch Intern Med.* 2007;167(22):2461-2468.

9. Estruch R, Ros E, Salas-Salvado J, et al. Primary prevention of cardiovascular disease with a Mediterranean diet. *N Engl J Med.* 2013;368:1279-1290. doi:10.1056/NEJMoa1200303

10. Jenkins DJ, Jones PJ, Lamarche B, et al. Effect of a dietary portfolio of cholesterol-lowering foods given at 2 levels of intensity of dietary advice on serum lipids in hyperlipidemia: a randomized controlled trial. *JAMA.* 2011;306(8):831-839. doi:10.1001/jama.2011.1202

11. *The Portfolio Diet Fact Sheet.* Heart UK-The Cholesterol Charity. Available at: http://heartuk.org.uk/images/uploads/healthylivingpdfs/huk_factsheet_d01_portd.pdf. Accessed April 19, 2016; 2008.

12. Chapman MJ, Ginsberg HN, Amarenco P, et al. For the European Atherosclerosis Society Consensus Panel. Triglyceride-rich lipoproteins and high-density lipoprotein cholesterol in patients at high risk of cardiovascular disease: evidence and guidance for management. *Eur Heart J.* 2011;32:1345-1361.

13. Trombold JR, Christmas KM, Machin DR, Kim IY, Coyle EF. Acute high-intensity endurance exercise is more effective than moderate- intensity exercise for attenuation of postprandial triglyceride elevation. *J Appl Physiol.* 2013;114:792-800.

14. Felando M. *Lower Your Triglycerides with Lifestyle.* Learn Your Lipids Web site. Available at: http://www.learnyourlipids.com/wp-content/uploads/2014/02/TrigsTearSheet.pdf. Accessed March 20, 2016.

15. Ogden CL, Carroll MD, Kit BK, Flegal KM. *Prevalence of Obesity in the United States, 2009–2010.* NCHS data brief no. 82. Hyattsville, MD: National Center for Health Statistics; 2012.

16. Sikand G, Kashyap ML, Yang I. Medical nutrition therapy lowers serum cholesterol and saves medication costs in men with hypercholesterolemia. *J Am Diet Assoc.* 1998;98(8):889-894.

17. McCoin M, Sikand G, Johnson EQ, et al. The effectiveness of medical nutrition therapy delivered by registered dietitians for disorders of lipid metabolism: a call for further research. *J Am Diet Assoc.* 2008;108(2):233-239.

18. Sikand G, Kashyap ML, Wong ND, Hsu JC. Dietitian intervention improves lipid values and saves medication costs in men with combined hyperlipidemia and a history of niacin noncompliance. *J Am Diet Assoc.* 2000;100(2):218-224.

19. U.S. Department of Health and Human Services. *The Health Consequences of Smoking—50 Years of Progress: A Report of the Surgeon General.* Atlanta, GA: U.S. Department of Health and Human Services, Centers for Disease Control and Prevention, National Center for Chronic Disease Prevention and Health Promotion, Office on Smoking and Health; 2014.

20. U.S. Department of Health and Human Services. *A Report of the Surgeon General: How Tobacco Smoke Causes Disease: What It Means to You.* Atlanta, GA: U.S. Department of Health and Human Services, Centers for Disease Control and Prevention, National Center for Chronic Disease Prevention and Health Promotion, Office on Smoking and Health; 2010.

21. *Nicotine Replacement Therapy.* American Cancer Society Web site. Available at: http://www.cancer.org/healthy/stayawayfromtobacco/guidetoquittingsmoking/guide-to-quitting-smoking-nicotine-replacement-therapy. Published February 6, 2014. Accessed March 8, 2016.

22. *Prescription Drugs to Help You Quit Smoking.* American Cancer Society Web site. Available at: http://www.cancer.org/healthy/stayawayfromtobacco/guidetoquittingsmoking/guide-to-quitting-smoking-help-phys-rx-drugs. Published February 6, 2014. Updated 2014. Accessed March 5, 2016.

23. Drygas W, Jegler A, Kunski H. Study on threshold dose of physical activity in coronary heart disease prevention. Part I. Relationship between leisure time physical activity and coronary risk factors. *Int J Sports Med.* 1988;9:275-278.

24. Kokkinos P, Myers J. Exercise and physical activity: clinical outcomes and applications. *Circulation.* 2010;122:1637-1648.

25. Costa RR, Lima Alberton C, Tagliari M, Martins Kruel LF. Effects of resistance training on the lipid profile in obese women. *J Sports Med Phys Fitness.* 2011;51:169-177.

26. Sheikholeslami Vatani D, Ahmadi S, Ahmadi Dehrashid K, Gharibi F. Changes in cardiovascular risk factors and inflammatory markers of young, healthy, men after six weeks of moderate or high intensity resistance training. *J Sports Med Phys Fitness.* 2011;51:695-700.

27. Eckel RH, Jakicic JM, Ard JD, et al. American College of Cardiology/American Heart Association Task Force on Practice Guidelines. 2013 AHA/ACC guideline on lifestyle management to reduce cardiovascular risk: a report of the American College of Cardiology/American Heart Association Task Force on Practice Guidelines. *J Am Coll Cardiol.* 2014;63(25 Pt B):2960-2984.

28. Gordon D, Chen S, Durstine L. The effects of exercise training on the traditional lipid profile and beyond. *Curr Sports Med Rep.* 2014;13:253-259.

29. Durstine JL, Grandjean PW, Davis PG, Ferguson MA, Alderson NL, DuBose KD. Blood lipid and lipoprotein adaptations to exercise: a quantitative analysis. *Sports Med.* 2001;31:1033-1062.

30. American College of Sports Medicine. In: Pescatello LS, senior ed. *ACSM's Guidelines for Exercise Testing and Prescription.* 9th ed. Philadelphia, PA: Lippincott Williams & Wilkins; 2014.

31. Leon A, Sanchez O. Response of blood lipids to exercise training alone or combined with dietary intervention. *Med Sci Sports Exerc*. 2001;33(6 suppl):S502-S515 (discussion S528–S529).
32. *American Heart Association Recommendations for Physical Activity in Adults*. American Heart Association Web site. Available at: http://www.heart.org/HEARTORG/HealthyLiving/PhysicalActivity/FitnessBasics/American-Heart-Association-Recommendations-for-Physical-Activity-in-Adults_UCM_307976_Article.jsp#.VvrPetIrLs0. Published August 17, 2015. Updated 2015. Accessed March 20, 2016.
33. American College of Sports Medicine. *ACSM's Guidelines for Exercise Testing and Prescription*. Philadelphia, PA: Lippincott Williams & Wilkins; 2013.
34. Toeffler GH. Psychosocial factors in coronary and cerebral vascular disease. In: Silver JM, ed. *Up To Date*. Available at: UpToDate.com. Accessed March 20, 2016; January 21, 2016.
35. Hansen AS, Marckmann P, Dragsted L, Nielsen IF, Nielsen S, Grønbaek M. Effect of red wine and red grape extract on blood lipids, haemostatic factors, and other risk factors for cardiovascular disease. *Eur J Clin Nutr*. 2005;59(3):449-455.
36. Goldberg IJ, Mosca L, Piano MR, Fisher EA. Wine and your heart: a science advisory for healthcare professionals from the Nutrition Committee, Council on Epidemiology and Prevention, and Council on Cardiovascular Nursing of the American Heart Association. *Circulation*. 2001;103(3):472-475.
37. Kaplan NM, Douglas PS. Clinical implications and treatment of left ventricular hypertrophy in hypertension. In: Bakris GL, ed. *Up To Date*. Available at: UpToDate.com. Published August 2015. Accessed March 8, 2016; August 2015.
38. Sacks FM, Moore TJ, Appel LJ, et al. A dietary approach to prevent hypertension: A review of the dietary approaches to stop hypertension (DASH) study. *Clin Cardiol*. 1999;22(S3):6-10.
39. *What is Metabolic Syndrome?* National Institutes of Health Web site. Available at: http://www.nhlbi.nih.gov/health/health-topics/topics/ms. Published November 6, 2015. Updated 2015. Accessed March 20, 2016.
40. Ohlson LO, Larsson B, Svardsudd K, et al. The influence of body fat distribution on the incidence of diabetes mellitus. 13.5 years of follow-up of the participants in the study of men born in 1913. *Diabetes*. 1985;34(10):1055-1058.

CHAPTER 7

Lipid Medications Overview: Prescription and Nonprescription Preparations

Joyce L. Ross and Kenneth Kellick

> ### Key Points
>
> - Statins are the first-line therapy for lowering atherogenic cholesterol.
> - Nonstatin medications have a role in lowering both LDL-C as well as triglycerides.
> - PCSK9 inhibitors are a potent new class of LDL-C lowering medication but at present are limited to very-high-risk patients.
> - Many patients use over-the-counter preparations or supplements, and the clinician should be familiar with the risks and benefits of these products.

PRESCRIPTION MEDICATIONS

I. Introduction

This chapter provides an overview of lipid medications and highlights the characteristics of each class. Chapter 8 provides in-depth discussion on the statin drugs, and Chapter 9 discusses the nonstatin drugs. Discussion on the newer LDL-lowering drugs is provided in Chapter 12 on Familial Hypercholesterolemia. Side-effect and safety issues are detailed in Chapter 11.

II. Historical Background

A. Discovery of the LDL receptor In 1973, Drs. Michael Brown and Joseph Goldstein revolutionized the lipid world with the discovery of the LDL receptor and the theory of regulation of cholesterol metabolism, which has informed treatment from that period of time and persists today. Their work resulted in the reception of the 1985 Nobel Prize in Physiology for "the regulation of cholesterol management of cholesterol metabolism."[1,2] The key findings were that liver cells contain receptors located on their surface that are necessary to mediate the uptake of LDL particles that circulate in the bloodstream.

B. Genetic hypercholesterolemia Their discovery provided the key to understanding hereditary forms of hypercholesterolemia, in particular familial hypercholesterolemia. They found that in persons with average cholesterol levels, ample number and function of receptors existed resulting in acceptable levels of LDL-C. Conversely, those with inherited forms of hypercholesterolemia did not have adequate number or function of LDL-C receptors to clear cholesterol from the blood resulting in persistent increased LDL-C often with premature coronary artery disease.

C. Early drugs The first lipid drugs were niacin, found to lower cholesterol in higher doses in the mid 1950s, and cholestyramine, a bile acid sequestrant developed by Merck in the late 1950s.

The discovery of HMG-CoA reductase inhibitors, known as statins, provided the greatest revolution in treatment of elevated cholesterol. In November 1986, Merck Pharmaceuticals sent a new drug application (NDA) to the U.S. Federal Drug Administration, and lovastatin (Mevacor) was given FDA approval to become the first commercial statin in September 1987.

III. Statins

A. Benefits The most researched and widely used class of medications are the statin drugs. There has been consistent evidence of their benefit to reduce morbidity and mortality from cardiovascular disease shown by randomized controlled trials, observational studies, and basic science investigation. While statins have the greatest potential for LDL-C lowering with reduction of the incidence of recurrent cardiovascular events and all-cause mortality, other studies have suggested other, non-LDL-C lowering (pleiotropic) effects from statin therapy.

B. Guidelines The 2013 ACC/AHA Guidelines[3] as well as the NLA Recommendations[4] are consistent and reinforce that the statin drugs should be first line for LDL-C lowering and intensive treatment with statins should be implemented in those with the highest risk and therefore the most likely to benefit from therapy. To be successful, the management plan should be individualized and consider the degree of ASCVD risk, nature of the patients' lipoprotein abnormality, mechanism of action of classes of medication, side effects, and personal medication history of the patient.

C. Statins and familial hypercholesterolemia It should be noted that the efficacy of statins in familial hypercholesterolemia (FH) is often lower than in the general population.[5,6] This attenuated effectiveness in FH is related to the mechanism of action of the statins, which is based on their ability to up-regulate LDL receptors. Because clearance of LDL-C by the LDL receptor is compromised in those with FH, a variation in responsiveness is found from one patient to another, specifically related to the genetic mutation.[5,6]

D. Doses and potency The statins are potent LDL-C lowering drugs with greatest potency at higher doses. Table 7.1 lists the percentage of LDL-C lowering that can be expected with the different statin drugs.

E. Summary Overall, statins are uncomplicated to take and are generally very well tolerated; however, research and patient subjective reports with statin therapy demonstrate that some patients on statins exhibit side effects that may lead to discontinuation of the therapy. See Chapter 11 for discussion on statin safety and side effects.

Table 7.1. 2013 ACC/AHA Guidelines—Statin Intensity		
ACC/AHA 2013 Blood Cholesterol Guideline: Statin Intensity		
High-Intensity	**Moderate-Intensity**	**Low-Intensity**
Daily dose lowers LDL-C on average, by ~ ≥ 50%	Daily dose lowers LDL-C on average, by ~ 30 to <50%	Daily dose lowers LDL-C on average, by <30%
Atorvastatin (40)–80 mg **Rosuvastatin 20 (40) mg**	**Atorvastatin 10 (20) mg** **Rosuvastatin (5) 10 mg** **Simvastatin 20-40 mg** **Pravastatin 40 (80) mg** **Lovastatin 40 mg** *Fluvastatin XL 80 mg* **Fluvastatin 40 mg bid** *Pitavastatin 2-4 mg*	*Simvastatin 10 mg* **Pravastatin 10-20 mg** **Lovastatin 20 mg** *Fluvastatin 20-40 mg* *Pitavastatin 1 mg*

Specific statins and doses are noted in bold that were evaluated in randomized controlled trials.
Statins and doses that are approved by the U.S. FDA but were not tested in the RCTs reviewed are listed in *italics*.
(Data from Stone NJ, et al. *Circulation.* 2013;01.cir.0000437738.63853.7a, originally published November 12, 2013. https://doi.org/10.1161/01.cir.0000437738.63853.7a.)

IV. The Nonstatin Medications

A. Overview

1. **Use of additional classes of lipid-lowering medication** The use of additional drugs may be necessary for patients who do not reach target LDL-C goals on maximum-dose statin regimens or in those who do not tolerate doses necessary to bring the LDL-C to goal. When this occurs, recommendations reinforce the need to intensify drug therapy by combining maximally tolerated statin dosages with a bile acid sequestrant, a cholesterol absorption inhibitor, or PCSK9 inhibitors. In addition, hypertriglyceridemia may require using nonstatin medications such as fish oil and fibrates. Classes of available lipid therapy options are illustrated in Table 7.2. The 2013 ACC/AHA Guidelines did not address use of nonstatins as they focused on evidence from randomized clinical trials; however, in 2016, the ACC published an Expert Consensus outlining pathways for the role of nonstatin therapies for LDL-C lowering.

   Most recently (April 2016), the FDA has withdrawn approval for use of niacin in combination with statin therapy for the reduction of cardiovascular risk. The 2016 ACC Expert Consensus Decision Pathway statement does not include niacin in their algorithms; limited indications for this medication can be considered in special circumstances.

2. **Evidence to support use of nonstatins** While the 2013 ACC/AHA Guidelines panel did not find data to support routine use of nonstatins, the recent IMPROVE-IT study, a trial of patients who had been hospitalized for an acute coronary syndrome who were randomized to either simvastatin and ezetimibe or simvastatin alone, showed that the addition of ezetimibe resulted in lower LDL-C and improved cardiovascular outcomes. This study gave support to the role of nonstatins for lipid lowering.

B. Bile acid resins or sequestrants

1. The bile acid resins or sequestrants (BAS) are one of the first lipid-lowering agents, but are less potent than other classes of medication now available and are not always well

Table 7.2. Overview of Lipid Medications			
Drug Class, Agents, and Daily Doses	Lipid/Lipoprotein Effects	Side Effects	Contraindications
Statins	LDL-C ↓18%-55% HDL-C ↑5%-15% TG ↓7%-30%	Myopathy, increased liver enzymes	Absolute: active or chronic liver disease Relative: concomitant use of certain drugs
Bile acid sequestrants	LDL-C ↓15%-30% HDL-C ↑3%-5% TG No Δ or ↑	Gastrointestinal distress, constipation, decreased absorption of other drugs	Absolute: dysbetalipoproteinemia, TG ≥ 400 mg/dL Relative: TG ≥ 200 mg/dL
Nicotinic acid	LDL-C ↓5%-25% HDL-C ↑15%-35% TG ↓20%-50%	Flushing, hyperglycemia, hyperuricemia (or gout), upper gastrointestinal distress, hepatotoxicity	Absolute: chronic liver disease, severe gout Relative: diabetes, hyperuricemia, peptic ulcer disease
Fibric acids	LDL-C ↓5%-20% HDL-C ↑10%-20% TG ↓20%-50%	Dyspepsia, gallstones, myopathy, unexplained non-CHD deaths in WHO study	Absolute: severe renal disease, severe hepatic disease
Cholesterol absorption inhibitor	LDL-C ↓13%-20% HDL-C ↑3%-5% TG ↓5%-11%	Gastrointestinal disorders (diarrhea), arthralgia, pain in extremities	When combined with a statin: active liver disease or unexplained persistent elevations in hepatic transaminases
Long-chain omega-3 fatty acid drugs	LDL-C ↓6%-↑25% HDL-C ↓5%-↑7% TG ↓19%-44%	Gastrointestinal disorders (eructation, dyspepsia), taste perversion	Hypersensitivity to components of the drug

tolerated. BAS decrease LDL-C levels by an average of 13%-21%.[5] They can be used as monotherapy when patients cannot tolerate statin therapy, but primarily these drugs are used as an addition to a statin to further lower LDL-C (Table 7.3).

2. **Mechanism of action** BAS's highly positively charged molecules bind to the negatively charged bile acids in the intestine, inhibiting their lipid-solubilizing activity and thus blocking cholesterol absorption. BAS further inhibit the reabsorption of bile acids and thus cause a contraction of the bile acid pool, leading to increased bile acid synthesis that competes with cholesterol synthesis in the liver, further contributing to the lowering of serum cholesterol levels.

3. **Evidence of benefits** Although they have not been shown to decrease overall mortality in patients with FH, studies of colestipol and cholestyramine have demonstrated a reduction in CHD events, directly proportional to the degree of LDL reduction obtained.[7,8] The Lipid Research Clinics Coronary Primary Prevention Trial,[7] with 3000 patients enrolled, showed cardiovascular event reduction. The Familial Atherosclerosis Treatment Study (FATS), although small, also revealed reductions in the incidences of myocardial infarction and other cardiovascular events[8]; both of these trials support data showing that these drugs have some long-term benefits.

4. **Side effects** As they are not systemically absorbed, their overall risk profile is very favorable. They have a Pregnancy Class B. The same affinity of the BAS to bind also have the potential to bind to important vitamins, hormones, or medications in the intestine and can result in subtherapeutic serum levels; therefore, caution is indicated in the dosing schedule to avoid ingestion around meals and times when other medications are taken. Caution is necessary in use with patients with TG levels ≥500 mg/dL since they have been found to dramatically further increase TG levels.

5. **Adherence** The principal limiting factor to broader use of these medications is patient adherence, which may be hindered by drug interactions and gastrointestinal side effects.[5] Colesevelam (Welchol), the most recently approved bile acid sequestrant, has a more favorable side-effect profile and is considered the medication of choice within the class. Formulations include six large capsules or an oral suspension that can be mixed in water and other liquids.

C. **Cholesterol absorption inhibition**

1. The cholesterol absorption inhibitor ezetimibe (Zetia) is another option for LDL-C reduction in patients with FH or those who may be unable to obtain LDL-C goals with maximally tolerated statin therapy. Because it also blocks absorption of other sterols, it is the only drug that can effectively treat sitosterolemia.

2. **Mechanism of action** Ezetimibe lowers LDL-C by blocking the Niemann-Pick C1–like 1 (NPC1L1) protein, thereby reducing absorption of cholesterol from the intestine. Polymorphisms affecting NPC1L1 are associated with both lower levels of LDL cholesterol and a lower risk of cardiovascular events.

3. **Evidence** Recent data from The IMPROVE-IT trial,[8] which compared cardiovascular outcomes of ezetimibe/simvastatin combination therapy with simvastatin alone, concluded that when added to statin therapy, ezetimibe resulted in incremental lowering of LDL cholesterol levels and improved cardiovascular outcomes. When added to statins, it was found to reduce LDL-C on average by an additional 23%-24%.

4. **Side effect** There is minimal systemic absorption of the drug resulting in a favorable risk profile.

Table 7.3.	Characteristics of Lipid Medications							
	Mechanism of Action	Lipoprotein Effects	Dose	Contraindications	Adverse Reactions	Drug Interactions	Advantages	Disadvantages
HMGCoA Reductase Inhibitors	Inhibit the rate limiting enzyme in cholesterol synthesis, thereby reducing hepatic cholesterol production and up-regulating hepatic LDL receptors	↓LDL 31%–60% ↓TG 7%–30% ↑HDL 5%–15%	Oral administration once per day	Absolute: Active or chronic liver disease Pregnancy Breast-feeding Relative: Concomitant use with certain medications (eg, strong CYP 3A4 inhibitors)	Myopathy ↑liver enzymes; baseline testing recommended but monitoring no longer required ↑plasma glucose Possible cognitive impairment	Interactions due to CYP 450, drug transporters, glucuronidation Caution with fibrates, antifungals, protease inhibitors, macrolides, antiarrhythmics, cyclosporine, grapefruit juice	Observational data from large cohorts suggest that statin treatment decreases the excess lifetime risk of CVD due to FH to a level similar to that of the general population	No large CV end point trials available in FH Less effective in FH Pregnancy category X
Bile Acid Sequestrants	Prevent reabsorption of bile acids in the intestine, thereby increasing fecal loss of bile acid–bound LDL; also up-regulate LDL	↓LDL 13%–21% ↔/↑TG ↑HDL 3%–5%	Oral administration granules for suspension once per day or tablets twice per day	Absolute: Dysbetalipoproteinemia TG > 400 mg/dL Relative: TG > 200 mg/dL	Gastrointestinal side effects (particularly constipation)	Other medications should be administered 1 h before or 4 h after bile acid sequestrants	Colesevelam is pregnancy category B	Not proven to decrease overall mortality in FH
Cholesterol Absorption Inhibitor Ezetimibe (Zetia)	Inhibits cholesterol absorption in the intestine, thereby increasing hepatic LDL receptors	↓LDL 15%–20% ↓TG 10% ↑HDL 1%–2%	10 mg orally once/day	None	Myalgia (rare) ↑LFTs Upper respiratory infection Diarrhea	May increase cyclosporine levels Should be administered 2 h before or 4 h after bile acid sequestrant	Combination product available with simvastatin and atorvastatin	Not proven to decrease long-term CV outcomes compared with statin monotherapy Pregnancy category C
Nicotinic Acid (Niacin)	Inhibits the synthesis of VLDL and LDL May also increase the rate of chylomicron TG removal from plasma	↓LDL 5%–25% ↓TG 20%–50% ↑HDL 15%–35%	Oral administration 1-3 times/day	Absolute: Unexplained hepatic dysfunction Active peptic ulcer Arterial bleeding Relative: Diabetes Hyperuricemia Peptic ulcer disease	Flushing, hot flashes Hyperglycemia Hepatotoxicity Hyperuricemia, gout Dyspepsia	Risk of muscle toxicity increased when given with statins (typically seen at niacin doses > 1 g and high-dose statins)	Combination products available with simvastatin and lovastatin OTC products available	Not proven to decrease long-term CV outcomes compared with statin monotherapy Pregnancy category C

Drug	Mechanism	Lipid effects	Dosing	Contraindications	Adverse effects	Drug interactions	FDA/Administration	Special considerations
Omega-3 Fatty Acids	Reduces hepatic very-low-density lipoprotein triglycerides (VLDL-TG) synthesis and/or secretion and enhances TG clearance from circulating VLDL particles	LDL-C ↓6%–↑25% HDL-C ↓5%–↑7% TG ↓19%–44%	Oral administration 4 g caps per day	Hypersensitivity to components of the drug	Gastrointestinal disorders (eructation, dyspepsia), taste perversion Arthralgia	Should be used with caution in patients with known sensitivity or allergy to fish and/or shellfish No drug-drug interactions were observed in medications that are typical substrates of cytochrome P-450 enzymes	FDA approved for purity and consistency in dosing	Potential for prolongation of bleeding time risk for pancreatitis has not been determined. The effect on cardiovascular mortality and morbidity has not been determined
Antisense Oligonucleotide Mipomersen (Kynamro)	Binds to apoB-100 mRNA resulting in RNase H–mediated degradation of the cognate mRNA thereby inhibiting translation of the apoB-100 protein	↓LDL 25% ↓TG 18% ↑HDL 15%	200 mg s.c. once per week Not recommended in severe renal impairment	Moderate or severe hepatic impairment Active liver disease	Injection-site reactions Influenzalike symptoms Increased ALT Increased hepatic fat Nausea Headache Angina Palpitations	No clinically relevant drug interactions reported with warfarin, simvastatin, or ezetimibe	Pregnancy category B Elimination half-life 1-2 mo	s.c. administration Black box warning: Hepatotoxicity REMS program Must be refrigerated Not yet evaluated in patients on LDL apheresis
MTP Inhibitor Lomitapide (Juxtapid)	Inhibits MTP in the endoplasmic reticulum, thereby preventing the assembly of apoB-containing lipoproteins in hepatocytes and enterocytes	↓LDL 40% ↓TG 45% ↓HDL 7%	5-60 mg orally once per day without food, 2 h after the evening meal Maximum dose of 40 mg/d in patients with renal impairment	Concomitant use with strong or moderate CYP 3A4 inhibitors Pregnancy Moderate or severe hepatic impairment Active liver disease	Diarrhea Nausea Vomiting Dyspepsia Abdominal pain Increased hepatic fat Increased LFTs Low-fat diet should be initiated to minimize GI side effects	Should not exceed 30 mg/d when taken with weak CYP 3A4 inhibitors including atorvastatin and oral contraceptives Interacts with P-gp substrates, warfarin, and bile acid sequestrants	Oral administration	Drug-drug interactions Black box warning: hepatotoxicity REMS program Reduced absorption of fat-soluble vitamins and fatty acids
PCSK9 Inhibitors	Inhibit circulating PCSK9 from binding to low-density lipoprotein (LDL) receptor (LDLR), preventing PCSK9-mediated LDLR degradation, permitting LDLR to recycle back to the liver cell surface. By inhibiting the binding increases the number of LDLRs available to clear LDL from the blood, thereby lowering LDL-C levels	LDL ↓ 29%–70% in LDL	Injection generally q2wk 75-420 mg filled syringes	Contraindicated in patients with a history of a serious hypersensitivity reaction to components of the drug	Rash, urticaria Upper respiratory tract infection Influenza Gastroenteritis Nasopharyngitis 1%–1½% of patients experienced treatment-related neurocognitive effects, mainly confusion and some memory loss	No known drug-drug interactions reported	Subcutaneous injection either once or twice per month; prefilled syringes easily administered at home	Must be refrigerated and warmed to room temperature 30 min prior to use Patient cost varies by insurance company The effect on cardiovascular mortality has not been determined

Adapted from Marbach J, McKeon JL, Ross J, Duffy D. Novel treatments for familial hypercholesterolemia: pharmacogenetics at work. Pharmacotherapy. September 2014;34(9):961-972.

D. Omega-3 fatty acids

1. Long-chain omega-3 polyunsaturated fatty acids are often referred to as "fish oils" when found as a dietary supplement in over-the-counter preparations. The bioactives in marine oil are eicosapentaenoic acid (EPA) and docosahexaenoic acid (DHA), which when taken in high doses (4 g daily) can lower TG in patients with dyslipidemia.

   A prescription formulation of EPA and DHA omega-3 fatty acids, Lovaza,[9] has been available since 2004 and is prescribed primarily to lower TGs in patients with TGs ≥ 500 mg/dL. This combination of omega-3 fatty acid esters provides significant TG reduction but is noted to result in elevations in LDL-C, which can be substantial. However, research has shown that non-HDL-C and apolipoprotein B are not significantly increased.[10] An all-EPA formulation, icosapent (Vascepa) is the second FDA-approved omega-3 fatty acid. Each 1-g icosapent capsule contains at least 96% EPA and no DHA and may not change LDL.

2. **Mechanism of action** The mechanism of action is not completely understood; however, possible explanations include inhibition of acyl-CoA: 1,2-diacylglycerol acyltransferase, increased mitochondrial and peroxisomal β-oxidation in the liver, decreased lipogenesis in the liver, and increased plasma lipoprotein lipase activity. It may reduce the synthesis of TGs in the liver because EPA and DHA are poor substrates for the enzymes responsible for TG synthesis, and EPA and DHA inhibit esterification of other fatty acids.[9]

3. **Evidence** There is continuing discussion regarding benefit of omega 3 fatty acids.[11]

4. **Nonprescription formulations** Patients can also purchase nonprescription fish oil and should be instructed to take the equivalent dose of prescription formulations. These formulations are labeled as "supplements" and are not FDA approved. The purity of the compounds may not be known, and often the number of pills needed exceed that of the prescription formulation.

5. **Side effects** Omega-3 fatty acids are generally considered very safe. In large doses there may be platelet aggregation inhibition, but whether this is a clinically significant effect is not known.

E. Niacin therapy

1. Niacin, also known as nicotinic acid, is one of the first lipid-lowering medications.[12] Niacin is an essential, water-soluble, B-3 vitamin that, when given in high doses, is effective in lowering total cholesterol, LDL-C, and TG and raising HDL-C. See Part 2 of this chapter for discussion on nonprescription formulations.

2. **Mechanism of action** The mechanisms of niacin in hyperlipidemia is not well understood, but there are several actions felt to favorably influence lipid levels. Niacin lowers VLDL formulation in the liver by blocking release of free fatty acids and may also up-regulate ABCA-1, which is involved in reverse cholesterol transport.

3. **Evidence** Initial evidence for the effectiveness of niacin comes from the pre-statin era when the Coronary Drug Project demonstrated a significantly lower incidence of nonfatal myocardial infarction and decreased mortality.[13,7] Although favorable effects of niacin on lipoproteins have been demonstrated in several trials, both the AIM-HIGH trial[14] and the HPS-2 THRIVE trial[15] failed to demonstrate a reduction in cardiovascular end points when niacin was added to simvastatin.

4. **Side effects** Niacin can cause mild-to-moderate serum aminotransferase elevations with high doses and certain formulations linked to acute liver injury, which can be severe as well as fatal. They are often poorly tolerated due to flushing and pruritus.

5. **Current use** The role of niacin has lessened in recent years. In April 2016, the FDA withdrew approval of this class of lipid-lowering medication in combination with statin therapy. The 2016 ACC Expert Consensus on the role of nonstatins has not included niacin in their treatment algorithms. Further, although niacin can raise HDL-C, this is not recommended as a target for therapy. See Chapter 11 on drug safety for discussion regarding current use of niacin.

F. Fibric acid derivatives

1. The first fibrates were synthesized in the mid-1950s. There are two common formulations, gemfibrozil and fenofibrate. They reduce TG by 30%-50%.

2. **Mechanism** Fibrates lower TG by stimulating PPAR α. They also inhibit apolipoprotein C III and stimulate lipoprotein lipase, both of which reduce TG levels. Fibrates raise HDL-C and have slight LDL-C lowering effects.

3. **Evidence**
   a. Results of several clinical trials such as the Veterans Affairs High-Density Lipoprotein Cholesterol Intervention Trial (VA-HIT) study,[16] demonstrated the efficacy of gemfibrozil, a fibrate, on cardiovascular events. Beneficial effects on microvascular complications with fenofibrate were shown in the Fenofibrate Intervention and Event Lowering in Diabetes (FIELD).[17]
   b. A more recently published fibrate trial, the Action to Control Cardiovascular Risk in Diabetes (ACCORD) lipid-lowering trial was disappointing because it did not show the intended benefit.[18] Conclusions from the trial found that the combination of fenofibrate and simvastatin did not reduce the rate of fatal cardiovascular events, nonfatal myocardial infarction, or nonfatal stroke, as compared with simvastatin alone. These results do not support the routine use of combination therapy with fenofibrate and simvastatin to reduce cardiovascular risk in the majority of high-risk patients with type 2 diabetes.

4. **Side effects** Fibrates are contraindicated in patients with active liver or gallbladder disease. There is greater risk for rhabdomyolysis when used in combination with statins. Fenofibrates should have dose adjustment for patients with renal disease; however, gemfibrozil does not require adjustment. Gemfibrozil must be taken twice a day and has more drug interactions. It should be used with caution with statins.

G. Proprotein convertase subtilisin kexin type 9 inhibitors

1. In 2015, proprotein convertase subtilisin/kexin type 9 inhibitors (PCSK9 inhibitors) (a new, monoclonal antibody given in a subcutaneous injection) were approved for use for limited indications as an adjunct to diet and maximally tolerated statin therapy for the treatment of adults with heterozygous familial hypercholesterolemia (HeFH) or clinical atherosclerotic CVD, who require additional lowering of LDL-C. Two formulations have been approved, alirocumab[19] and evolocumab.[20] They can reduce LDL-C by 50%-60% and also lower Lp(a). Cost for these drugs is very high, approximately $15,000 a year. Access to these drugs is currently heavily regulated by insurance carriers.

2. **Mechanism of action** Carriers of mutations in the PCSK9 gene result in lifelong reductions in levels of LDL-C[21,22] and a 50%-90% reduction in the incidence of coronary events, even in populations with a high prevalence of non-lipid-related cardiovascular risk factors. PCSK9 is a serine protease synthesized in the liver prior to being secreted into systemic circulation where it binds to hepatic LDL receptors, targeting them for degradation.[23] PCSK9 causes the degradation of LDL receptors, so a loss of function mutation means that the PCSK9 does not degrade the LDL receptors, leaving many LDL receptors on the liver cells so that more LDL-C is removed from the bloodstream, which dramatically lowers LDL-C levels.

3. **Evidence** PCSK9 inhibitors are monoclonal antibodies and must be injected on a routine basis. At present, there have been no clinical trials providing evidence that PCSK9 inhibitors reduce cardiovascular events and death. Studies are now under way that will provide this information. Evolucumab vs placebo reduced LDL, decreased composite of major and nonfatal CV events; no effect on CV mortality or other secondary endpoints.

4. **Side effects** Premarketing trials have shown that these drugs were well tolerated; however, further information on safety and side effects will be provided by ongoing trials.

H. Mipomersen

1. Mipomersen (Kynamro)[24] was approved by the FDA in 2013, for limited access through a Risk Evaluation and Mitigation Strategy (REMS) program. Mipomersen is an adjunct to standard lipid-lowering medications and diet to reduce LDL-C, apoB, and TC in patients with homozygous familial hypercholesterolemia (HoFH).

2. **Mechanism** Mipomersen is a second-generation antisense oligonucleotide complementary to the human apoB-100 mRNA, which was developed based on a known genetically inherited mutation of the apoB gene that leads to hypobetalipoproteinemia.[5]

   It is given as a subcutaneous injection. Once injected, it is transported to the liver where it binds the target mRNA, leading to selective degradation of the mRNA strand by RNase enzymes, thereby inhibiting apoB-100 translation.[25] This ultimately leads to decreased production of all apoB-containing lipoproteins including VLDL-C, LDL-C, and lipoprotein (a).

I. Lomitapide

1. Lomitapide (Juxtapid)[26] is an oral once per day microsomal triglyceride transfer protein (MTP) inhibitor approved by the FDA in 2012, for patients with HoFH as add-on therapy to a low-fat diet and medications that reduce LDL-C, apoB, and TC. As with mipomersen, access is granted through a REMS program.

2. **Mechanism** Lomitapide inhibits MTP, which is located in both the hepatocyte and enterocyte endoplasmic reticula, and is responsible for incorporating triglycerides into nascent apoB, ultimately developing into nascent apoB, VLDL-C, and chylomicrons[27] Complete inhibition of this process occurs in abetalipoproteinemia, a rare inherited disorder marked by failure of MTP production, thereby impeding hepatic VLDL-C secretion. Patients with abetalipoproteinemia have extremely low TC, LDL-C, and apoB levels and fat malabsorption, fat-soluble vitamin deficiencies, and hepatic steatosis.[28,29]

V. Summary: Prescription Medications

This section has provided an overview of all medications to treat dyslipidemia. The statins remain the cornerstone of therapy, but the role of nonstatin medications is well recognized. New and powerful LDL-C lowering medications are now available; however, they are restricted to a small percent of patients who are at very high risk.

NONPRESCRIPTION FORMULATIONS

I. Introduction: Nonprescription Formulations

According to the Consumer Healthcare Products Association, the average US household spends about $338 per year on over-the-counter (OTC) products including diet and dietary supplements.[30] The dollar amount spent on OTC products for cholesterol is not published due to wide variance between households. Data on most products that are nonprescription are limited.

The FDA defines "supplement" as:

- A dietary ingredient such as a vitamin, mineral, herb, or other botanical amino acid for use by man to supplement the diet
- Supplements are not intended to treat, diagnose, prevent, or cure diseases and cannot make claims to do so

The FDA defines "over the counter" as:

- Drugs that are safe and effective for use by the general public without seeking treatment by a health professional

The FDA review of all available OTC drugs is completed by the Center for Drug Evaluation's Office of Drug Evaluation IV. OTC medications are developed under the OTC Monograph Process or through the New Drug Application (NDA) Process. Any company or sponsor seeking to market or produce their product as OTC applies to the Division of Nonprescription Drug Products (DNDP) in the Office of Drug Evaluation IV. The DNDP reviews consumer studies and postmarketing safety data as well as original efficacy data, drug development, labeling, and any regulatory issues. The DNDP is also responsible for the development of OTC drug monographs. Once a final monograph is implemented, companies can make and market an OTC produce without need for FDA preapproval if the produce conforms to the acceptable ingredients, doses, formulations, and labeling outlined in the monograph.[31]

With supplements, the FDA does not regulate them, nor do they require going through any type of drug approval process. Any company or sponsor, prior to marketing a dietary supplement, is required to confirm that their product (whether manufactured or distributed) is safe, any claims made about the product are not false or misleading, and the product complies with the Federal Food, Drug, and Cosmetic Act and FDA regulations in all other respects.

The focus of this review will be limited to some of the available OTC products and dietary supplements that have proven benefit in lowering serum cholesterol levels. The amounts of cholesterol lowering may vary by product, dosage form, and dose utilized. The following products may be considered as an adjunct or, in some cases, a supplement to conventional pharmacotherapy. Before starting any of these products, it is recommended that patients have a discussion with their physician.[32]

As many patients read about and use OTC products and supplements, it is helpful for the provider to be familiar with these medications and their benefits and risks. Because they are not FDA approved, safety and efficacy may vary as well as consistency for any particular product preparation. Tables 7.4-7.7 provide information on the use of these products with respect to their ability to lower cholesterol. OTC medications differ from dietary supplements in terms of their FDA regulatory requirements.

Table 7.4. Nonprescription Products With Strong or Good Evidence[33]	
Strong Evidence	**Good Evidence**
Garlic	Arginine Betaine
Niacin	Chitosan
Omega-3 Fatty Acids (EPA/DHA)	Guggul
Psyllium	Phytoestrogens
Red Yeast Rice	Policosanol Ribose

Table 7.5.   Nonprescription Products With Unclear or Poor Evidence

Acacia	Goldenseal	Pyruvate
Alfalfa	Grape seed	Qi-gong
Amalaki	Grapefruit seed extract	Quercetin
Amaranth oil	Green Coffee/Tea	Red clover
American hellebore	Gymnema	Red yeast rice
Aortic acid	Hawthorn	Reishi
Arabinogalactan	Honey (manuka honey)	Resveratrol
Ashwagandha	Horny goat weed	Rhubarb
Astaxanthin	Hydroxymethylbutyrate (HMB)	Riboflavin
Astragalus	Inositol nicotinate	Safflower
Ayurveda	Kefir	Savory
Betaine	Krill oil	Scotch broom
Biotin	Kudzu	Sea buckthorn
Brewers' yeast	Lecithin	Selenium
Carrageenan	L-Carnitine	Sesame
Chondroitin	Lecithin	Shea butter
Chromium	Lecithin	Soy
Cinnamon	Lemongrass	Spirulina
CoEnzyme Q10	Lignans	Squill
Conjugated linoleic acid	Lutein	Sulfur
Copper	Lycopene	Sunflower
Corydalis	Melatonin	Taurine
Cordyceps	Milk thistle	Thiamine
Creatine	Monterey pine	Thymus extract
Danshen	Mustard oil	Tocotrienols
DHEA	NAC (N-acetyl cysteine)	Tribulus
Docosahexaenoic acid	Nopal	Turmeric
Dong quai	Onion	Vitamin B_6, B_{12}, C, D, E, K
Elderberry	Oregano	Whey protein
Fenugreek	Palm oil	White horehound
Flaxseed	Pantothenic acid	Wild yam
Gamma-aminobutyric acid:	Peony	Yucca
Gamma-oryzanol	Phosphatidylcholine	Zinc
Ginger	Polydextrose	
Ginkgo	Pomegranate	
Ginseng	Probiotics	
	Pycnogenol	

Table 7.6.	Nonprescription Products With Negative Evidence
Negative Evidence	
Acacia	Evening primrose oil
Acidophilus	Glucosamine
Arginine	Sunflower oil
Beta-carotene	

Adapted from the Natural Medicines Monograph. http://www.naturalmedicines.com. 2016: Natural Medicines.

II. Products

A. **Arginine** Arginine can be found naturally in wheat germ and certain nuts as well as being biochemically synthesized. This product has been shown useful for weight loss and subsequent lipid lowering.

1. **Evidence** A study of 90 obese patients with BMI values >29.9 were randomized to receive either L-arginine 3 or 6 g 3 times a day or placebo for 8 weeks. Statistically significant weight loss in addition to decrease in blood pressure, LDL, and triglycerides as well as an increase in HDL were noted in the intervention group. There were no notable adverse reactions.[35] In a study of younger individuals, 27 patients with baseline LDL levels 238 ± 43 mg/dL were given a 4-week trial of L-arginine (7 g 3 times daily or placebo 3/day) or placebo powder. In this study, lipid levels were unchanged after L-arginine or placebo, but measures of endothelium dependent dilation were improved.[36]

2. **Safety** Arginine is generally regarded as safe in lower doses.

B. **Garlic**

1. Garlic is chemically known as *Allium sativum* and found in the common garlic plant. Garlic has been often been associated with blood pressure herbal treatment but has also been studied for cardiovascular disease benefits specifically in terms of cholesterol reduction.

2. **Mechanism** The proposed mechanism of action for cholesterol reduction includes enzyme inhibition involved in lipid synthesis, increase in antioxidant properties within the body, decrease in platelet aggregation, and prevention of lipid peroxidation of LDL and erythrocytes.

3. **Evidence** In 2010, the U.S. Department of Health and Human Services released a report stating garlic produced short-term (~3 months), small reductions in both LDL and total cholesterol. A study published in 2007 in the Archives of Internal Medicine

Table 7.7.	Psyllium and Viscous Soluble Fibers[34]			
Product	**Metamucil Powder**	**Citrucel Powder**	**Benefiber Powder**	**Fibersure**
Active ingredient	Psyllium husk	Methylcellulose	Wheat dextrin	Inulin
Natural	Natural	Semisynthetic		Natural
Lowers cholesterol	Yes	Minimal	No	No
Product	**Metamucil Capsules**	**Citrucel Caplets**	**Fibercon Caplets**	**Fiberchoice**
Active ingredient	Psyllium husk	Methylcellulose	Calcium polcarbophyl	Inlyl
Natural	Natural	Semi-synthetic	Synthetic	Natural
Lowers cholesterol	Yes	Minimal	No	No

completed a parallel design study of 192 patients with LDL levels ranging from 130 to 190 mg/dL to receive four of the possible treatment groups: raw garlic, powdered garlic supplement, aged garlic extract supplement, or placebo. They concluded that none of the garlic supplements had any significant effects on LDL, as well as HDL, total cholesterol, and triglycerides after 6 months.

There is also concern regarding the bioavailability, potency of active ingredient, and variety of dosage forms of garlic. Based on the lack of any significant evidence, it appears that garlic has little to no effect on cholesterol levels and should not be recommended for use.[37-41]

C. Guggul

1. Guggul is scientifically known as *Commiphora wightii* and comes from the Indian bdellium tree bark. The extract of the gum has been used in nontraditional medicine for centuries.

2. Evidence
   a. In one study, a specific Italian product that contains plant extracts of several naturally occurring substances—*Curcuma longa*, silymarin, guggul, chlorogenic acid, and inulin—was given to 78 patients with metabolic syndrome at a dose of 2 pills per day for 4 months. Fasting glucose dropped from the average of 117 mg/dL to 115 mg/dL, $P = .014$, and total cholesterol from 186 to 174 mg/dL, $P = .03$. No other significant changes were noted, and no adverse reactions were described.[42] In a small Norwegian general practice study, 43 women and men, age 27-70, with elevated cholesterol were given a guggul product four capsules daily or placebo for 12 weeks. The study noted drops in total cholesterol and HDL-C with no change in LDL and triglycerides between the active and placebo group. Gastrointestinal discomfort was noted in several of the patients. Guggul supplementation did not achieve the desired effects in human patients in this trial.[43]
   b. A recent review of guggul suggested that while promising results in other trials have been shown, more studies are needed.[44] At this time, it is not recommended for treatment of dyslipidemia.

III. Niacin Nonprescription Formulations

A. Over-the-counter preparations of niacin are available; however, the efficacy and safety are unclear. Preparations that are felt to be effective include immediate-release niacin and some sustained-release formulations. Inositol nicotinate (sold as "no-flush") niacin is slowly converted to free nicotinic acid, but blood levels of free niacin are 20-200 times lower than the commercial niacin products and thus not reaching clinically effective hypolipidemic blood levels. Niacinamide is made in vivo from niacin but due to differences in chemical structure has no lipid-lowering effects.

B. As indications for use of prescription formulations of niacin are lessening, there would appear to be few reasons to use a nonprescription product.

IV. Omega-3 Fatty Acids Nonprescription Formulations

A. Omega-3 fatty acids, known as "fish oil," have been extensively studied for its activity of triglyceride reduction.[45] Omega-3 fatty acids are largely composed of EPA and DHA.

B. There are several prescription products that are FDA approved with standardized composition as well as multiple OTC supplements that may vary in composition, purity, and quality. The capsules are generally large and require four capsules for prescription formulations and often more for OTC preparations. For triglyceride lowering, advise patients who take an OTC preparation to either look on the product label for EPA/DHA content or ask the pharmacist to assist. They should take enough capsules to equal approximately 2000 mg EPA + 2000 mg DHA daily.

C. Krill oil supplements contain omega-3 fatty acid as well, but studies supporting their use are lacking.[45]

V.   Psyllium and Other Viscous Soluble Fibers

A. Psyllium is a soluble fiber used primarily as a gentle bulk-forming laxative in products and to increase gastric emptying time and lower cholesterol. Psyllium comes from a shrublike herb called Plantago ovata that grows worldwide but is most common in India. The Plantago plant can produce up to 15 000 tiny, gel-coated seeds, from which psyllium husk is derived.

  1. Psyllium has been used to treat constipation, diarrhea, irritable bowel syndrome, hemorrhoids, and other intestinal problems. The soluble fiber in psyllium and similar fibers have long been a recognized therapy in cholesterol-lowering regimens.[46–48]

  2. There are a multitude of commercial fiber products on the market, and the consumer is often confused as to their use and clinical benefit. The National Fiber Council periodically updates its information on common commercially available fiber supplements in both power and solid dosage forms (Table 7.7). Given the differences in cholesterol lowering between various commercial products, the consumer should read package labels and carefully consult the literature and evidence-based recommendations before consuming a fiber product for cholesterol lowering.

B. Mechanism When psyllium husk comes in contact with water, it swells and forms a gelatinlike mass that helps transport waste including cholesterol esters through the intestinal tract and removal through defecation.

C. Evidence

  1. In a 250-patient study, subjects were given either 5.1 g psyllium husk twice daily or a placebo for 26 weeks. There were small changes in total cholesterol (–2.1% vs +2.6%), LDL cholesterol (–2.9% vs + 3.9%), and triglycerides (+3.2% vs +2.8%) in the psyllium group when compared to placebo.[49]

  2. A commercial hydroxypropyl methylcellulose fiber product was compared to placebo cohort of 165 individuals with primary hypercholesterolemia. The product was given as a bar or a drink in three different concentrations (3, 5, or 10 g). Patients were tested for a total of 6 weeks and demonstrated LDL-C reductions ranging from 6.1% to 13.3% in all but one individual patient grouping. Adverse events, mostly gastrointestinal, were similar in both drug and placebo groups.[49]

  3. These and other data suggest a small effect in most patients who use viscous soluble fiber as part of their daily diet. It should be considered a part of the heart-healthy diet, along with other modalities in patients with hypercholesterolemia not brought to goal with lifestyle modification.

VI.   Phytoestrogens

A. A number of nonprescription phytoestrogen products are available. These are largely soy-isoflavone sources and often contain bean extract, black cohosh, and dong quai, the latter being used to relieve menopausal symptoms. Side effects of these products are often gastrointestinal upsets, but other reactions may occur.

Phytoestrogens are a diverse group of naturally occurring nonsteroidal plant compounds that are structural similar to estradiol and have the ability to cause estrogenic and/or antiestrogenic effects, by sitting in and blocking receptor sites against estrogen. Phytoestrogens exert their effects primarily through binding to estrogen receptors.

B. Evidence

1. A study randomized 50 obese postmenopausal women to receive four isoflavone capsules or placebo for 6 months. The isoflavone capsule contained 17.5 mg of isoflavones extracted from natural soy with the total dose 70 mg/d (the isoflavone composition was 44 mg of daidzein, 16 mg of glycitein, and 10 mg of genistein). Both groups participated in a 3-times-weekly exercise program in the second 6 months of the program. This study was unable to demonstrate any significant change in plasma lipids; however, the sample size was small.[50]

2. In another trial, 120 postmenopausal women were randomized to receive pure genistein 54 mg or placebo daily for 12 months. The patients all had metabolic syndrome. All patients followed a Mediterranean diet and received the pure supplement or placebo. In this trial, total cholesterol decreased from 187 to 160 mg/dL, LDL dropped from 108.8 to 78.7 mg/dL, the triglyceride change was from 159 to 129 mg/dL, and HDL increased from 46.4 to 56.8 mg/dL. Systolic and diastolic blood pressures were also reduced in genistein recipients.[51]

3. Given the modest effect of isoflavones on the lipid profile, it is difficult to make a strong recommendation for consumption.

VII. Policosanol

A. Policosanols are long chain alcohols originally extracted from sugarcane, but more recently from beeswax, cereal grains, grasses, leaves, fruits, nuts, and other seeds. They have been sold commercially as a dietary adjunct to lower cholesterol. Early studies showed some promise when these products were added as a part of the healthy heart diet or in conjunction with various hypolipidemic agents.[52,53] Recent reviews have questioned their role in cholesterol lowering.[37]

B. **Evidence** In a small trial, 36 patients taking chronic statin therapy were randomized to receive a modified policosanol product or placebo. A third arm took an open-label policosanol supplement. While it was safe as a supplement, there were no noted changes in plasma lipids.[54]

1. Based on all recent evidence, there appears to be no role for policosanol supplementation in a cholesterol-lowering regimen.

VIII. Red Yeast Rice

A. Red yeast rice is the fermented rice product from the growth of the yeast, *Monascus purpureus*. An active product of the fermented rice is called monacolin and is a naturally produced form of the prescription medication lovastatin.

B. **Mechanism** Due to this chemical structure similarity to lovastatin, the proposed mechanism of action of red yeast rice is through inhibition of HMG CoA reductase and inhibition of cholesterol synthesis, as well as up-regulation of LDL receptors, and increased excretion of bile acids in the liver.

C. Evidence

1. In a study done by Becker et al., 62 patients were included with dyslipidemia and past history of statin-related myalgias. The patients were randomized to receive either 1800 mg twice daily of red yeast rice or placebo for a total of 24 weeks. The results produced a significant LDL-C reduction in patients taking red yeast rice at 12 weeks and 24 weeks of 42 mg/dL and 35 mg/dL, respectively. Triglycerides and HDL cholesterol had no significant changes between the groups. Additional studies have produced similar results in LDL-C reductions.

2. Results from some studies suggest that red yeast rice may be used as an effective supplement for lowering LDL-C in patients that have had history of statin-related myalgias or intolerance.[55–57]

D. Safety

1. There is concern about the safety of red yeast products available on the market currently. In an article that addressed current FDA oversight over red yeast rice products, the authors recommended caution in use of red yeast rice products due to lack of FDA regulation over production. They found that a number of red yeast products had additional active ingredients such as CoQ10, fish oil, niacin, as well as citrinin, known to cause nephrotoxicity. Recommendations include caution and thorough investigation of additional active ingredients in red yeast rice supplements before use.

2. Given the lack of data with currently available red rice yeast products, they are not recommended as part of a cholesterol-lowering regimen.

IX. Plant Sterols and Stanols

Plant sterols and stanols have long been supported as a part of the heart-healthy diet. These products compete for cholesterol absorption in the gut as well as possibly compete with ATP-binding cassette proteins and shunt cholesterol back into the intestinal lumen for excretion. Evidence shows that addition of 2-3 g/day of sterols or stanols lowers LDL by 6%-13%.[41] The strength of the evidence supporting their use has given spreadlike products to be used in place of butter as part of dietary recommendations to lower cholesterol.

X. Summary: Nonprescription Formulations

Most practitioners of lipid management have some patients who take supplements or nonprescription preparations for their hypolipidemic actions. It is therefore important for practitioners to be familiar with these products in order to properly advise their patients.

Strong evidence to support these practices is lacking, and existing studies are often poorly designed and controlled. While agents generally are nontoxic, the safety of many products is unclear. Clinicians should discuss the risks and benefits of using nonprescription products with patients who express interest in using them as part of a lipid management plan.

References

1. Press Release. Physiology or Medicine 1985—Nobelprize.org. *Nobel Media AB 2014.* Web March 16, 2016.
2. Brown MS, Goldstein JL. A receptor-mediated pathway for cholesterol homeostasis. *Science.* 1986;232:34-47.
3. Stone NJ, Robinson J, Lichtenstein AH, et al. 2013 ACC/AHA guideline on the treatment of blood cholesterol to reduce atherosclerotic cardiovascular risk in adults: a report of the American College of Cardiology/American Heart Association Task Force on Practice Guidelines. *Circulation.* 2014;129(25 suppl 2):S1-S45.
4. Jacobson TA, Ito MK, Maki KC, et al. National Lipid Association recommendations for patient-centered management of dyslipidemia: Part 1—full report. *J Clin Lipidol.* 2015;9:129-169.

5. Marbach J, McKeon J, Ross J, Duffy D. Novel treatments for familial hypercholesterolemia: pharmacogenetics at work. *Pharmacotherapy*. September 2014;34(9):961-972.
6. Goldberg AC, Hopkins PN, Toth PP, et al. Familial hypercholesterolemia: screening, diagnosis and management of pediatric and adult patients: clinical guidance from the National Lipid Association Expert Panel on familial hypercholesterolemia. *J Clin Lipidol*. 2011;5(3):133-140.
7. Brown G, Albers JJ, Fisher LD, et al. Regression of coronary artery disease as a result of intensive lipid-lowering therapy in men with high levels of apolipoprotein B. *N Engl J Med*. 1990;323:1289-1298.
8. Cannon CP, Blazing MA, Giugliano RP; for the IMPROVE-IT Investigators. Ezetimibe added to statin therapy after acute coronary syndromes. *N Engl J Med*. 2015;372:2387-2397.
9. Lovaza Prescribing Information. GlaxoSmithKline, Triangle Park, NC.
10. Brown WV, Bays H, Harris W, Miller M. Using omega-3 fatty acids in the practice of clinical lipidology. *J Clin Lipidol*. 2011;5:424-433.
11. Bowe KS, Harris WS, Kris-Etherton PM. Omega-3 fatty acids and cardiovascular disease: are there benefits? *Curr Treat Options Cardiovasc Med*. 2016;18(11):69.
12. Endo A. A historical perspective on the discovery of statin. *Proc Jpn Acad Ser B Phys Biol Sci*. May 11, 2010;86(5):484-493.
13. The Lipid Research Clinics Coronary Primary Prevention Trial results. I. Reduction in incidence of coronary heart disease. *JAMA*. 1984;251:351-364.
14. AIM-High Trial. Safety profile of extended-release niacin in the AIM-HIGH Trial. *N Engl J Med*. 2014;371:288-290.
15. HPS-2 THRIVE Collaborative Group. Effects of extended-release niacin with laropiprant in high-risk patients. *N Engl J Med*. 2014;371:203-212.
16. Rubins HB, Collins D, Robbins SJ. The VA HDL Intervention Trial: clinical implications. *Eur Heart J*. July 2000;21(14):1113-1115.
17. The FIELD study investigators. Fenofibrate intervention and event lowering in diabetes (FIELD) trial. *Lancet*. 2005;366:1849-1861.
18. The ACCORD Study Group. Effects of combination lipid therapy in Type 2 diabetes mellitus. *N Engl J Med*. 2010;362:1563-1574.
19. Regeneron Pharmaceuticals, Tarrytown, NY.
20. Amgen, Thousand Oaks, CA.
21. Cohen J, Pertsemlidis A, Kotowski IK, Graham R, Garcia CK, Hobbs HH. Low LDL cholesterol in individuals of African descent resulting from frequent nonsense mutations in PCSK9. *Nat Genet*. 2005;37(2):161-165.
22. Cohen JC, Boerwinkle E, Mosley TH Jr, Hobbs HH. Sequence variations in PCSK9, low LDL, and protection against coronary heart disease. *N Engl J Med*. 2006;354:1264-1272.
23. Qian YW, Schmidt RJ, Zhang Y, et al. Secreted PCSK9 downregulates low density lipoprotein receptor through receptormediated endocytosis. *J Lipid Res*. 2007;48:1488-1498.
24. Genzyme Corporation. Kynamro (mipomersen sodium) injection. Prescribing Information. 2013; Cambridge, MA.
25. Yu RZ, Lemonidis KM, Graham MJ, et al. Cross-species comparison of in vivo PK/PD relationships for second-generation antisense oligonucleotides targeting apolipoprotein B-100. *Biochem Pharmacol*. 2009;77:910-919.
26. Aegerion Pharmaceuticals, Inc. Juxtapid (lomitapide) capsules. *Prescribing Information*. Cambridge, MA; 2013.
27. Wetterau JR, Lin MCM, Jamil H. Microsomal triglyceride transfer protein. *Biochim Biophys Acta*. 1997;1345:136-150.
28. Wetterau JR, Aggerbeck LP, Bouma ME, et al. Absence of microsomal triglyceride transfer protein in individuals with abetalipoproteinemia. *Science*. 1992;258:999-1001.
29. Di Leo E, Lancellotti S, Penacchioni JY, et al. Mutations in MTP gene in abeta- and hypobeta-lipoproteinemia. *Atherosclerosis*. 2005;180:311-318.
30. Consumer Healthcare Products Association. Statistics on OTC use. Available at: http://www.chpa.org/market-stats.aspx. Accessed on March 19, 2016.
31. FDA. OTC (nonprescription) drugs: development and regulation of OTC (nonprescription) drug products. Available at: http://www.fda.gov/Drugs/DevelopmentApprovalProcess/HowDrugsareDevelopedandApproved/ucm209647.htm. Accessed on March 19, 2016.
32. FDA. Are dietary supplements approved by the FDA? Available at: http://www.fda.gov/aboutfda/transparency/basics/ucm194344.htm. Accessed on March 19, 2016.
33. Adapted from the Natural Medicines Monograph. http://www.naturalmedicines.com. 2016 Natural Medicines.
34. http://www.nationalfibercouncil.org/supplement_chart.shtml. Accessed on March 16, 2016.
35. Dastabi A. Oral L-arginine administration improves anthropometric and biochemical indices associated with cardiovascular diseases in obese patients: a randomized, single blind placebo controlled clinical trial. *Res Cardiovasc Med*. December 29, 2015;5(1):e29419.
36. Clarkson P, Adams MR, Powe AJ, et al. Oral L-arginine improves endothelium-dependent dilation in hypercholesterolemic young adults. *J Clin Invest*. April 15, 1996;97(8):1989-1994.
37. Nijjar PS, Burke FM, Bloesch A, et al. Role of dietary supplements in lowering low-density lipoprotein cholesterol: a review. *J Clin Lipidol*. 2010;4:248-258.

38. Rahman K, Lowe GM. Garlic and cardiovascular disease: a critical review. *J Nutr.* 2006;136(3):736-740.
39. US Department of Health & Human Services, AHRQ. Garlic: effects on cardiovascular risks and disease, protective effects against cancer, and clinical adverse effects summary. Available at: http://archive.ahrq.gov/clinic/epcsums/garlicsum.htm. Accessed on March 19, 2016.
40. Gardner CD, Lawson LD, Block E, et al. Effect of raw garlic vs. commercial garlic supplements on plasma lipid concentrations in adults with moderate hypercholesterolemia. *Arch Intern Med.* 2007;167:346-353.
41. Nijjar PS, Burke FM, Bloesch A, Rader DJ. Role of dietary supplements in lowering low-density lipoprotein—a review. *J Clin Lipidol.* 2010;4:248-258.
42. Patti AM. Effect of a natural supplement containing curcuma longa, guggul, and chlorogenic acid in patients with metabolic syndrome. *Angiology.* October 2015;66(9):856-861.
43. Nohr LA, Rasmussen LB, Straand J. Resin from the mukul myrrh tree, guggul, can it be used for treating hypercholesterolemia? A randomized, controlled study. *Complement Ther Med.* January 2009;17(1):16-22.
44. Deng R. Therapeutic effects of guggul and its constituent guggulsterone: cardiovascular benefits. *Cardiovasc Drug Rev.* 2007;25(4):375-390.
45. Harris WS. N-3 fatty acids and serum lipoproteins: human studies. *Am J Clin Nutr.* 1997;65(5):1645-1654.
46. Anderson JW. Dietary fibre, complex carbohydrate and coronary artery disease. *Can J Cardiol.* 1995;11(suppl): 55G-62G.
47. Anderson JW, Zettwoch N, Feldman T, et al. Cholesterol-lowering effects of psyllium hydrophilic mucilloid for hypercholesterolemic men. *Arch Intern Med* 1988;148:292-296.
48. Sprecher DL, Harris BV, Goldberg AC, et al. Efficacy of psyllium in reducing serum cholesterol levels in hypercholesterolemic patients on high- or low-fat diets. *Ann Intern Med.* 1993;199:545-554.
49. Maki KC, Carson ML, Kerr Anderson WH, et al. Lipid-altering effects of different formulations of hydroxypropylmethylcellulose. *J Clin Lipidol.* 2009;3:159-166.
50. Aubertin-Leheudre M, Lord C, Khalil A, Dionne IJ. Effect of 6 months of exercise and isoflavone supplementation on clinical cardiovascular risk factors in obese postmenopausal women: a randomized, double-blind study. *Menopause.* 2007;4:624-629.
51. Squadrito F, Marini H, Bitto A, et al. Genistein in the metabolic syndrome: results of a randomized clinical trial. *Endocrinol Metab.* 2013;98:3366-3374.
52. Castano G, Fernandez L, Mas R, et al. Effects of addition of policosanol to omega-3 fatty acid therapy on the lipid profile of patients with type II hypercholesterolaemia. *Drugs R D.* 2005;6:207-219.
53. Castano G, Fernandez L, Mas R, Illnait J, Mesa M, Fernandez JC. Comparison of the effects of policosanol and atorvastatin on lipid profile and platelet aggregation in patients with dyslipidaemia and type 2 diabetes mellitus. *Clin Drug Investig.* 2003;23:639-650.
54. Backes JM, Gibson CA, Ruisinger JF, Moriarty PM. Modified-policosanol does not reduce plasma lipoproteins in hyperlipidemic patients when used alone or in combination with statin therapy. *Lipids.* 2011;46:923-929.
55. Heber D, Yip I, Ashley JM, Elashoff DA, Elashoff RM, Go VL. Cholesterol-lowering effects of a proprietary Chinese red-yeast-rice dietary supplement. *Am J Clin Nutr.* 1999;69(2):231-236.
56. Becker DJ, Gordon RY, Halbert SC, French B, Morris PB, Rader DJ. Red yeast rice for dyslipidemia in statin-intolerant patients: a randomized trial. *Ann Intern Med.* 2009;150(12):830-839.
57. Childress L, Gay A, Zargar A, Ito MK. Review of red yeast rice content and current Food and Drug Administration oversight. *J Clin Lipidol.* 2013;7:117-122.

Statins

Wayne S. Warren and Michelle L. Warren

> ### Key Points
>
> ■ Statin medications are one of the most well-studied and commonly used medications.
>
> ■ The most important aspect of statins is their ability to lower LDL-C.
>
> ■ Statins also have important "pleiotropic" effects, which may be important, in addition to lowering LDL-C.
>
> ■ While all statins are HMG-CoA–reductase inhibitors, there are pharmacokinetic differences among the various statins.
>
> ■ Statins, while considered to be relatively safe drugs, can have side effects and drug-drug interactions. Muscle symptoms are commonly reported; however, the true prevalence is unclear due to varying definition of muscle symptoms and presence of symptoms due to causes other than statins.

I.   Introduction

Inhibitors of the enzyme 3-hydroxy-3-methylglutaryl coenzyme A (HMG-CoA) reductase, commonly referred to as statins, have to be near the top of the list of most important pharmacologic advances of the second half of the 20th century. They are by far the most studied (>170 000 patients in clinical outcomes trials alone)[1] class of medications in history.

Beyond improving a wide range of lipid parameters, they have unequivocally been shown to reduce a variety of adverse cardiovascular outcomes and cardiovascular mortality as well. Trials have shown a linear correlation between percent lipid lowering and event reduction,[2] as well as a linear correlation between achieved LDL-C and event rates.[3] The low adverse event rates and overall safety shown explain the fact that they are among the most prescribed class of medications in the United States and world.

Since approval of the first statin, lovastatin (Mevacor, Merck) in 1987, six others have been approved and remain on the market today (Fig. 8.1). While varying in pharmacokinetics, pharmacodynamics, and lipid-lowering efficacy at approved doses, each of these agents owe much, if not all of their efficacy to a reduction in concentrations of circulating atherogenic lipoproteins. Differences between the various compounds and additional potential therapeutic effects will be outlined in the pages that follow.

II.   Mechanism

A. Lipid lowering/event reduction

1. Statins' best understood mechanism is as competitive inhibitors of HMG-CoA reductase. This enzyme catalyzes the rate-limiting step in cholesterol biosynthesis, the conversion of HMG-CoA to mevalonate.

2. Structurally, they all share a dihydroxy heptanoic acid group, which links to the binding site of the enzyme, HMG-CoA reductase (Fig. 8.1). The various agents have been grouped according to derivation [fungal (simvastatin, lovastatin, pravastatin) vs synthetic (fluvastatin, atorvastatin, rosuvastatin, and pitavastatin)] or solubility

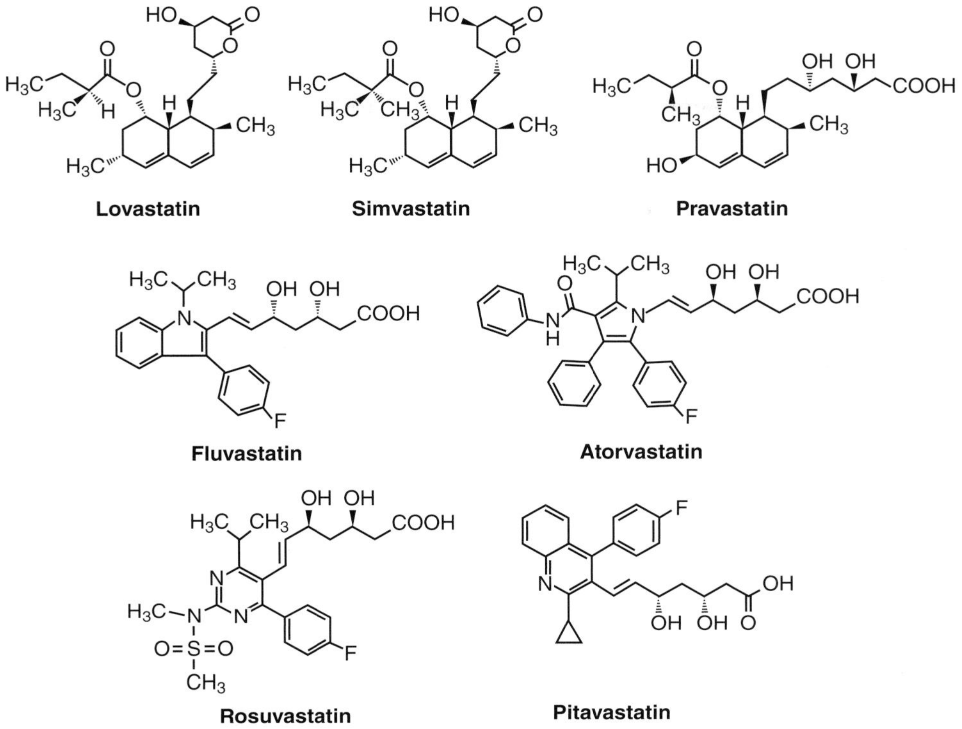

FIGURE 8.1: Statin structures.

[lipophilic (simvastatin and lovastatin being most lipid soluble, with fluvastatin, pitavastatin, and atorvastatin less so) vs hydrophilic (pravastatin and rosuvastatin)], but neither classification has yet been shown to be clinically relevant.

3. Reduced activity of the HMG-CoA–reductase enzyme leads to depletion of the hepatic cholesterol pool and subsequent upregulation of sterol regulatory element–binding proteins (SREBPs). SREBPs are nuclear transcription factors that lead to increased transcription/translation of LDL receptors. With more receptors on the surface of the hepatocyte, more circulating LDL and VLDL particles are bound via their apoB and apoE moieties and therefore taken up by the liver.[4] Somewhat unexpectedly (perhaps as a counterregulatory mechanism), statins also upregulate proprotein convertase subtilisin-kexin type 9 (PCSK9) expression by the liver and therefore increase its circulating level as well. Circulating PCSK9 attaches to the LDL/LDL receptor (LDLR) complex and, after its internalization by the hepatocyte, promotes degradation of LDLR, preventing its recycling back to the surface of the hepatocyte.

4. A final (nonreceptor-mediated) lipid effect of these medications is to reduce assembly and secretion of VLDL particles from the liver by reducing rates of apoB production.[5,6] This helps explain their efficacy in patients with heterozygous and homozygous familial hypercholesterolemia, who have limited or no functional LDL receptors.

5. While cholesterol is a necessary precursor of steroid hormones and bile acids, LDL reduction has not resulted in any specific negative systemic effects. Studies have shown steady levels of sex and adrenal gland hormones in spite of statin therapy.

B. Statin-associated muscle symptoms

1. The most frequently reported side effects of statins are muscle complaints. Muscle toxicity seen with these agents have been theorized to be related to reduction in ubiquinone (coenzyme Q10, CoQ10), which also has mevalonate as a precursor and is known to stabilize cell membranes and play a key role in the mitochondrial electron transport system. Several studies have reported reduced serum CoQ10 levels in statin-treated patients, and others have detected evidence consistent with mitochondrial dysfunction.[7]

2. Other theories of myotoxicity include the reduction of cholesterol synthesis in muscle cells leading to a lower cholesterol content in cell membranes and resulting instability, or reduced synthesis of farnesyl pyrophosphate and geranylgeranyl pyrophosphate resulting in apoptosis of muscle cells.[7]

III. Pleiotropic Effects

A. Statins owe the majority of their ability to decrease cardiovascular events and mortality to a reduction of atherogenic lipoproteins. Studies of LDL reduction by nonstatin agents and partial ileal bypass surgery lend further evidence to the essentially confirmed "LDL hypothesis," the concept that excess LDL is a major cause of the development and progression of atherosclerosis and that reducing LDL by any means will reduce the frequency of cardiovascular events.[8–10] In spite of this, numerous additional properties of statins, so-called pleiotropic effects, have been demonstrated. These include reducing synthesis of certain isoprenylated proteins, which control a variety of cellular functions, as well as anti-inflammatory and antithrombotic effects, and enhancement of the endothelium. Whether any of these effects contribute to the beneficial clinical outcomes remain a source of controversy.

B. Evidence Supporting Pleiotropic Effects: Survival and Coronary Events

1. Strong evidence supporting at least an indirect contribution of these pleiotropic effects to efficacy is the early separation of survival curves in several acute coronary syndrome (ACS) clinical trials. In the Myocardial Ischemia Reduction with Aggressive Cholesterol Lowering (MIRACL) trial, atorvastatin reduced recurrent ischemic events within 16 weeks.[11] In the Pravastatin or Atorvastatin Evaluation and Infection Therapy (PROVE-IT) study, separation of the Kaplan-Meier curves appeared to occur within 30 days and achieved statistical significance by 4 months.[12] This would be expected to take longer if attributed solely to lipid-lowering effects, and indeed, this is what occurred in most trials of patients with *stable* CAD.

2. In the West of Scotland Coronary Prevention (WOSCOP) Study of primary prevention, high-risk patients with similar on-treatment LDL-C levels had a 36% lower event rate if they were taking pravastatin, compared to placebo.[13] Similarly, in the Cholesterol and Recurrent Events (CARE) secondary prevention trial, pravastatin-treated patients had a significantly lower risk of events than their placebo-controlled counterparts with comparable lipid levels.[14]

3. Review of angiographic trials show event reduction which is more impressive than what would be expected from relatively modest changes in plaque burden/volume.[15,16] Statins reduce inflammation as evidenced by reductions in high sensitivity C-reactive protein, NF-KB, and cellular adhesion molecule (E-selectin and ICAM-1) expression.[17–19]

C. **Vascular and thrombotic benefits**

1. Statins have vasodilatory properties, enhancing production of endothelium-derived nitric oxide. Improvement in flow-mediated dilation has been observed as early as 3 hours, long before any effects are seen in plasma LDL-C.[20] Studies have shown a restoration of endothelial function in young smokers independent of changes in LDL.[21]

2. Lipid independent antioxidant effects have been demonstrated, among these being the inhibition of reactive oxygen species production[22] and reduction of angiotensin II–mediated free radical production in vascular smooth muscle cells.[23]

3. Antithrombotic effects such as increased thrombomodulin expression on the cell surface and reduced tissue factor expression occur via inhibition of the Rho/Rho kinase pathway.[24,25]

D. **Plaque stabilization** Additional potentially plaque-stabilizing features include inhibition of vascular smooth muscle proliferation,[26,27] reduced macrophage accumulation in plaque, and inhibition of matrix metalloproteinase (MMP) production by these macrophages,[28] thereby protecting the fibrous cap and preventing plaque rupture.

IV. Pharmacokinetics

A. **Pharmacokinetic profile** Table 8.1 outlines the pharmacokinetic profiles of currently available statins. A comprehensive review of statin drug-drug interactions is available in the National Lipid Association (NLA) Task Force on Statin Safety.[29] All statins are substrates for the organic anion transporting polypeptide (OATP1B1, encoded by the SLCO1B1 gene), which mediates hepatocyte uptake. Metabolism can then occur via various cytochrome P450 (CYP) enzymes and glucuronidation (via uridine glucuronosyl transferase, UGT). Efflux transporters such as breast cancer resistance protein (BCRP, also known as ABCG2) and P-glycoprotein (P-gp, also known as ABCB1) are involved in transport out of the hepatocyte and therefore biliary excretion.

B. **Statins in Asian populations** Numerous studies in Asian patients have shown LDL lowering similar to Westerners at significantly lower statin doses.[30–33] As for outcome studies, the Primary Prevention of Cardiovascular Disease with Pravastatin in Japan (MEGA) study reported a 33% event reduction with low-dose pravastatin in spite of a modest 18% (15% compared to control) LDL reduction.[34] On the other hand, some studies in Asians have shown additional benefits at even the highest dosing strengths of statins, with no significant increase in adverse events.[30,31,35] In HPS2-THRIVE, the incidence of myopathy in Chinese patients assigned to either treatment arm (niacin/laropiprant plus simvastatin or simvastatin alone) was increased compared to European patients.[36] Genetic variability in drug metabolism via CYP450, P-gp, and possibly OATP1B1 may all play a role. Statins are considered to be safe in the Asian population. However, using lower than usual doses of statins for initial therapy in Asian and Asian-American patients and then titrating upward is advisable.

C. **Prescribing information** Tables 8.2 and 8.3 compare data from the prescribing information of all available statins regarding altered pharmacokinetics in patients with hepatic and renal impairment, as well as LDL-C lowering across the dosing range. All statins are contraindicated in patients with acute liver disease or unexplained persistent elevations of hepatic aminotransferase levels. Notable clinically relevant factors specific to particular statins are highlighted below.

Table 8.1.   Pharmacokinetics of Statins

Variable	Lovastatin	Pravastatin	Simvastatin	Fluvastatin XL	Atorvastatin	Rosuvastatin	Pitavastatin
Lipophilicity (log D at pH 7.4)	a	(−0.75)-(−1.00)	1.50-1.75	1.00-1.25	1.00-1.25	(−0.25)-(0.50)	a
Tmax (time to peak plasma concentration)	2 h	1-1.5 h	4 h	3 h	1-2 h	3-5 h	1 h
Hepatic first-pass metabolism	High	High	High	High	High	Minimal	Minimal
Bioavailability	<5%	17%	<5%	29%	14%	20%	51%
Protein binding	>95%	50%	95%	98%	>98%	88%	99%
Major metabolic enzyme	CYP3A4	No significant metabolism by CYP450	CYP3A4	CYP2C9 CYP3A4 ~ 20% CYP2C8 ~ 5%	CYP3A4	CYP2C9-minimal	CYP2C9, CYP2C8 Both minimal
Renal excretion	10%	20%	13%	5%	<2%	10%	15%
T½	1.1-1.7 h	1.8 h	1.9 h	9 h	14 h	19 h	12 h

[a]Lipophilicity: Log D is the partition coefficient (water/n-octanol) for unionized drugs. The higher the number, the more lipophilic. Value for lovastatin is unknown, though it is felt to be similar to simvastatin. Value for pitavastatin also unknown, considered to be between atorvastatin and rosuvastatin.

(Data from Shitara Y, Sugiyama Y. Pharmacokinetic and pharmacodynamic alterations of 3-hydroxy-3-methylglutaryl coenzyme A (HMG-CoA) reductase inhibitors: Drug–drug interactions and interindividual differences in transporter and metabolic enzyme functions. Pharmacol Ther. 2006;112(1):71-105. doi:10.1016/j.pharmthera.2006.03.003; and package inserts.)

Table 8.2. Statins in Patients With Hepatic and/or Renal Impairment

Drug	Hepatic Impairment	Renal Impairment
Lovastatin	Unknown	CrCl 10-30 mL/min (severe): concentration = 2-fold greater
Pravastatin	The lowest starting dose should be used Cirrhosis (class not specified): Cmax = 1.34-fold greater AUC = 1.52-fold greater	Severe impairment: Cmax = 27% increase AUC = 69% increase Starting dose of 10 mg/d
Simvastatin	Unknown	Mild-moderate impairment = no adjustment necessary Severe impairment = start dosing at 5 mg/d and closely monitor
Fluvastatin XL	Cirrhosis: Cmax & AUC = 2.5-fold greater	Data unknown; however, systemic exposures are significantly lower with extended-release fluvastatin vs immediate release
Atorvastatin	Child Pugh A: Cmax & AUC = 4-fold greater Child Pugh B: Cmax = 16-fold greater AUC = 11-fold greater	No dose adjustment necessary
Rosuvastatin	Child Pugh A: Cmax = 60% greater AUC = 5% greater Child Pugh B: Cmax = 100% greater AUC = 21% greater	Severe impairment (CrCl < 30 mL/min): Concentration = ~3-fold greater Starting dose 5 mg/d (maximum 10 mg)
Pitavastatin	Child Pugh A: Cmax = 1.3 to 1-fold greater AUC = 1.6 to 1-fold greater Child Pugh B: Cmax = 2.7 to 1-fold greater AUC = 3.8 to 1-fold greater	CrCl 30-59 mL/min: Cmax = 60% greater AUC = 102% greater CrCl 15-29 mL/min: Cmax = 18% greater AUC = 36% greater Starting dose 1 mg (maximum 2 mg)

All statins are contraindicated in patients with acute or unexplained liver disease.
Data from package inserts.

Table 8.3. Comparison of LDL Cholesterol Reductions of Each Statin in Various Doses, per Prescribing Information

Statin	Dosage and LDL Reduction
Lovastatin	20 mg (−27%) 40 mg (−31%) 40 mg bid (−40%)
Pravastatin	40 mg (−34%) 80 mg (−37%)
Simvastatin	20 mg (−38%) 40 mg (−41%) 80 mg (−47%)
Fluvastatin XL	80 mg XL (−35%)
Atorvastatin	10 mg (−39%) 20 mg (−43%) 40 mg (−50%) 80 mg (−60%)
Rosuvastatin	5 mg (−45%) 10 mg (−52%) 20 mg (−55%) 40 mg (−63%)
Pitavastatin	1 mg (−32%) 2 mg (−36%) 4 mg (−43%)

V. Pharmacokinetics of Individual Statin Drugs

A. Lovastatin

1. **Half-life, bioavailability, and dosing** Lovastatin is a lipophilic statin with a half-life of about 1-2 hours. The short half-life might translate to increased effectiveness if taken in the evening near the time of peak cholesterol synthesis. Maximum bioavailability is demonstrated when immediate-release lovastatin (Mevacor) is administered with an evening meal[37]; in contrast, extended-release tablets exhibit better absorption when administered without food.[38] These differences are relatively minor and should not be major factors regarding timing of administration. High adherence rates to therapy are much more important for long-term efficacy. The dosing range for lovastatin is 10-80 mg/d, resulting in LDL reductions from 27% to 40%.

2. **Metabolism and interactions**
   a. Lovastatin is metabolized by CYP3A4; therefore, inhibitors or inducers of this enzyme system can result in meaningful drug interactions. Most notably, concurrent use of strong inhibitors of CYP3A4 such as macrolide antibiotics (excluding azithromycin), azole antifungals (excluding fluconazole), cyclosporine, HIV protease inhibitors, cobicistat-containing products, and nefazodone is contraindicated. Reduced elimination of lovastatin due to these interactions may result in an increased potential for toxicity.
   b. Grapefruit juice (but not orange juice) is also an inhibitor of CYP3A4 and should be avoided in large quantities. Up to 240 mL (about an 8 oz glass) per day would not be expected to result in clinically noticeable effects. This effect is dose-dependent and appears to have a limited duration of action. Separating a dose of lovastatin by at least 2 hours from grapefruit juice intake seems prudent. When lovastatin or simvastatin were administered in the evening, one glass of grapefruit juice in the morning had no clinically relevant effects.[46]
   c. Patients taking verapamil, diltiazem, dronedarone, or danazol should not exceed a dose of lovastatin of 20 mg/d. With amiodarone, the dose should not exceed 40 mg/d. Gemfibrozil, due to the OATP1B1 interactions and interference with glucuronidation by UGT, should be avoided. Care should be taken with other fibrates and niacin (≥1 g/d), which are known to increase the risk of myopathy on their own. Dose adjustments may be necessary when using lovastatin with colchicine and ranolazine.

3. **Renal dosing** In patients with severe renal impairment (CrCl < 30 mL/min), dosing >20 mg/d should be used cautiously.

B. Pravastatin

1. **Half-life, bioavailability, dosing** Pravastatin is a hydrophilic statin with a half-life of about 2 hours. The difference between taking pravastatin in the morning and the evening is small, and the recommendation about timing of administration discussed above for lovastatin also applies to pravastatin. Pravastatin may be administered with or without food. The dosing range for pravastatin is 10-80 mg/d. LDL reductions of 20%-37% have been shown.[39]

2. **Metabolism and interactions**
   a. Pravastatin is not metabolized by cytochrome P450 isoenzymes, which makes this drug a nice option for patients taking other medications of concern. Pravastatin is primarily metabolized via glucuronidation (UGT) in the liver and is a substrate of the transporters OATP1B1, P-gp, and BCRP.

b. In patients taking cyclosporine, a starting dose of 10 mg is appropriate. Doses of 20 mg/d should not be exceeded. If taken with clarithromycin, the pravastatin dose should not exceed 40 mg/d. Interactions with colchicine, fenofibrate, and niacin are possible. Gemfibrozil should be avoided. Pravastatin should be taken 1 hour before or 4 hours after the use of a bile acid sequestrant.

3. **Renal** Patients with severe renal impairment should use a starting dose of 10 mg/d.

C. Simvastatin

1. **Half-life, bioavailability, and dosing** Simvastatin is a lipophilic statin with a half-life of about 2 hours. Absorption is not affected by food. As with lovastatin and pravastatin, evening doses are ideal but not critical. The dosing range for simvastatin is 5-40 mg (80 mg is no longer recommended due to risk for interactions but may be continued for patients who have been stable on this dose for more than 1 year). This results in LDL reductions of 28%-47%.[40]

2. **Metabolism and interactions**
   a. Like lovastatin, simvastatin is metabolized by CYP3A4; therefore, they share the precautions regarding interactions with other drugs and grapefruit juice caused by inhibitors or inducers of this isoenzyme (see lovastatin).
   b. Additionally, patients taking verapamil, diltiazem, or dronedarone should not exceed a simvastatin dose of 10 mg/d. With amlodipine, amiodarone, and ranolazine, the simvastatin dose should not exceed 20 mg/d. Use of gemfibrozil and danazol is contraindicated. Close monitoring of INR is advised when simvastatin is coadministered with warfarin or if dosage adjustments are made. Digoxin concentrations may increase if taken with simvastatin and should be monitored. Niacin, fenofibrate, and colchicine should be coadministered cautiously.

3. **Renal** In patients with severe renal impairment, a starting dose of 5 mg/d is recommended.

D. Fluvastatin XL

1. **Half-life, bioavailability, and dosing** Fluvastatin is a medication that had been initially approved in a range of doses; however, an extended-release formulation provides improved efficacy and safety and will be the sole focus of this discussion. Fluvastatin XL is moderately lipophilic, possibly causing slower and less penetration into muscle cells.[47] It has a half-life of about 9 hours and can be taken at any time of the day with or without food. Fluvastatin XL 80 mg once daily has demonstrated LDL reductions of 35%.[41]

2. **Metabolism and interactions** Metabolism of fluvastatin XL takes place predominantly by CYP2C9 but also uses CYP3A4 and CYP2C8 to lesser degrees. Due to the CYP2C9 metabolic pathway (fluvastatin also competitively inhibits CYP2C9), phenytoin should be administered with caution and plasma phenytoin levels should be monitored when therapy is initiated or doses are adjusted. An increase in the concentrations of both drugs has been reported, especially in patients with particular CYP2C9 polymorphisms. Blood glucose levels should be monitored when fluvastatin is used in combination with glyburide. When taken with cyclosporine in the Assessment of Lescol in Renal Transplantation (ALERT) trial,[48] no increase in adverse effects were seen using the 40-mg dose. Recommendations for use with fluconazole, a CYP2C9 inhibitor, limit the dose of fluvastatin to 20 mg twice daily, so fluvastatin XL 80 mg should probably be avoided.

Fluvastatin was shown in an early study to not be affected by gemfibrozil,[49] though there are still warnings regarding concomitant use with fibrates in general, as well as niacin. In combination with warfarin, fluvastatin has increased prothrombin times. Therefore, when combined, prothrombin time/INR should be monitored closely.

3. **Renal** In patients with mild-moderate renal impairment, dosage adjustments are not necessary. While doses >40 mg/d have not been studied in patients with severe renal disease, the KDIGO (Kidney Disease: Improving Global Outcomes) group[50] considers fluvastatin XL 80 mg an acceptable dose based on the ALERT trial.[48]

E. Atorvastatin

1. **Half-life, bioavailability, and dosing** Atorvastatin is a lipophilic statin with a half-life of ~14 hours, permitting dosing at any time of the day. Food may mildly decrease the rate and extent of absorption, but efficacy is not significantly affected. The dosing range is 10-80 mg/d, resulting in typical LDL reductions of 39%-60%.[42]

2. **Metabolism and interactions** Atorvastatin is metabolized by CYP3A4, but to a lesser extent than lovastatin and simvastatin. As a result, the concomitant use with calcium channel blockers, amiodarone, dronedarone, and ranolazine is not restricted. However, in patients taking cyclosporine or the protease inhibitors tipranavir plus ritonavir or telaprevir, use of atorvastatin should be avoided. When coadministering atorvastatin with other protease inhibitors, it is advisable to use the lowest dose that will achieve the degree of LDL lowering desired. Warnings about coadministration of macrolide antibiotics, azole antifungals, and certain antidepressants previously noted with lovastatin and simvastatin also apply to atorvastatin. There is also a potential interaction with grapefruit juice (see lovastatin and simvastatin).

No clinically meaningful interactions with warfarin have been reported. Though studies are not available, gemfibrozil would be expected to increase Cmax of atorvastatin, and fenofibrate would certainly be considered a safer alternative. Digoxin, niacin, and colchicine in combination with atorvastatin may also result in adverse effects.

3. **Renal** Atorvastatin does not require dosing adjustment due to renal insufficiency.

F. Rosuvastatin

1. **Half-life, bioavailability, and dosing** Rosuvastatin is a hydrophilic statin that has the longest half-life of all statins at about 19 hours. It can be taken at any time of the day, with or without food. Patients taking antacids containing aluminum and magnesium hydroxide should be advised to take the antacid at least two hours after rosuvastatin. The dosing range of rosuvastatin is 5-40 mg/d, and it has the ability to reduce LDL by 45%-63%.[43]

2. **Metabolism and interactions** Metabolism takes place by CYP2C9, but hepatic metabolism is only a minor elimination pathway. This limits drug interactions caused by CYP isoenzyme inducers or inhibitors. Inhibitors of transporter proteins OATP1B1 and BCRP, such as cyclosporine and HIV protease inhibitors, have the potential to increase the risk of side effects and should be coadministered with caution. With cyclosporine, doses should be limited to 5 mg/d.

Patients combining rosuvastatin with gemfibrozil, lopinavir/ritonavir (Kaletra), or atazanavir and ritonavir should be started at doses of 5 mg/d and should not exceed 10 mg/d. Rosuvastatin can have a potentiating effect on coumarin-type anticoagulants and can prolong prothrombin time; therefore, careful monitoring is necessary with initiation or change in dose. As with other statins, the potential exists for interactions with fenofibrate, colchicine, and niacin.

3. **Renal** For patients with severe renal impairment (CrCl ≤ 30 mL/min) and not on hemodialysis, dosing should be started at 5 mg and should not exceed 10 mg.

G. Pitavastatin

1. **Half-life, bioavailability, and dosing** Pitavastatin, the newest of all statins, possesses a moderate lipophilicity placing it between atorvastatin and rosuvastatin when evaluating by water/*n*-octanol partition coefficients. Although it has a half-life of ~12 hours, LDL reduction is slightly greater following evening administration. Pitavastatin may be administered with or without meals. The dosing range is 1-4 mg/d yielding LDL reductions of 32%-43%.[44]

2. **Metabolism and interactions** Pitavastatin is marginally metabolized by CYP2C9 and even less by CYP2C8. Interactions as a result of effects on these isoenzymes are not significant.

   In patients taking cyclosporine, use of pitavastatin is contraindicated, likely due to OATP1B1 interactions. This is also a potential a problem with rifampicin, rifamycin SV, clarithromycin, and indinavir. While some references suggest avoiding pitavastatin in patients taking lopinavir/ritonavir, a study of 24 healthy adults found the pitavastatin/antiretroviral combination to be safe and well tolerated [REF][51]. Coadministration with gemfibrozil should be avoided. Standard warnings apply to concurrent administration with colchicine, fibrates, or high doses of niacin. Due to increased pitavastatin exposure when taken with erythromycin, the dose should not exceed 1 mg/d. Likewise, doses of 2 mg/d should not be exceeded with rifampin. No interactions have been seen with highly protein-bound drugs including warfarin.

3. **Renal** Patients with moderate or severe renal impairment (GFR = 15-59 mL/min) or end-stage renal disease on hemodialysis should start pitavastatin at doses of 1 mg/d and not exceed 2 mg/d.

VI. Statin Effects on Lipids

A. LDL

1. As stated in the introduction, there is a linear relationship between achieved LDL and event rates, supporting the concept of "lower is better." Statins, until the recent availability of PCSK9 inhibitors, were the most potent LDL-lowering medications available. This fact, combined with extensive data regarding their safety and outcomes, make them the treatment of choice when lifestyle changes alone have not resulted in sufficient risk reduction.

2. **Guidelines and recommendations** Numerous guidelines have been published by various professional societies over the last few years, most notably ACC/AHA (2013) and NLA (2014). The ACC/AHA focused on the use of fixed dose statins of various lipid-lowering intensities in four major patient benefit groups. This was the only approach evaluated in multiple RCTs, the only studies the writing group considered. Lipid targets and goals were eliminated. The NLA recommendations were patient-centered and used evidence from RCTs and subgroup analyses, observational studies, and genetic studies. Treatment targets and goals for LDL-C and non–HDL-C were maintained as they were felt to be important tools as part of a successful treatment strategy, and the use of additional agents (nonstatins) was endorsed when goals were not attained with maximally tolerated statin therapy. See Chapter 3 for a more detailed discussion of guidelines.

Table 8.4. STELLAR Trial				
Daily Statin Dose	**LDL Cholesterol**	**HDL Cholesterol**	**Triglycerides**	**Non-HDL Cholesterol**
Pravastatin 10 mg	−20%	3%	−8%	−19%
20 mg	−24%	4%	−8%	−22%
40 mg	−30%	6%	−13%	−27%
80 mg	N/A	N/A	N/A	N/A
Simvastatin 10 mg	−28%	5%	−12%	−26%
20 mg	−35%	6%	−18%	−33%
40 mg	−39%	5%	−15%	−35%
80 mg	−46%	7%	−18%	−42%
Atorvastatin 10 mg	−30%	6%	−20%	−34%
20 mg	−43%	5%	−23%	−40%
40 mg	−48%	4%	−27%	−45%
80 mg	−51%	2%	−28%	−48%
Rosuvastatin 10 mg	−46%	8%	−20%	−42%
20 mg	−52%	10%	−24%	−48%
40 mg	−55%	10%	−26%	−51%
80 mg	N/A	N/A	N/A	N/A

(Reprinted with permission from Jones PH, Davidson MH, Stein EA, et al. Comparison of the efficacy and safety of rosuvastatin versus atorvastatin, simvastatin, and pravastatin across doses (STELLAR Trial). *Am J Cardiol.* 2003;92:152-160.)

3. The Statin Therapy for Elevated Lipid Levels Compared Across Doses of Rosuvastatin (STELLAR) trial[52] was a randomized, open label trial comparing the effects of the four most commonly prescribed statins at a range of doses over a 6-week period. The results are given in Table 8.4. This shows the ability of statins to reduce LDL-C from 30% to 55% at commonly used doses, depending on the particular agent chosen. With various guidelines suggesting specific goal levels for LDL-C or, alternatively, reduction of ~50% from baseline in high-risk patients, many patients will require either atorvastatin or rosuvastatin at their two highest doses ("high-intensity statin therapy"). For a variety of reasons, treatment goals cannot be attained in all patients. Therefore, combination therapy with other lipid-lowering agents will be necessary for those with high "residual risk."

B. **Triglycerides** Statins have also been shown to lower triglycerides and, therefore, have beneficial effects on non-HDL cholesterol, as well as the atherogenic dyslipidemia seen in patients with metabolic syndrome and diabetes. As shown in STELLAR, triglycerides are typically decreased from 15% to 28%. While the percent lowering is less than that seen for LDL-C, the effects are similar in that higher doses or more potent statins yield the greatest triglyceride reduction. As with other triglyceride-lowering agents (omega-3 fish oil and fibrates), the percent reductions are greater with higher baseline triglyceride levels.

C. **HDL** Statins can also increase HDL-C-C by up to 10%, but that effect is inconsistent and HDL-C is not currently a target of therapy.

D. Residual risk

1. Residual risk refers to remaining atherogenic dyslipidemia after goals for LDL-C are met. For most clinical purposes, LDL-C is calculated (using the Friedewald Calculation). This represents the cholesterol content of the LDL particle; however, numerous trials have shown that measures of apolipoprotein B (ApoB) or LDL particle number (LDL-P) are better measures of total atherosclerotic particle burden and risk for CVD.[53,54] There is one ApoB on every VLDL, IDL, LDL, and Lp(a).

2. ApoB and LDL-P can be measured but calculation of non–HDL-C (total cholesterol – HDL-C) is an approximation of ApoB and LDL-P and can be derived from the basic lipid panel without additional cost above a standard lipid profile, and with no requirement for the patient to be fasting.

3. Statins, by upregulating LDL receptors and reducing assembly and secretion of VLDL particles, lower levels of all atherogenic lipoproteins. Therefore, particle numbers for both LDL and VLDL, as well as their cholesterol and triglyceride contents, are all reduced. While all LDL particles are considered atherogenic, statins seem to preferentially reduce the number of small dense LDL particles, a theoretical advantage as these may be more harmful than their number alone suggests. The 2013 ACC/AHA guidelines do not recommend specific targets of therapy beyond LDL-C; however, NLA guidelines support using treatment goals for both LDL-C and non–HDL-C.

VII. Clinical Outcome Trials

A. As mentioned in the introduction, statins have been evaluated in more than 170 000 patients participating in clinical outcome trials over the last 25 years.[1] Most of the early trials were placebo controlled, but since 2005, a number of large studies compared specific statins/doses of varying "intensities." Taken as a whole, they provide incontrovertible evidence that statins reduce all cardiovascular events which are a consequence of atherosclerosis, as well as coronary heart disease death and total mortality. A summary of these trials is shown in Tables 8.5 and 8.6.[13,14,34,44,55–77]

B. **Event reduction** Event reduction has been linear and consistent with observed epidemiologic studies that estimate a 1% event reduction for every 1% decrease in LDL. The linear relationship between on-treatment LDL-C and coronary heart disease events is seen in both primary prevention (patients with risk factors but no known vascular disease) and secondary prevention (patients with pre-existing vascular disease).[3] Since the risk is substantially greater in the secondary prevention patients, the number needed to treat (NNT) to prevent one cardiovascular event is obviously much smaller. This effect is seen in both men and women, even in those patients more than 80 years old.[61]

C. **Effectiveness** Statin effectiveness spans a wide range of pretreatment LDL levels. Since most studies recruited patients based on their overall cardiovascular risk and not a specific LDL level at baseline, many guidelines recommend assessing an individual patient's absolute risk to guide therapy. It is worth noting that in each of the trials comparing different intensities of statins, the higher-intensity regimen resulted in a statistically significant benefit[12,73–76] compared to the lower intensity. As achieved LDL becomes lower, the benefits of further lowering with more intense regimens do seem to be attenuated. The issue of treatment goals for LDL-C and non–HDL-C is addressed in Chapter 3.

Table 8.5.   Placebo-Control Trials

Trial Name	Number of Patients	Patient Characteristics	Treatment	Median Follow-up (y)	Baseline LDL (mg/dL)	LDL Change	Composite End Point
SSSS	4444	Adults with angina or prior MI	Simvastatin 20-40 mg vs placebo	5.4	190.32	−35%	−34%
WOSCOPS	6595	Men with no CHD (HTN 15%, smoker 44%, DM 1%)	Pravastatin 40 mg vs placebo	4.8	193.44	−26%	−31%
CARE	4159	Adults with prior MI	Pravastatin 40 mg vs placebo	5.0	139.62	−32%	−24%
Post-CABG	1351	Adults 21-74 y old bypass 1-11 y previous	Lovastatin 40-80 mg vs lovastatin 2.5-5 mg	4.3	156.78	−24.5%	−18% (NS)
AFCAPS/TexCAPS	6605	Adults with no CHD, HDL cholesterol <35 mg/dL in men, <40 mg/dL in women (HTN 22%, smokers 13%)	Lovastatin 20-40 mg vs placebo	5.2	151.71	−25%	−40%
LIPID	9014	Adults with history of prior MI or UA (smokers 10%, DM 9%, HTN 42%, obese 18%)	Pravastatin 40 mg vs placebo	6.0	151.32	−25%	−24%
GISSI-P	4271	Acute MI patients (≤6 mo) with total blood cholesterol ≥200 mg/dL	Pravastatin 20 mg vs no treatment	2.0	152.88	−16%	−10% (NS)
LIPS	1677	Adults post PCI (MI history 44%, smokers 25%, DM 14%, PAD 6%)	Fluvastatin 80 mg vs placebo	3.9	133.38	−27%	−31% ($P = .07$)
HPS	20 536	Adults with CHD, arterial disease, or diabetes (HTN 41%, no CHD 35%)	Simvastatin 40 mg vs placebo	5.4	131.82	−32%	−27%
PROSPER	5804	Adults age 70-82 (smokers 26%, DM 11%, PAD 7%, CHD 13%, TIA 11%, vascular disease 44%)	Pravastatin 40 mg vs placebo	3.3	147.81	−27%	−19%
ALLHAT-LLT	10 355	Adults (smokers 23%, DM 35%, HTN 100%, CHD 14%)	Pravastatin 40 mg vs usual care	4.9	146.64	−17%	−9% (NS)
ASCOT-LLA	10 305	Adults with HTN + ≥3 RF (DM 25%, smokers 32%, CVA/TIA 10%, PAD 5%)	Atorvastatin 10 mg vs placebo	3.3	134.16	−35%	−36%
ALERT	2102	Renal transplant patients (smokers 19%, DM 19%, HTN 76%)	Fluvastatin 40 mg vs placebo	5.5	161.46	−32%	−35%
CARDS	2838	Adults with DM + 1 RF, no CVD (smokers 23%, HTN 84%, obese 37%)	Atorvastatin 10 mg vs placebo	4.1	118.17	−31%	−35%
ALLIANCE	2442	Adults with known CHD	Atorvastatin 10-80 mg vs usual care	4.7	148.2	−11%	−17%
4D	1255	Adults with diabetes on hemodialysis	Atorvastatin 20 mg vs placebo	4.0	126.75	−18%	−8% (NS)
ASPEN	2410	Type II DM age 40-75	Atorvastatin 10 mg vs placebo	4.0	114.27	−29%	−10%
MEGA	8214	Age 40-70 no CHD or stroke	Pravastatin 10-20 mg vs usual care	5.0	157.95	−15%	−33%
JUPITER	17 802	Healthy adults, LDL < 130, hsCRP ≥ 2.0	Rosuvastatin 20 mg vs placebo	2.0	105.3	−50%	44%
GISSI-HF	4574	Adults with NYHA class II-IV CHD	Rosuvastatin 10 mg vs placebo	4.2	119.34	−27%	+1% (NS)
AURORA	2773	Adults 50-80 y old on hemodialysis	Rosuvastatin 10 mg vs placebo	4.6	100.62	−31%	−4% (NS)

Data from Refs. [1,13,14,34,44,53–70]

Table 8.6.	Active-Control Trials						
Trial Name	Number of Patients	Patient Characteristics	Treatment	Median Follow-up (y)	Baseline LDL (mg/dL)	LDL Change	Composite End Point
PROVE-IT	4162	Adults with ACS	Atorvastatin 80 mg vs pravastatin 40 mg	2.1	102.18	−35%	−16%
A to Z	4497	Adults with ACS	Simvastatin 40 mg then simvastatin 80 mg vs placebo then simvastatin 20 mg	2.0	81.51	−18%	−11%
TNT	10 001	Adults with stable CHD	Atorvastatin 80 mg vs atorvastatin 10 mg	5.0	98.28	−24%	−22%
IDEAL	8888	Adults with stable CHD	Atorvastatin 40-80 mg vs simvastatin 20-40 mg	4.8	102.96	−22%	−16%
SEARCH	12 064	History of MI in patients age 15-80	Simvastatin 80 mg vs simvastatin 20 mg	7.0	97.5	−14%	−6%

Data from Refs.[1,12,71–74]

VIII. Statin Treatment for Special Populations

A. Diabetes

1. Patients with diabetes are at high risk for coronary heart disease and often have an abnormal lipid profile including low HDL and elevated triglycerides, yet a "normal" or only mildly elevated LDL.

2. **Evidence** Subgroup analysis of numerous studies and perhaps most notably the Collaborative Atorvastatin Diabetes Study (CARDS), which was a trial specifically looking at diabetics without a previous history of cardiovascular disease, have all shown marked benefits of statins in patients with diabetes. In CARDS, a 37% relative risk reduction for cardiovascular events was seen after a median follow-up of 3.9 years, resulting in termination of the study 2 years earlier than anticipated. Risk reduction was also shown for elderly patients[78] and even for patients with pretreatment LDLs as low as 100.

3. **Management** The 2013 ACC/AHA Guidelines advise treatment with statins for diabetics (type 1 or 2) aged 40-75 years with an LDL 70-189 regardless of other risk factors. Treatment should be with a moderate-intensity statin unless 10-year ASCVD risk is ≥7.5%, in which case a high-intensity statin should be used.[79] The NLA Recommendations risk assessment algorithm places diabetes as a "very high-risk" feature with the most stringent LDL-C goal.

B. Pediatrics

1. Detailed information on diagnosis and management of dyslipidemia in the pediatric population is covered in Chapter 14. Current recommendations are for universal lipid assessment of children between the ages of 9 and 11 (consider earlier if family history is unknown), and if normal, repeat every 5 years thereafter.[80] Screening at age 2 is advised if either parent has familial hypercholesterolemia (FH) or a history of premature coronary heart disease. An LDL > 160 indicates possible FH, and appropriate diagnostic criteria should be applied to more formally evaluate. Cascade screening (testing all first-degree relatives) of a child with FH should be carried out.

Table 8.7.	Use of HMG-CoA–Reductase Inhibitors in Children and Adolescents	
Medication	**Age Approved**	**Dosing**
Lovastatin	Age 10-17 years old	10-40 mg/d
Pravastatin	Age 8-18 years old	20-40 mg/d
Simvastatin	Age 10-17 years old	10-40 mg/d
Fluvastatin (XL)	Age 10-16 years old	20-80 mg/d
Atorvastatin	Age 10-17 years old	10-20 mg/d
Rosuvastatin	Age 10-17 years old	5-20 mg/d
Pitavastatin[a]	Age 6-17 years old*	1-4 mg/d

[a]Not FDA approved in pediatric patients. Safety and dosing based on results of the PASCAL study in children 6-17 years old.
(Data from Braamskamp MJ, Stefanutti C, Langslet G, et al. Efficacy and safety of pitavastatin in children and adolescents at high future cardiovascular risk. *J Pediatr*. 2015;167:338-343.)

2. **Management**
   a. Lifestyle changes should always be the initial intervention, as they are in adults. If LDL remains ≥190 or non–HDL-C ≥ 220 mg/dL, patient should be referred to a pediatric lipid specialist for treatment. Treatment for boys, but not until the onset of menses in girls, has not shown any interference with growth or sexual maturation.[81]
   b. All currently marketed statins except pitavastatin are FDA approved for pediatric patients with heterozygous FH. Pitavastatin has been studied in children and adolescents and was also found to be safe and efficacious.[82] Table 8.7 summarizes pediatric indications and dosing guidelines for these medications.[83] Statin-treated children with high LDL-C have been shown to have a reduction in carotid intima-medial thickness, a marker of atherosclerosis, compared to placebo.[84]

3. **Evidence** A Cochrane meta-analysis of 1074 children in eight randomized controlled trials showed a 32% decrease in LDL with low-intensity statin treatment.[85] Follow-up of the Dutch pediatric pravastatin trial (214 patients) revealed only 1.5% discontinuing the medication due to side effects. Eighty-two percent remained on therapy over the 10 years of follow-up, and there were no serious adverse events reported.[86] See Chapter 14 for a more detailed discussion of pediatric lipid management.

C. **Hepatic dysfunction** Evidence regarding the use of statins in patients with various forms of chronic liver disease is summarized in 2014 update by the National Lipid Association (NLA) Statin Liver Safety Task Force.[87] Specific clinical issues are related to the individual disease states.

1. **Nonalcoholic fatty liver disease**
   a. Nonalcoholic fatty liver disease (NAFLD) is the most common cause of chronic liver disease in Western nations.[88] Patients with NAFLD include a subset at risk for progressive disease, those with nonalcoholic steatohepatitis (NASH). Patients with NAFLD commonly have insulin resistance with resulting hyperglycemia and atherogenic dyslipidemia, characterized by increased serum triglycerides, low HDL-C, and the presence of small, dense LDL particles. In fact, one view of pathogenesis identifies lipotoxicity as the primary driver of cellular injury and death in NASH.[89] There is also increased production of many proinflammatory markers such as uric acid, C-reactive protein, IL-6, and TNF-alpha.[90] As such, these patients are at increased risk of cardiovascular disease. Studies confirm that patients with NAFLD are more prone to early carotid atherosclerosis and

advanced high-risk coronary plaque, independent of additional cardiovascular risk factors.[90] Coronary artery disease is the most common cause of death in these patients.[92,93]

b. Statins and NAFLD

There is concern that patients with liver disease may be at increased risk for hepatotoxicity from statins. A 2010 survey of 937 primary care physicians revealed that only 50% would prescribe statins if baseline ALT values were 1.5 times the upper limit of normal.[94] A second study found that patients with NAFLD were less likely to receive appropriate statin treatment than those without NAFLD or those with undetected NAFLD and that many previously on a statin had their dose reduced or stopped when the diagnosis was made. A great deal of data is available to discredit these attitudes.

c. Evidence

Pravastatin 80 mg/d was studied prospectively in hypercholesterolemic patients with chronic liver disease and found to be safe and well tolerated.[95] ALT elevations occurred more frequently in the placebo group. A retrospective study of 71 patients with NAFLD revealed 15.4% of patients taking statins developed an increase in ALT, and in each case, the effect was transient, ALT returning to baseline without discontinuation of treatment.[96] Numerous small studies have shown improvement in aminotransferase levels with statin treatment.[97–100] These studies have included patients taking pitavastatin, atorvastatin, rosuvastatin, and simvastatin.

d. Efficacy

As for effects on cardiovascular events in these patients, posthoc analysis of the Greek Atorvastatin and Coronary Heart Disease Evaluation (GREACE),[101] Assessing the Treatment Effect in Metabolic Syndrome Without Perceptible Diabetes (ATTEMPT),[102] and IDEAL[103] trials, all looking at patients with abnormal LFTs (presumably due to NAFLD), suggests significant CV outcome benefits from statins. In GREACE and IDEAL, these benefits were significantly greater in the patients who had abnormal aminotransferases than those who did not.

e. Statin benefits for liver disease

As for the use of statins for treatment of the liver disease itself, data are extremely limited. Animal studies have reported a prevention of progression of hepatic inflammation and fibrosis, through anti-inflammatory, antiapoptotic, and antioxidant effects.[104,105] As noted above, studies in humans have shown reduction in aminotransferase levels. Several small trials have used ultrasound or computed tomography (CT) to evaluate statin effects on liver steatosis, and others have studied liver histology.[106] Most showed reduction in steatosis with inconsistent effects on inflammation. Fibrosis was not reduced in any studies except for a preliminary report using rosuvastatin in six patients.[107]

f. Conclusion

Statins are safe and effective treatment for hyperlipidemia and to reduce cardiovascular events in patients with NAFLD. Hepatotoxicity from these agents is not increased compared to those with normal liver enzyme levels[108] and serious liver injury is exceedingly rare. Obviously, reports of jaundice, constitutional symptoms, or worsening of liver enzymes or clotting studies in statin-treated patients should be promptly evaluated. Current guidelines do not recommend the use of statins to treat the liver disease seen in NAFLD. Any changes in this recommendation will require prospective randomized control trials of appropriate size and duration.[109]

2. **Primary biliary cholangitis**
   a. Primary biliary cholangitis, formerly known as primary biliary cirrhosis (PBC), is an autoimmune disease characterized by inflammation of small- and medium-sized bile ducts, resulting in chronic cholestasis. It primarily affects middle-aged women, and 75%-95% of patients have hypercholesterolemia. Though most PBC patients are not at increased cardiovascular risk, there appears to be a subgroup of patients who have specific disorders of lipid metabolism and who are at increased risk.[110,111]
   b. Evidence
   A review of 58 patients with PBC on statins, treated for a mean duration of 41 months (range 3-125 months), found no increase of ALT levels and no complaints of muscle pain or weakness.[112] This is consistent with two prospective trials, a 48-week study of 19 patients with atorvastatin[113] and a 12-month study of 21 patients with simvastatin.[110] Several small studies suggested benefits on biochemical markers and progression of cholestasis,[114–116] but this was not confirmed by a longer study with atorvastatin.[113]

3. **Other liver disease** Finally, statins are felt to be safe in patients with chronic stable autoimmune hepatitis[87] as well as viral hepatitis B and C.[117,118] In a well-matched cohort study, 166 patients with hepatitis C who received statin treatment had an improvement in median liver enzyme levels from baseline compared with those did not receive a statin. In the same study, statin therapy did not increase the risk of hepatotoxicity in hepatitis C patients compared to hepatitis C−negative individuals.[119] In a study from the Electronically Retrieved Cohort of HCV Infected Veterans (ERCHIVES) database, atorvastatin and fluvastatin were associated with a significant dose-dependent reduction in the development of cirrhosis and incidence of hepatocellular carcinoma.[120]

D. Chronic kidney disease

1. Chronic kidney disease (CKD) is associated with an increased risk of cardiovascular disease,[121] with death from cardiovascular disease being much more common than progression to dialysis. This may be explained by both traditional and uremia-related risk factors. Plasma lipid and lipoprotein profiles are changed in quantitative, but above all in qualitative, structural, and functional ways.[122] The Kidney Disease: Improving Global Outcomes (KDIGO) organization, whose founding sponsor is the National Kidney Foundation, released guidelines in late 2013,[50,123] which included 13 recommendations regarding lipid management in CKD. Detailed discussion on the management of dyslipidemia in patients with chronic kidney disease is covered in Chapter 15.

2. **Evidence**
   a. In the Study of Heart and Renal Protection (SHARP) trial, 9270 patients with CKD but without pre-existing cardiovascular disease were randomly assigned to receive simvastatin 20 mg plus ezetimibe 10 mg daily or placebo. The active treatment group experienced a 17% reduction in major atherosclerotic events after median of 4.9 years, despite adherence rates of only about two-thirds.[121] Suggested by this trial is greater benefit in patients with early CKD, where events and overall cardiovascular deaths are mostly due to conventional atherosclerotic disease. Unfortunately, the active treatment provided no benefit regarding decline in renal function.
   b. In the prospective Pravastatin Pooling Project, an analysis of three randomized trials, 22.8% of 19 700 patients had moderate CKD, defined as a GFR of

30-59.99 mL/min per 1.73 m².[124] These patients had the same benefits on the primary end point, a 23% relative risk reduction in cardiovascular events, as the patients with normal renal function. In a posthoc analysis of the Scandinavian Simvastatin Survival Study (4S) trial (secondary prevention), simvastatin patients with an eGFR of <75 mL/min had a 31% relative risk reduction of all-cause mortality and lower rates of major coronary events.

3. **Dialysis** It is worth noting that in the subgroup of patients in SHARP who entered the study already on dialysis, there was a minor trend toward benefit, but this result did not reach statistical significance. Previous trials of statin use in dialysis patients failed to show benefit as well. For the 1255 patients in the German Diabetes and Dialysis (4D) study, no cardiovascular event or mortality reduction was seen from atorvastatin 20 mg/d despite a median 42% reduction in LDL.[68] In the Study to Evaluate the Use of Rosuvastatin in Subjects on Regular Hemodialysis: An Assessment of Survival and Cardiovascular Events (AURORA) of 2776 patients, use of rosuvastatin 10 mg/d did not have any effect on cardiovascular events or mortality, in spite of a similar 43% LDL reduction.[72]

4. **Transplant** For patients who have undergone a kidney transplant, statin treatment is generally recommended. The Assessment of Lescol in Renal Transplantation (ALERT) trial studied 2102 renal transplant recipients. While the use of fluvastatin (Lescol) 40-80 mg/d, reduced the end point of coronary death or nonfatal MI by 17%, this was not statistically significant.[48] However, there was a significant 35% relative risk reduction in the risk of cardiac death or nonfatal MI in an unblinded extension study. Benefits seen in ALERT were felt by KDIGO to be consistent with those seen in the general population, though the strength of the recommendation for use of statins in these patients was graded as weak due to limited data.

5. **Summary** To summarize, the safety of statins in CKD has been shown, with the incidence of cancer, muscle pain, increased creatinine kinase or aminotransferases, hepatitis, and gallstones similar in both groups.

    KDIGO recommends using statins to treat most CKD patients with eGFR <60 mL/min per 1.73 m². Specific lipid goals are not supported by existing evidence. While patients on dialysis should not be treated for this indication alone, they should undergo the same cardiovascular risk assessment as patients in the general population. Statins should be continued in patients who are receiving them at the time of dialysis initiation. Kidney transplant recipients are very likely to benefit from statin treatment as well. Detailed information on managing renal patients with dyslipidemia is discussed in Chapter 15.

E. HIV

1. HIV has become a chronic disease and patients have an increased risk of CVD at all ages compared to the general population, even after controlling for other risk factors.[125] This is due to the virus itself, side effects of some antiretroviral medications, and the fact that patients are now living to an age where CVD is more prevalent. As such, diagnosis and management of dyslipidemia have become an important part of care for these patients.

2. **Antiretroviral therapy** Protease inhibitors can cause increases in triglycerides and LDL-C, decreases in HDL-C, and accumulation of ApoB and ApoCIII. They can also contribute to central obesity, lipoatrophy, and insulin resistance. With newer medications available, protease inhibitors are being used less. Nucleoside reverse transcriptase inhibitors are also associated with high triglycerides and lipoatrophy.

3. **Statin use in patients infected with HIV** Statins are safe and effective in HIV-infected patients; however, lovastatin and simvastatin should be avoided due to extensive CYP3A4 interactions with ART medications.[126] The choice among other statins should be determined by possible interactions with the patient's current ART regimen and the statin intensity needed. Several thorough references are available to assist in navigating HIV therapy/statin interactions[127,128] as well as a systemic review of statin treatment in HIV infection.[129] Management of dyslipidemia in patients living with HIV is discussed in Chapter 15.

IX. Safety/Adverse Events

Safety and side effects of lipid medications are covered in detail in Chapter 12. We briefly present those safety and side effects specific to statins here.

A. Pregnancy and breastfeeding

All statins are currently pregnancy category X and should not be used in women who are pregnant or those who are of child-bearing age who are not using a reliable form of contraception. Given the potential for passage of statins into human milk and possible risk to infants, statins are not recommended for use in nursing mothers. Further discussion on this topic can be found in Chapter 15.

B. Liver concerns

1. **Hepatic enzymes** Isolated abnormalities of hepatic enzymes are commonly seen in the care of patients undergoing routine chemistry panel testing. However, elevations of aminotransferases to more than 3 times the upper limit of normal (ULN) are rare with statin therapy, occurring in <1% of patients receiving intermediate doses of any statin, and perhaps twice as often when the maximum dose of any statin is used.[130] This is true across the dosing spectrum for any given statin and not related to the degree of LDL reduction. These elevations are often transient, with 70% of cases resolving spontaneously by the time of follow-up testing.[131]

2. **Severe liver toxicity** The incidence of severe liver toxicity or liver failure in patients taking statins is no different from the rate of liver failure in the general population *not* taking a statin, about one case per million people.[132] Whether such an occurrence is statin related or not, it is exceptionally rare and likely idiosyncratic in nature. In spite of the steady increase in the use of statins since the late 1990s, there has not been a detectable increase in rates of severe liver injury causally associated with statin use. No data exist to show that periodic monitoring would be effective in identifying this rare occurrence at an early stage.

3. **Monitoring of liver enzymes** In 2012, the FDA concluded that routine periodic monitoring of liver enzymes in patients taking statins is not warranted. Statin labels now recommend these tests be performed before starting statin therapy and as clinically indicated thereafter. Patients taking statins should be routinely monitored for symptoms of hepatic dysfunction including malaise, fatigue, weakness, anorexia, and dark-colored urine, as well as physical findings of jaundice or hepatomegaly. Laboratory abnormalities of increased direct bilirubin or prothrombin time and decreased albumin are considered more accurate assessments of "liver function" than isolated elevations of ALT and/or AST.

4. **Management of elevated liver tests** If aminotransferase levels are greater than 3 times upper limit of normal (ULN) on repeat or if direct bilirubin is elevated (and

CK is normal, ruling out a muscle etiology), statin treatment should be withheld until a formal evaluation is done.[87] If a diagnosis of NAFLD seems likely in an asymptomatic patient after this evaluation, statin therapy may be restarted (with possible dose reduction) if aminotransferases are stable. If aminotransferases are less than 3 times ULN and direct bilirubin and CK are normal, there is no need to discontinue the statin, and doing so is likely to subject the patient to an unnecessarily high risk of cardiovascular events.

C. Muscle issues

1. Muscle complaints are now almost synonymous with the term "statin intolerance" due to the rarity of any other reported adverse events with these agents.

2. **Terminology**
   a. The terminology used to describe statin-associated muscle symptoms (SAMS) has been inconsistent over the past 30 years, causing much confusion. The definitions of SAMS are outlined in Chapter 11.
   b. Terms have also been defined by the NLA Statin Muscle Safety Task Force.[133] Myalgia describes unexplained discomfort with normal CK level: aches, stiffness, tenderness, or exercise associated cramping. Myopathy refers to muscle weakness but is not necessarily associated with elevated CK. Myositis denotes inflammation confirmed by biopsy or imaging. Myonecrosis refers to different grades of muscle damage with CK elevations, the most severe of which is clinical rhabdomyolysis.

3. Muscle soreness (myalgia) is by far the most common SAM, occurring in ~10%-25% of patients in clinical practice.[134,135]
   a. Incidence
   The incidence of myalgia in clinical trials has generally been much less, at least partially due to frequent prerandomization run-in periods to assess compliance and tolerability, with resulting exclusion of patients with muscle complaints. In most clinical trials, rates of muscle soreness in statin-treated patients are quite similar to those taking placebo, and in some studies, the placebo group had a higher rate.[62,66,136]
   b. Evidence
   In two retrospective studies, most statin-intolerant patients tolerated statins when rechallenged. In one, 92.2% of 2721 patients remained on treatment for 12 months when rechallenged.[137] In another, 72.5% of patients intolerant to at least two statins remained on treatment for at least 6 months.[138] In a recent prospective study of patients intolerant to at least two statins, patients who were symptom-free after 4 weeks of *placebo* were randomized to alirocumab, ezetimibe, or atorvastatin 20 mg/d. 6.9% of screened patients had muscle-related symptoms on placebo and were excluded. While 46% of patients (previously statin intolerant) taking atorvastatin reported a skeletal muscle-related adverse event, only 22.2% had discontinued treatment at 24 weeks, similar to the alirocumab- and ezetimibe-treated patients. Overall, the muscle-related adverse events were less in the alirocumab group.[139]
   c. Factors associated with SAMS
   Studies are fairly consistent in showing an increased incidence of muscle complaints in those who are the most physically active,[134,140,141] and exercise-induced increases of CK have been shown to be higher in statin-treated patients.[142] Other factors associated with more frequent myalgia include female gender, low body

mass index, excess alcohol intake, and, of course, the concomitant use of inter-acting medications[143,144] (as well as polypharmacy in general). In the Prediction of Muscular Risk in Observational conditions study (PRIMO), starting a new medication was identified as a trigger by 30% of individuals who had muscular symptoms. Certain polymorphisms of the SLCO1B gene that encodes the OATP1B1 have been associated with statin intolerance.[145]

d. Serious events

While statins can certainly cause SAMS, serious events are rare. A systemic review looked at data from trials as well as case reports and reports to regulatory authorities.[131] This included 21 trials and 180 000 patient years on statin therapy. Myopathy attributable to statins occurred at a rate of 11 per 100 000 patient years. In cohorts of 355 000 patients taking lipid-lowering medication (excluding the no-longer available cerivastatin), rhabdomyolysis was estimated at 3 per 100 000 patient years and unlikely to exceed 7 per 100 000 patient years.

e. In summary, the frequently reported myalgias often have nonstatin etiologies and may be influenced by patient expectations of negative effects.[138] The majority of patients, when rechallenged with a statin, are able to continue treatment. Single patient (N-of-1) trials have been advocated to evaluate individuals for true statin intolerance.[146]

f. Management of statin intolerance due to SAMS

Management of statin intolerance is summarized here and discussed in detail in Chapter 11. As a first step, it is important to stop the statin and see if symptoms resolve. If they do, a retrial of statin (different statin or the same one at a lower dose) is recommended to see if symptoms reoccur. Also, rule out other possible causes of SAMS. Avoiding interacting medications is a necessary step (see Section IV). If symptoms develop during treatment, checking a CK level and TSH is appropriate.

i. Coenzyme Q10

Supplementation with coenzyme Q10 has produced conflicting results in clinical trials.[147–149] However, some patients report benefit with doses of 100-200 mg daily.

ii. Vitamin D

Two cross-sectional studies and several case reports have linked vitamin D deficiency with statin-associated myalgia.[150–153] All of these studies were unblinded, but overall, the results suggest that vitamin D deficiency contributes to statin-induced myalgias and that supplementation is useful in many of these patients. No data exists regarding the use of vitamin D in nondeficient patients with myalgia.

iii. Fluvastatin and Pitavastatin

Much has been written about fluvastatin XL. Given its very slow release from the gastrointestinal tract, there is a greatly increased first-pass uptake, avoiding hepatic saturation and resulting in markedly reduced drug concentrations in the peripheral circulation and therefore low systemic exposure.[154,155] Many studies, some prospective, indicate that fluvastatin XL is less likely to cause muscle effects than other statins[134,156] and is well-tolerated in a majority of patients unable to remain on other statins.[154] Whether this is due to its previously described high first-pass extraction with minimal plasma concentrations, high protein binding, lack of the need of either CYP3A4 or UGT (glucuronidation) for metabolism (and therefore minimal drug interactions) is unknown. Pitavastatin, the newest statin, may also result in fewer SAMS than other similar potency statins.

iv. Switching to a low dose of a statin with a long half-life, typically rosuvastatin, and using it less frequently than usual (anywhere from alternate day to as rarely as once a week) is another option. Doses of rosuvastatin (5-20 mg) were tolerated in 72.5% of previously statin-intolerant patients when used on alternate days (35% LDL reduction).[157] 80% of patients tolerated twice weekly (26% LDL reduction),[158] and 75% of patients once weekly administration of rosuvastatin (23%-29% LDL reduction).[159,160]

v. Finally, alternate statin therapy has been successfully reintroduced even after an episode of rhabdomyolysis.[161]

D. New-onset diabetes

1. Over the last few years, attention has been given to the potential diabetogenic effect of statins. The JUPITER trial showed a small but statistically significant increase in the rate of type 2 diabetes with rosuvastatin. A closer analysis of this trial found that in patients with at least one of four major risk factors for developing diabetes (metabolic syndrome, impaired fasting glucose, BMI > 30 kg/m^2, or hemoglobin A1c >6%), incident diabetes increased by 28%.[162] In patients without any of these risk factors, there was no increase. It should be noted that all patients in the study had high sensitivity C-reactive protein levels of 2.0 mg/L or higher, itself an independent predictor for development of diabetes.[163]

2. **Evidence** Several meta-analyses have also addressed this question. When trials including 91 140 patients without diabetes at baseline were analyzed, a 9% increase for incident diabetes was noted with statin therapy.[164] There was no apparent difference between the various statins. It was calculated that treatment of 255 patients with statins for 4 years resulted in one extra case of diabetes. Another analysis compared the risk of new-onset diabetes in moderate- vs high-intensity statin therapy in 32 752 patients without diabetes at baseline.[165] This suggested a 12% increase of diabetes in the high-intensity group over a mean follow-up of 4.9 years.

3. **Biologic mechanisms** Several reasons for this mild but real increased risk of diabetes have been proposed but remain unproven.[166] Studies assessing the effects of statins on insulin sensitivity have been inconsistent. Data regarding effects on beta cell function, gluconeogenesis, incretin response, and renal tubular absorption of glucose are all lacking.[167] Differences in metabolic effects of various statins have been evaluated[168,169] with no firm conclusions.

4. Prospective head-to-head trials comparing all statins have not been done. One prospective trial found a significant 7.2% increase in fasting blood glucose with atorvastatin vs a nonsignificant 2.1% increase with pitavastatin.[170] Posthoc analysis found the difference between the two treatments to be statistically significant (P = .0054).

5. **Benefits far outweigh risks** Many patients taking statins who do not already have diabetes are at significantly increased risk for developing diabetes. The added risk from statins is low and dwarfed by the cardiovascular event reduction seen in patients across the spectrum from abnormal glucose tolerance to overt diabetes. Sources estimate prevention of 2.5 events per case of diabetes in primary prevention[162] and more than 5.4 events per diabetes case in secondary prevention.[164] High-intensity statin therapy resulted in two additional cases of diabetes and 6.5 fewer cardiovascular events per 1000 patient years compared to a moderate-intensity regimen.[165] Most patients who develop diabetes will do so regardless of statin therapy, and prevention through lifestyle changes is much preferred than avoidance of a medication with a proven track record of benefit.

E. Cognitive function

1. Numerous case reports and one randomized trial have suggested memory loss or cognitive impairment associated with statin use and reversed on discontinuation of therapy. Patients were generally over the age of 50 and time to onset varied from 1 day to years. Observational studies show cognitive benefit more often than decline.[171] In February 2012, the U.S. Food and Drug Administration (FDA) modified the warning section for all statins, noting these reports. The FDA stated that these changes were uncommon and did not lead to clinically significant cognitive decline.[172]

2. **Evidence from randomized clinical trials** There are two large randomized controlled trials to offer some insight, as this question was a prespecified secondary end point. The Patient-Centered Research into Outcomes Stroke Patients Prefer and Effectiveness Research (PROSPER) study of 5804 elderly patients assessed cognitive function at six different time points during the study.[173] Mean follow-up was 42 months. There was cognitive decline observed in all subjects, but no difference in any of the cognitive domains was found in pravastatin-treated patients compared to placebo. In the Heart Protection Study (HPS) using simvastatin, cognitive function was assessed by a questionnaire during a telephone interview at the end of the study.[174] After a mean follow-up of 5.3 years, no differences were seen between the simvastatin and placebo groups.

3. **Evidence from Observational Studies** Some observational studies are particularly reassuring. In one, elderly patients with normal cognition or mild cognitive impairment at baseline were followed annually. Statin users had significantly better cognition, and those with normal cognition at baseline had significantly slower decline compared with nonusers.[175] A long-term study of 4095 patients showed similar results of various cognitive measures between statin users and nonusers.[176]

4. Two recent reviews of this subject came to the same conclusion: that there is no evidence of detrimental effects of statins on cognitive function.[177] One of these, however, went on to point out that this does not exclude the possibility that for an individual patient, a rare side effect may occur, as is the case for any type of medication.[171]

F. Very Low LDL

1. A final concern among certain clinicians is the patient with a very low LDL-C on statin therapy.

2. Evidence

   a. Separate analyses of patients in the TNT, PROVE-IT, and JUPITER studies have been done. In the secondary prevention TNT trial, there was a highly significant reduction in the rate of major cardiovascular events with descending achieved on-treatment LDL-C, and no clinically important difference in adverse events across quintiles (the lowest being those with achieved LDL-C < 64 mg/dL), including a group of 98 patients with LDL-C < 40 mg/dL.[178]

   b. In PROVE-IT, patients with LDL-C of 40-60 mg/dL and those <40 mg/dL again had no worsening of any safety parameters.[179] Posthoc analysis from JUPITER found no increases in myalgias or myopathy, neuropsychiatric conditions, cancer, or diabetes in the rosuvastatin-treated patients with an LDL-C < 50 mg/dL.[180] In 767 patients (~9.4%) on rosuvastatin who achieved LDL-C < 30 mg/dL, increases in diabetes, hematuria, hepatobiliary disorders, and insomnia were noted when compared to the patients not achieving LDL-C < 30 mg/dL.[181] The absolute incidence rates of these events were low, however, ranging from ~1 to 3 cases per 100 person years of observation. A meta-analysis of statin trials supported the results of these previously mentioned studies.[182] A small (nonsignificant) increase in hemorrhagic stroke was outweighed by a much lower risk for other cerebrovascular events, yielding the lowest risk of overall major cerebrovascular events in the patients with the lowest achieved LDL-C.

X.   Summary

Cardiovascular disease is the leading cause of morbidity and mortality for both men and women in the United States. It accounted for nearly 787 000 deaths in 2011, nearly half of these from coronary heart disease alone. Despite a vast number of prospective clinical trials showing consistent cardiovascular event and mortality reduction, there are still inadequate numbers of appropriate patients receiving standard of care lipid-lowering therapy.[183] The cornerstone of this therapy, after suitable lifestyle changes, is the use of statins. Their long track record of safety while resulting in benefits across a wide range of patient populations justifies their place as the most prescribed class of medications in the United States. However, adherence to this potentially lifesaving therapy is low.[184] It is hoped that better understanding of the data will motivate both physicians and patients to initiate and continue this therapy in the appropriate target groups.

References

1. Cholesterol Treatment Trialists' (CTT) Collaboration. Efficacy and safety of more intensive lowering of LDL cholesterol: a meta-analysis of data from 170,000 participants in 26 randomised trials. *Lancet*. 2010;376:1670-1681.
2. Robinson JG, Smith B, Maheshwari N, et al. Pleiotropic effects of statins: benefit beyond cholesterol reduction? *J Am Coll Cardiol*. 2005;46:1855-1862.
3. Expert Dyslipidemia Panel of the International Artherosclerosis Society Panel members. An International Atherosclerosis Society Position Paper: global recommendations for the management of dyslipidemia-Full report. *J Clin Lipidol*. 2014;8:29-60.
4. Brown MS, Goldstein JL. A receptor-mediated pathway for cholesterol homeostasis. *Science*. 1986;232:34-47.
5. Ginsberg HN, Le NA, Short MP, Ramakrishnan R, Desnick RJ. Suppression of apolipoprotein B production during treatment of cholesteryl ester storage disease with lovastatin: implications for regulation of apolipoprotein B synthesis. *J Clin Invest*. 1987;80:1692-1697.
6. Arad Y, Ramakrishnan R, Ginsberg HN. Lovastatin therapy reduces low-density lipoprotein apoB levels in subjects with combined hyperlipidemia by reducing the production of apoB-containing lipoproteins: implications for the pathophysiology of apoB production. *J Lipid Res*. 1990;31:567-582.
7. Shitara Y, Sugiyama Y. Pharmacokinetic and pharmacodynamic alterations of 3-hydroxy-3-methylglutryl coenzyme A (HMG-CoA) reductase inhibitor: drug-drug interactions and interindividual differences in transporter and metabolic enzyme functions. *Pharmacol Ther*. 2006;112:71-105.
8. Buchwald H, Varco RL, Matts JP, et al. Effect of partial ileal bypass surgery on mortality and morbidity from coronary heart disease in patients with hypercholesterolemia. Report of the Program on the Surgical Control of the Hyperlipidemias (POSCH). *N Engl J Med*. 1990;323:946-955.
9. Lipid Research Clinics Program. The Lipid Research Clinics Coronary Primary Prevention Trial results. II. The relationship of reduction in incidence of coronary heart disease to cholesterol lowering. *JAMA*. 1984;251:365-374.
10. Cannon CP, Blazing MA, Giugliano RP, et al. Ezetimibe added to statin therapy after acute coronary syndromes. *N Engl J Med*. 2015;372:2387-2397.
11. Schwartz GG, Olsson AG, Ezekowitz MD, et al. Effects of atorvastatin on early recurrent ischemic events in acute coronary syndromes: the MIRACL study: a randomized controlled trial. *JAMA*. 2001;285:1711-1718.
12. Ray KK, Cannon CP. Early time to benefit with intensive statin treatment: could it be the pleiotropic effects? *Am J Cardiol*. 2005;96(suppl):54F-60F.
13. Packard CJ. Influence of pravastatin and plasma lipids on clinical events in the West of Scotland Coronary Prevention Study (WOSCOPS). *Circulation*. 1998;97:440-443.
14. Sacks FM, Pfeffer MA, Moye LA, et al. The effect of pravastatin on coronary events after myocardial infarction in patients with average cholesterol levels. Cholesterol and Recurrent Events Trial investigators. *N Engl J Med*. 1996;335:1001-1009.
15. Brown BG, Zhao XQ, Sacco DE, Albers JJ. Lipid lowering and plaque regression: new insights into prevention of plaque disruption and clinical events in coronary disease. *Circulation*. 1993;87:1781-1791.

16. Brown BG, Hillger L, Zhao XQ, Poulin D, Albers JJ. Types of change in coronary stenosis severity and their relative importance in overall progression and regression of coronary disease: observations from the FATS Trial: Familial Atherosclerosis Treatment Study. *Ann N Y Acad Sci*. 1995;748:407-418.
17. Bustos C, Hernandez-Presa MA, Ortego M, et al. HMG-CoA reductase inhibition by atorvastatin reduces neointimal inflammation in a rabbit model of atherosclerosis. *J Am Coll Cardiol*. 1998;32:2057-2064.
18. Musial J, Undas A, Gajewski P, Jankowski M, Sydor W, Szceklik A. Anti-inflammatory effects of simvastatin in subjects with hypercholesterolemia. *Int J Cardiol*. 2001;77:247-253.
19. Ridker PM, Rifai N, Pfeffer MA, Sacks F, Braunwald E. Long-term effects of pravastatin on plasma concentration of C-reactive protein: the Cholesterol and recurrent Events (CARE) Investigators. *Circulation*. 1999;100;230-235.
20. Ray KK, Cannon CP. The potential relevance of the multiple lipid-independent (pleiotropic) effects of statins in the management of acute coronary syndromes. *J Am Coll Cardiol*. 2005;46:1425-1433.
21. Beckman JA, Liao JK, Hurley S, et al. Atorvastatin restores endothelial function in normocholesterolemic smokers independent of changes in low-density lipoprotein. *Circ Res*. 2004;95:217-223.
22. Rikitake Y, Kawashima S, Takeshita S, et al. Anti-oxidative properties of fluvastatin, an HMG-CoA reductase inhibitor, contribute to prevention of atherosclerosis in cholesterol-fed rabbits. *Atherosclerosis*. 2001;154:87-96.
23. Wassmann S, Laufs U, Baumer AT, et al. HMG-CoA reductase inhibitors improve endothelial dysfunction in normocholesterolemic hypertension via reduced production of reactive oxygen species. *Hypertension*. 2001;37:1450-1457.
24. Masamura K, Oida K, Kanehara H, et al. Pitavastatin-induced thrombomodulin expression by endothelial cells acts via inhibition of small G proteins of the Rho family. *Arterioscler Thromb Vasc Biol*. 2003;23:512-517.
25. Eto M, Kozai T, Cosentino F, et al. Statin prevents tissue factor expression in human endothelial cells: role of Rho/Rho-kinase and Akt pathways. *Circulation*. 2002;105:1756-1759.
26. Huhle G, Abletshauser C, Mayer N, Weidinger G, Harenberg J, Heene DL. Reduction of platelet activity markers in type II hypercholesterolemic patients by a HMG-CoA-reductase inhibitor. *Thromb Res*. 1999;95: 229-234.
27. Schror K. Platelet reactivity and arachidonic acid metabolism in type II hyperlipoproteinaemia and its modification by cholesterol-lowering agents. *Eicosanoids*. 1990;3(2):67-73.
28. Aikawa M, Rabkin E, Sugiyama S, et al. An HMG-CoA reductase inhibitor, cerivastatin, suppresses growth of macrophages expressing matrix metalloproteinases, and tissue factor in vivo, and in vitro. *Circulation*. 2001;103:276-283.
29. Jacobson TA. National Lipid Association task force on Statin safety-2014 Update. *J Clin Lipidol*. 2014;8:3S.
30. Wu C-C, Sy R, Tanphaichitr V, Hin ATT, Suyono S, Lee Y-T. Comparing the efficacy and safety of atorvastatin and simvastatin in Asians with elevated low-density lipoprotein-cholesterol: a multinational, multicenter, double-blind study. *J Formos Med Assoc*. 2002;101:478-487.
31. Morales D, Chung N, Zhu J-R, et al. Efficacy and safety of simvastatin in Asian and non-Asian coronary heart disease patients: a comparison of the GOALLS and STATT studies. *Curr Med Res Opin*. 2004;20:1235-1243.
32. Itoh T, Matsumoto M, Hougaku H, et al.; on behalf of the Simvastatin Study Group. Effects of low-dose simvastatin therapy on serum lipid levels in patients with moderate hypercholesterolemia: a 12-month study. *Clin Ther*. 1997;19:487-497.
33. Tomlinson B, Mak TWL, Tsui JYY, et al. Effects of fluvastatin on lipid profile and apolipoproteins in Chinese patients with hypercholesterolemia. *Am J Cardiol*. 1995;76(suppl):136A-139A.
34. Nakamura H, Arakawa K, Itakura H, et al.; for the MEGA Study Group. Primary prevention of cardiovascular disease with pravastatin in Japan (MEGA Study): a prospective randomized controlled trial. *Lancet*. 2006;368:1155-1163.
35. Chung N, Cho S-Y, Choi D-H, et al. STATT: a titrate-to-goal study of simvastatin in Asian patients with coronary heart disease. *Clin Ther*. 2001;23:858-870.
36. HPS2-THRIVE Collaborative Group. HPS2-THRIVE randomized placebo-controlled trial in 25,673 high risk patients of ER niacin/laropiprant: trial design, pre-specified muscle and liver outcomes, and reasons for stopping study treatment. *Eur Heart J*. 2013;34:1279-1291.
37. *Mevacor (Lovastatin) [package insert]*. Whitehouse Station, NJ: Merck & Co. Inc.; 2005.
38. *Altoprev (Lovastatin Extended-Release Tablets) [package insert]*. Florham Park, NJ: Andrx Labs, Inc.; 2002.
39. *Pravastatin Sodium [package insert]*. North Wales, PA: TEVA Pharmaceuticals USA, Inc.; 2014.
40. *Simvastatin [package insert]*. Dayton, NJ: Aurobindo Pharma USA, Inc.; 2014.
41. *Lescol (fluvastatin) [package insert]*. East Hanover, NJ: Novartis; 2003.
42. *Atorvastatin Calcium [Package Insert]*. Morgantown, WV: Mylan Pharmaceuticals; 2015.
43. *Crestor [Package Insert]*. Wilmington, DE: AstraZeneca Pharmaceuticals LP; 2014.
44. *Livalo [Package Insert]*. Montgomery, AL: Kowa Pharmaceuticals America, Inc.; 2009.
45. Wright AP, Adusumalli S, Corey KE. Statin therapy in patients with cirrhosis. *Frontline Gastroenterol*. 2015;6(4): 255-261.
46. Lilja JJ, Kivisto KT, Neuvonen PJ. Duration of effect of grapefruit juice on the pharmacokinetics of the CYP 3A4 substrate simvastatin. *Clin Pharmacol Ther*. 2000;68:384-390.

47. Tekeda M, Noshiro R, Onozato ML, et al. Evidence for a role of human organic anion transporters in the muscular side effects of HMG-CoA reductase inhibitors. *Eur J Pharmacol.* 2004;483:133-138.
48. Holdass H, Fellstrom B, Jardine AG, et al. Effect of fluvastatin on cardiac outcomes in renal transplant recipients: a multicentre, randomized, placebo-controlled trial. *Lancet.* 2003;361:2024-2031.
49. Spence JD, Munoz CE, Hendricks L, et al. Pharmacokinetics of the combination of fluvastatin and gemfibrozil. *Am J Cardiol.* 1995;76:80A-83A.
50. Tonelli M, Wanner C; for the Kidney Disease: Improving Global Outcomes Lipid Guideline Development Work Group Members. Lipid Management in Chronic Kidney Disease. Synopsis of the kidney disease: improving global outcomes 2013 clinical practice guideline. *Ann Intern Med.* 2014;160:182-189.
51. Morgan RE, Campbell SE, Suehira K, et al. Effects of steady-state lopinavir/ritonavir on the pharmacokinetics of pitavastatin in healthy adult volunteers. *J Acquir Immune Defic Syndr.* 2012;60(2):158-164.
52. Jones PH, Davidson MH, Stein EA, et al. Comparison of the efficacy and safety of rosuvastatin versus atorvastatin, simvastatin, and pravastatin across doses (STELLAR Trial). *Am J Cardiol.* 2003;92:152-160.
53. Liu J, Sempos CT, Donahue RP, et al. Non-high-density lipoprotein and very-low-density lipoprotein cholesterol and their risk predictive values in coronary heart disease. *Am J Cardiol.* 2006;98:1363-1368.
54. Cromwell WC, Otvos JD, Keyes MF, et al. LDL particle number and risk of future cardiovascular disease in the Framingham Offspring Study—Implications for LDL management. *J Clin Lipidol.* 2007;1:583-592.
55. Scandinavian Simvastatin Survival study Group. Randomised trial of cholesterol lowering in 4444 patients with coronary heart disease: the Scandinavian Simvastatin Survival Study (4S). *Lancet.* 1994;344:1383-1389.
56. Shepherd J, Cobbe SM, Ford I, et al. Prevention of coronary heart disease with pravastatin in men with hypercholesterolemia. *N Engl J Med.* 1995;333:1301-1307.
57. The Post Coronary Artery Bypass Graft Trial Investigators. The effect of aggressive lowering of low-density lipoprotein cholesterol levels and low-dose anticoagulation on obstructive changes in saphenous-vein coronary-artery bypass grafts. *N Engl J Med.* 1997;336:153-162.
58. Downs JR, Clearfield M, Weiss S, et al. Primary prevention of acute coronary events with lovastatin in men and women with average cholesterol levels: results of AFCAPS/TexCAPS. *JAMA.* 1998;279:1615-1622.
59. The long-Term Intervention with Pravastatin in Ischaemic Disease (LIPID) Study Group. Prevention of cardiovascular events and death with pravastatin in patients with coronary heart disease and a broad range of initial cholesterol levels. *N Engl J Med.* 1998;339:1349-1357.
60. GISSI Prevenzione Investigators (Gruppo Italiano per lo Studio della Sopravvivenza nell'Infarto Miocardico). Results of low dose (20 mg) pravastatin GISSI Prevenzione trial in 4271 patients with recent myocardial infarction: do stopped trials contribute to overall knowledge? *Ital Heart J.* 2000;1:810-820.
61. Serruys PWJC, de Feyter P, Macaya C, et al.; for the Lescol Intervention Study (LIPS) Investigators. Fluvastatin for prevention of cardiac events following successful first percutaneous coronary intervention. *JAMA.* 2002;287:3215-3222.
62. Heart Protection Study Collaborative Group. MRC/BHF Heart Protection Study of Cholesterol lowering with simvastatin in 20 536 high-risk individuals: a randomized placebo-controlled trial. *Lancet.* 2002;360:7-22.
63. Shepherd J, Blauw GJ, Murphy MB, et al.; on behalf of the PROSPER study group. Pravastatin in elderly individuals at risk of vascular disease (PROSPER): a randomized controlled trial. *Lancet.* 2002;360:1623-1630.
64. The ALLHAT Officers and Coordinators for the ALLHAT Collaborative Research Group. Major outcomes in moderately hypercholesterolemic, hypertensive patients randomized to pravastatin vs usual care. *JAMA.* 2002;288:2998-3007.
65. Sever PS, Dahlof B, Poulter NR, et al. Prevention of coronary and stroke events with atorvastatin in hypertensive patients who have average or lower-than-average cholesterol concentrations, in the Anglo-Scandinavian Cardiac Outcomes Trial-Lipid Lowering Arm (ASCOT-LLA): a multicentre randomized controlled trial. *Lancet.* 2003;361:1149-1158.
66. Colhoun HM, Betteridge DJ, Durrington PN, et al. Primary prevention of cardiovascular disease with atorvastatin in type 2 diabetes in the Collaborative Atorvastatin Diabetes Study (CARDS): multicentre randomized placebo-controlled trial. *Lancet.* 2004;364:685-696.
67. Koren MJ, Hunninghake DB. Clinical outcomes in managed-care patients with coronary heart disease treated aggressively in lipid-lowering disease management clinics: the ALLIANCE study. *J Am Coll Cardiol.* 2004;44:1772-1779.
68. Wanner C, Krane V, Marz W, et al. Atorvastatin in patients with type 2 diabetes mellitus undergoing hemodialysis. *N Engl J Med.* 2003;353:238-248.
69. Knopp RH, d'Emden M, Smilde JG, Pocock SJ. Efficacy and safety of atorvastatin in the prevention of cardiovascular end points in subjects with type 2 diabetes: the atorvastatin Study for Prevention of Coronary Heart Disease Endpoints in non-insulin-dependent diabetes mellitus (ASPEN). *Diabetes Care.* 2006;29:1478-1485.
70. Ridker PM, Danielson E, Fonseca FAH, et al.; for the JUPITER Study Group. Rosuvastatin to prevent vascular events in men and women with elevated C-reactive protein. *N Engl J Med.* 2008;359:2195-2207.
71. GISSI-HF investigators. Effect of rosuvastatin in patients with chronic heart failure (the GISSI-HF trial): a randomized, double-blind, placebo-controlled trial. *Lancet.* 2008;372:1231-1239.

72. Fellstrom BC, Jardine AG, Schmieder RE, et al.; for the AURORA Study Group. Rosuvastatin and cardiovascular events in patients undergoing hemodialysis. *N Engl J Med.* 2009;360:1395-1407.

73. de Lemos JA, Blazing MA, Wiviott SD, et al. Early intensive vs a delayed conservative simvastatin strategy in patients with acute coronary syndromes: phase Z of the A to Z trial. *JAMA.* 2004;292:1307-1316.

74. LaRosa JC, Grundy SM, Waters DD, et al. Intensive lipid lowering with atorvastatin in patients with stable coronary disease. *N Engl J Med.* 2005;352:1425-1435.

75. Pedersen TR, Faergeman O, Kastelein JJ, et al. High-dose atorvastatin vs usual-dose simvastatin for secondary prevention after myocardial infarction: the IDEAL study: a randomized controlled trial. *JAMA.* 2005;294:2437-2445.

76. Study of the Effectiveness of Additional Reductions in Cholesterol and Homocysteine (SEARCH) Collaborative Group. Intensive lowering of LDL cholesterol with 80 mg versus 20 mg simvastatin daily in 12 064 survivors of myocardial infarction: a double-blind randomized trial. *Lancet* 2010;376(9753):1658-1669. doi:10.1016/S0140-6736 (10)60310-8.

77. Cannon CP, Braunwald EB, McCabe CH, et al. Intensive versus moderate lipid lowering with statins after acute coronary syndromes. *N Engl J Med.* 2004;350:1495-1504.

78. Neil HA, DeMicco DA, Luo DJ, et al. Analysis of efficacy and safety in patients aged 65-75 years at randomization. Collaborative Atorvastatin Diabetes Study(CARDS). *Diabetes Care.* 2006;29:2378-2384.

79. Stone NJ, Robinson JG, Lichtenstein AH, et al. 2013 ACC.AHA guideline on the treatment of blood cholesterol to reduce atherosclerotic cardiovascular risk in adults: a report of the American College of Cardiology/American Heart Association Task Force on Practice Guideline. *J Am Coll Cardiol.* 2014;63(25 Pt B):2889-2934.

80. Expert Panel on Integrated Guidelines for Cardiovascular Health and Risk Reduction in Children and Adolescents; National Heart, Lung, and Blood Institute. Expert Panel on Integrated Guidelines for cardiovascular health and risk reduction in children and adolescents: summary report, *Pediatrics.* 2011;128(suppl 5):S213-S256.

81. McCrindle BW, Urbina EM, Dennison BA, et al. Drug therapy of high-risk lipid abnormalities in children and adolescents: a scientific statement from the American Heart Association Atherosclerosis, Hypertension, and Obesity in Youth Committee, Council of Cardiovascular Disease in the Young, with the Council on Cardiovascular Nursing. *Circulation.* 2007;115:1948-1967.

82. Braamskamp MJAM, Stefanutti C, Langslet G, et al. Efficacy and safety of pitavastatin in children and adolescents at high future cardiovascular risk. *J Pediatr.* 2015;167:338-343.

83. Miller ML, Wright CC, Browne B. Lipid-lowering medications for children and adolescents. *J Clin Lipidol.* 2015;9:S67-S76.

84. Wiegman A, Hutten BA, de Groot E, et al. Efficacy and safety of statin therapy in children with familial hypercholesterolemia: a randomized controlled trial. *JAMA.* 2004;292(3):331-337.

85. Vuorio A, Kuoppala J, Kovanen PT, et al. Statins for children with familial hypercholesterolemia. *Cochrane Database Syst Rev.* 2014;(7):CD006401.

86. Kusters DM, Avis HJ, de Groot E, et al. Ten year follow-up after initiation of statin therapy in children with familial hypercholesterolemia. *JAMA.* 2014;312(10):1055-1057.

87. Bays H, Cohen DE. An assessment by the Statin Liver Safety Task Force. *J Clin Lipidol.* 2014;8:547-557.

88. Loomba R, Sanyal AJ. The global NAFLD epidemic. *Nat Rev Gastroenterol Hepatol.* 2013;10:686-690.

89. Spengler EK, Loomba R. Recommendations for diagnosis, referral for liver biopsy, and treatment of nonalcoholic fatty liver disease and nonalcoholic Steatohepatitis. *Mayo Clin Proc.* 2015;90(9):1233-1246.

90. Ndumele CE, et al. Hepatic steatosis, obesity, and the metabolic syndrome are independently and additively associated with increased systemic inflammation. *Arterioscler Thromb Vasc Biol.* 2011;31(8):1927-1932.

91. Puchner SB, et al. High-risk coronary plaque at coronary CT angiography is associated with nonalcoholic fatty liver disease, independent of coronary plaque and Stenosis Burden: results from the ROMICAT II trial. *Radiology.* 2015;274(3):693-701.

92. Ballestri S, Lonardo A, Bonapace S, et al. Risk of cardiovascular, cardiac and arrhythmic complications in patients with non-alcoholic fatty liver disease. *World J Gastroenterol.* 2014;20:1724-1745.

93. Oni ET, Agatston AS, Blaha MJ, et al. A systemic review: burden and severity of subclinical cardiovascular disease among those with nonalcoholic fatty liver; should we care. *Atherosclerosis.* 2013;230:258-267.

94. Rzouq FS, Volk ML, Hatoum HH, et al. Hepatotoxicity fears contribute to under-utilization of statin medications by primary care physicians. *Am J Med Sci.* 2010;340:89-93.

95. Lewis JH, Mortensen ME, Zweig S, et al. Efficacy and safety of high-dose pravastatin in hypercholesterolemic patients with well-compensated chronic liver disease: results of a prospective, randomized, double-blind, placebo-controlled, multicenter trial. *Hepatology.* 2007;46:1453-1463.

96. Riley P, Sudarshi D, Johal M, et al. Weight loss, dietary advice and statin therapy in non-alcoholic fatty liver disease: a retrospective study. *Int J Clin Pract.* 2008;62:374-381.

97. Han KH, Rha SW, Kang HJ, et al. Evaluation of short-term safety and efficacy of HMG-CoA reductase inhibitors in hypercholesterolemic patients with elevated serum alanine transaminase concentrations: PITCH study (PITavastatin versus atorvastatin to evaluate the effect on patients with hypercholesterolemia and mild to moderate hepatic damage). *J Clin Lipidol.* 2012;6:340-351.

98. Gomez-Dominquez E, Gisbert JP, Moreno-Monteagudo JA, et al. A pilot study of atorvastatin treatment in dyslipemid, non-alcoholic fatty liver patients. *Aliment Pharmacol Ther*. 2006;23(11):1643-1647.
99. Antonopoulos S, Mikros S, Mylonopoulou M, et al. Rosuvastatin as a novel treatment of non-alcoholic fatty liver disease in hyperlipidemic patients. *Atherosclerosis*. 2006;184:233-234.
100. Abel T, Feher J, Dinya E, et al. Safety and efficacy of combined ezetimibe/simvastatin treatment and simvastatin monotherapy in patients with non-alcoholic fatty liver disease. *Med Sci Monit*. 2009;12:MS6-MS11.
101. Athyros VG, Tziomalos K, Grossios TD, et al. Safety and efficacy of long-term statin treatment for cardio-vascular events in patients with coronary heart disease and abnormal liver tests in the Greek Atorvastatin and Coronary Heart Disease Evaluation (GREACE) Study: a post-hoc analysis. *Lancet*. 2010;376:1916-1922.
102. Athyros VG, Giouleme O, Ganotakis ES, et al. Safety and impact on cardiovascular events of long-term multi-factorial treatment in patients with metabolic syndrome and abnormal liver function tests: a post hoc analysis of the randomized ATTEMPT study. *Arch Med Sci*. 2011;7:796-805.
103. Tikkanen MJ, Fayyad R, Faergeman O, et al. Effect of intensive lipid lowering with atorvastatin on cardiovas-cular outcomes in coronary heart disease patients with mild-to moderate baseline elevations in alanine amino-transferase levels. *Int J Cardiol*. 2013;168:3846-3852.
104. Wang W, Zhao C, Zhou J, et al. Simvastatin ameliorates liver fibrosis via mediating nitric oxide synthase in rats with non-alcoholic steatohepatitis-related liver fibrosis. *PLoS One*. 2013;8:e76538.
105. Van Rooyen DM, Gan LT, Yeh MM, et al. Pharmacological cholesterol lowering reverses fibrotic NASH in obese, diabetic mice with metabolic syndrome. *J Hepatol*. 2013;59:144-152.
106. Tziomalos K, Athyros VG, Paschos P, et al. Nonalcoholic fatty liver disease and statins. *Metabolism*. 2015;64:1215-1229.
107. Kargiotis K, Katsiki N, Athyros VG, et al. Effect of rosuvastatin on non-alcoholic steatohepatitis in patients with metabolic syndrome and hypercholesterolaemia: a preliminary report. *Curr Vasc Pharmacol*. 2014;12:505-511.
108. Chalasani N, Aljadhey H, Kesterson J, et al. Patients with elevated liver enzymes are not at higher risk for statin hepatotoxicity. *Gastroenterology*. 2004;126:1287-1292.
109. Pastori D, Polimeni L, Baratta F, et al. The efficacy and safety of statins for the treatment of non-alcoholic fatty liver disease. *Dig Liver Dis*. 2015;47:4-11.
110. Cash WJ, O'Neill S, O' Donnell ME, et al. Randomized controlled trial assessing the effect of simvastatin in primary biliary cirrhosis. *Liver Int*. 2013;33(8):1166-1174 .
111. Longo M, Crosignani A, Battezzati PM, et al. Hyperlipidaemic state and cardiovascular risk in primary biliary cirrhosis. *Gut*. 2002;51:265-269.
112. Rajab MA, Kaplan MM. Statins in primary biliary cirrhosis: are they safe? *Dig Dis Sci*. 2010;55:2086-2088.
113. Stojakovic T, Claudel T, Putz-Bankuti C, et al. Low-dose atorvastatin improves dyslipidemia and vascular function in patients with primary biliary cirrhosis after one year of treatment. *Atherosclerosis*. 2010;209:178-183.
114. Ritzel U, Leonhardt U, Nather M, et al. Simvastatin in primary biliary cirrhosis: effects on serum lipids and distinct disease markers. *J Hepatol*. 2002;36:454-458.
115. Kamisako T, Adachi Y. Marked improvement in cholestasis and hypercholesterolemia with simvastatin in a patient with primary biliary cirrhosis. *Am J Gastroenterol*. 1995;90:1187-1188.
116. Kurihara T, Akimoto M, Abe K, et al. Experimental use of pravastatin in patients with primary biliary cirrhosis associated with hypercholesterolemia. *Clin Ther*. 1993;15(5):890-898.
117. Kalaitzakis E, Bjornsson ES. Use of statins in patients with liver disease. *Minerva Gastroenterol Dietol*. 2014;60(1):15-24.
118. Gibson K, Rindone JP. Experience with statin use in patients with chronic hepatitis C infection. *Am J Cardiol*. 2005;96:1278-1279.
119. Khorashadi S, Hasson NK, Cheung RC. Incidence of statin hepatotoxicity in patients with hepatitis C. *Clin Gastroenterol Hepatol*. 2006;4:902-907.
120. Simon TG, Bonilla H, Yan P, et al. Atorvastatin and fluvastatin are associated with dose-dependent reductions in cirrhosis and hepatocellular carcinoma, among patients with hepatitis C Virus: results from ERCHIVES. *Hepatology*. 2016;64(1):47-57. doi:10.1002/hep.28506.
121. Baigent C, Landray MJ, Reith CR, et al. The effects of lowering LDL cholesterol with simvastatin plus ezetimibe in patients with chronic kidney disease (Study of Heart and Renal Protection): a randomized placebo control trial. *Lancet*. 2011;377(9784):2181-2192.
122. Scarpioni R, Ricardi M, Albertazzi V, et al. Treatment of dyslipidemia in chronic kidney disease: effectiveness and safety of statins. *World J Nephrol*. 2012;1(6):184-194.
123. Wanner C, Tonelli M; the Kidney Disease: Improving Global Outcomes Lipid Guideline Development Work Group Members. KDIGO Clinical Practice Guideline for Lipid Management in CKD: summary of recommen-dation statements and clinical approach to the patient. *Kidney Int*. 2014;85:1303-1309.
124. Tonelli M, Isles C, Curhan GC, et al. Effect of pravastatin on cardiovascular events in people with chronic kidney disease. *Circulation*. 2004;110:1557-1563.
125. Triant VA, Lee H, Hadigan C, et al. Increased acute myocardial infarction rates and cardiovascular risk factors among patients with human immunodeficiency virus disease. *J Clin Endocrinol Metab*. 2007;92(7):2506-2512.

126. Husain NE, Ahmed MH. Managing dyslipidemia in HIV/AIDS patients: challenges and solutions. *HIV AIDS (Auckl)*. 2014;7:1-10.
127. Myerson M, Malvestutto C, Aberg JA. Management of lipid disorders in patients living with HIV. *J Clin Pharmacol*. 2015;55:957-974.
128. U.S. Food and Drug Administration. FDA Drug Safety Communication: interactions between certain HIV or hepatitis C drugs and cholesterol-lowering statin drugs can increase the risk of muscle injury. 2012. Available at: http://www.fda.gov/Drugs/DrugSafety/ucm293877.htm. Accessed March 4, 2016.
129. Feinstein MJ, Achenbach CJ, Stone NJ, Lloyd-Jones DM. A systematic review of the usefulness of statin therapy in HIV-infected patients. *Am J Cardiol*. 2015;115:1760-1766.
130. Cohen DE, Anania FA, Chalasani N. An assessment of statin safety by hepatologists. *Am J Cardiol*. 2006;97(suppl):77C-81C.
131. Law M, Rudnicka AR. Statin safety: a systematic review. *Am J Cardiol*. 2006;97(suppl):52C-60C.
132. Tolman KG. The liver and lovastatin. *Am J Cardiol*. 2002;89:1374-1380.
133. Rosenson R, Baker S, Jacobson T, et al. An assessment by the statin muscle safety task force: 2014 update. *J Clin Lipidol*. 2014;8:S58-S71.
134. Bruckert E, Hayem G, Dejager S, et al. Mild to moderate muscular symptoms with high-dosage statin therapy in hyperlipidemic patients—the PRIMO study. *Cardiovasc Drugs Ther*. 2005;6:403-414.
135. Cohen JD, Brinton EA, Ito MK, et al. Understanding statin use in America and gaps in patient education (USAGE): an internet-based survey of 10,138 current and former statin users. *J Clin Lipidol*. 2012;3:208-215.
136. The Stroke Prevention by Aggressive Reduction in Cholesterol Levels (SPARCL) Investigators. High-dose atorvastatin after stroke or transient ischemic attack. *N Engl J Med*. 2006;355:549-559.
137. Zhang H, Plutzky J, Skentzos S, et al. Discontinuation of statins in routine care settings: a cohort study. *Ann Intern Med*. 2013;158:526-534.
138. Mampuya WM, Frid D, Rocco M, et al. Treatment strategies in patients with statin intolerance: the Cleveland Clinic experience. *Am Heart J*. 2013;166:597-603.
139. Moriarty PM, Thompson PD, Cannon CP, et al. Efficacy and safety of alirocumab vs ezetimibe in statin-intolerant patients, with a statin rechallenge arm: the ODYSSEY ALTERNATIVE randomized trial. *J Clin Lipidol*. 2015;9:758-769.
140. Sinzinger H, O'Grady J. Professional athletes suffering from familial hypercholesterolaemia rarely tolerate statin treatment because of muscular problems. *Br J Clin Pharmacol*. 2004;57:525-528.
141. Sinzinger H, Schmid P, O'Grady J. Two different types of exercise-induced muscle pain without myopathy and CK-elevation during HMG-Co-enzyme-A-reductase inhibitor treatment. *Atherosclerosis*. 1999;143:459-460.
142. Thompson PD, Zmuda JM, Domalik LJ, et al. Lovastatin increases exercise-induced skeletal muscle injury. *Metabolism*. 1997;46:1206-1210.
143. Pasternak RC, Smith SC, Bairey-Merz CN, et al. ACC/AHA/NHLBI clinical advisory on statins. *Circulation*. 2002;106:1024-1028.
144. Moßhammer D, Schaeffeler E, Schwab M, et al. Mechanisms and assessment of statin-related muscular adverse effects. *Br J Clin Pharmacol*. 2014;78:454-466.
145. Ghatak A, Faheem O, Thompson PD. The genetics of statin-induced myopathy. *Atherosclerosis*. 2010;210:337-343.
146. Joy TR, Monjed A, Zou GY, et al. N-of-1 (single-patient) trials for statin-related myalgia. *Ann Intern Med*. 2014;160(5):301-310.
147. Marcoff L, Thompson PD. The role of coenzyme Q10 in statin-associated myopathy: a systematic review. *J Am Coll Cardiol*. 2007;49:2231-2237.
148. Young JM, Florkowski CM, Molyneux SL, et al. Effect of coenzyme Q(10) supplementation on simvastatin-induced myalgia. *Am J Cardiol*. 2007;100:1400-1403.
149. Caso G, Kelly P, McNurlan MA, Lawson WE. Effect of coenzyme q10 on myopathic symptoms in patients treated with statins. *Am J Cardiol*. 2007;99:1409-1412.
150. Gupta A, Thompson PD. The relationship of vitamin D deficiency to statin myopathy. *Atherosclerosis*. 2011;215(1):23-29.
151. Lee P, Greenfield JR, Campbell LV. Vitamin D insufficiency—a novel mechanism of statin-induced myalgia? *Clin Endocrinol (Oxf)*. 2009;71:154-155.
152. Ahmed W, Khan N, Glueck CJ, et al. Low serum 25 (OH) vitamin D levels (<32 ng/mL) are associated with reversible myositis-myalgia in statin-treated patients. *Transl Res*. 2009;153(1):11-16.
153. Glueck CJ, Budhani SB, Masineni SS, et al. Vitamin D deficiency, myositis-myalgia, and reversible statin intolerance. *Curr Med Res Opin*. 2011;27(9):1683-1690.
154. Stein EA, Ballantyne CM, Windler E, et al. Efficacy and tolerability of fluvastatin XL 80 mg alone, ezetimibe alone, and the combination of fluvastatin XL 80 mg with ezetimibe in patients with a history of muscle-related side effects with other statins. *Am J Cardiol*. 2008;101(4):490-496.
155. Barilla D, Prasad P, Hubert M, Gumbhir-Shah K. Steady-state pharmacokinetics of fluvastatin in healthy subjects following a new extended release fluvastatin tablet, Lescol XL. *Biopharm Drug Dispos*. 2004;25:51-59.

156. Silva MA, Swanson AC, Gandhi PJ, Tataronis GR. Statin-related adverse events: a meta-analysis. *Clin Ther.* 2006;28:26-35.
157. Backes JM, Venero CV, Gibson CA, et al. Effectiveness and tolerability of every-other-day rosuvastatin dosing in patients with prior statin intolerance. *Ann Pharmacother.* 2008;42:341-346.
158. Gadarla M, Kearns AK, Thompson PD. Efficacy of rosuvastatin (5 mg and 10 mg) twice a week in patients intolerant to daily statins. *Am J Cardiol.* 2008;101:1747-1748.
159. Backes JM, Moriarty PM, Ruisinger JF, Gibson CA. Effects of once weekly rosuvastatin among patients with a prior statin intolerance. *Am J Cardiol.* 2007;100:554-555.
160. Ruisinger JF, Backes JM, Gibson CA, Moriarty PM. Once-a-week rosuvastatin (2.5 to 20 mg) in patients with a previous statin intolerance. *Am J Cardiol.* 2009;103:393-394.
161. Simons JE, Holbrook AM, Don-Wauchope AC. Successful reintroduction of statin therapy after statin-associated rhabdomyolysis. *J Clin Lipidol.* 2015;9(4):594-596.
162. Ridker PM, Pradhan A, MacFadyen JG, et al. Cardiovascular benefits and diabetes risks of statin therapy in primary prevention: an analysis from the JUPITER trial. *Lancet.* 2012;380:565-571.
163. Freeman DJ, Norrie J, Caslake MJ, et al. C-reactive protein is an independent predictor of risk for the development of diabetes in the West of Scotland Coronary Prevention Study. *Diabetes.* 2002;51:1596-1600.
164. Sattar N, Preiss D, Murray HM, et al. Statins and risk of incident diabetes: a collaborative meta-analysis of randomized trials. *Lancet.* 2010;375:735-742.
165. Preiss D, Seshasai SRK, Welsh P, et al. Risk of incident diabetes with intensive-dose compared with moderate-dose statin therapy. *JAMA.* 2011;305(24):2556-2564.
166. Sampson UK, Linton MF, Fazio S. Are statins diabetogenic? *Curr Opin Cardiol.* 2011;26(4):342-347.
167. Maki KC, Ridker PM, Brown WV, et al. An assessment by the Statin Diabetes Safety Task Force: 2014 update. *J Clin Lipidol.* 2014;8:S17-S29.
168. Baker WL, Talati R, White CM, et al. Differing effect of statins on insulin sensitivity in non-diabetics: a systematic review and meta-analysis. *Diabetes Res Clin Pract.* 2010;87:98-107.
169. Koh KK, Sakuma I, Quon MJ. Differential metabolic effects of distinct statins. *Atherosclerosis.* 2011;215:1-8.
170. Gumprecht J, Gosho M, Budinski D, et al. Comparative long-term efficacy and tolerability of pitavastatin 4 mg and atorvastatin 20–40 mg in patients with type 2 diabetes mellitus and combined (mixed) dyslipidaemia. *Diabetes Obes Metab.* 2011;13:1047-1055.
171. Jukema JW, Cannon CP, De Craen AJM, et al. The controversies of statin therapy. *J Am Coll Cardiol.* 2012;60:875-881.
172. U.S. Food and Drug Administration. FDA Drug Safety Communication: important safety label changes to cholesterol-lowering statin drugs. Available at: http://www.fda.gov/drugs/drugsafety/ucm293101.htm. Accessed March 12, 2016.
173. Trompet S, Vliet PV, De Craen AJM, et al. Pravastatin and cognitive function in the elderly. Results of the PROSPER study. *J Neurol.* 2010;257:85-90.
174. Collins R, Armitage J, Parish S, Sleight P, Peto R; Heart Protection Study Collaborative Group. Effects of cholesterol-lowering with simvastatin on stroke and other major vascular events in 20536 people with cerebrovascular disease or other high risk conditions. *Lancet.* 2004;363:757-767.
175. Steenland K, Zhao L, Goldstein FC, et al. Statins and cognitive decline in older adults with normal cognition or mild cognitive impairment. *J Am Geriatr Soc.* 2013;61:1449-1455.
176. Joosten H, Visser ST, van Eersel ME, et al. Statin use and cognitive function: population-based observational study with long-term follow-up. *PLoS One.* 2015;10:e0118045.
177. Swiger KJ, Manalac RJ, Blumenthal RS, et al. Statins and cognition: a systematic review and meta-analysis of short- and long-term cognitive effects. *Mayo Clin Proc.* 2013;88(11):1213-1221.
178. LaRosa JC, Grundy SM, Kastelein JJP, et al. Safety and efficacy of atorvastatin-induced very low-density lipoprotein cholesterol levels in patients with coronary heart disease (a Post Hoc Analysis of the Treating to New Targets [TNT] Study). *Am J Cardiol.* 2007;100:747-752.
179. Wiviott SD, Cannon CP, Morrow DA, et al. Can low-density lipoprotein be too low? the safety and efficacy of achieving very low low-density lipoprotein with intensive statin therapy. *J Am Coll Cardiol.* 2005;46:1411-1416.
180. Hsia J, MacFadyen JG, Monyak J, et al. Cardiovascular event reduction and adverse events among subjects attaining low-density lipoprotein cholesterol <50 mg/dL with rosuvastatin. *J Am Coll Cardiol.* 2011;57:1666-1675.
181. Everett BM, Mora S, Glynn RJ, et al. Safety profile of subjects treated to very low low-density lipoprotein cholesterol levels (<30 mg/dL) with rosuvastatin 20 mg daily (from JUPITER). *Am J Cardiol.* 2014;114:1682-1689.
182. Boekholdt SM, Hovingh GK, Mora S, et al. Very low levels of atherogenic lipoproteins and the risk for cardiovascular events. *J Am Coll Cardiol.* 2014;64:485-494.
183. Morris PB, Ballantyne CM, Birtcher KK, et al. Review of clinical practice guidelines for the management of LDL-related risk. *J Am Coll Cardiol.* 2014;64:196-206.
184. Kumbhani DJ, Steg PG, Cannon CP, et al. Adherence to secondary prevention medications and four-year outcomes in outpatients with atherosclerosis. *Am J Med.* 2013;126:693-700.

Nonstatin Medications: Omega-3 Fatty Acids, Fibrates, Bile Acid Sequestrants, Niacin, and Cholesterol Absorption Inhibitors

Marina Kawaguchi-Suzuki

Key Points

- Nonstatin medications are used to supplement or augment statin therapy in patients with severe hypercholesterolemia or mixed dyslipidemia.
- Nonstatin medications may be used as an alternative if patients are statin intolerant.
- Omega-3 fatty acids are primarily used to lower TG levels in patients with hypertriglyceridemia and are well tolerated.
- Prescription omega-3 fatty acid products should be preferentially used to ensure eicosapentaenoic acid and docosahexaenoic acid contents and to minimize pill burden.
- Fibric acid derivatives (fenofibrate, fenofibric acid, and gemfibrozil) are primarily used to lower TG levels and are also indicated for primary hypercholesterolemia and mixed dyslipidemia.
- Use of gemfibrozil should be avoided in combination with a statin; fenofibrate should be the choice of fibrates in this case.
- Bile acid sequestrants (cholestyramine, colestipol, and colesevelam) are primarily used to lower LDL-C in combination with another lipid-lowering agent, while its drug-binding property (drug-drug interactions) may complicate the regimen.
- Bile acid sequestrants are not systemically absorbed and may be used in pregnant women or children.
- Niacin in higher doses lowers LDL-C and triglycerides and raises HDL-C but is often poorly tolerated. Recent research has shown that in combination with statins, there is no incremental clinical benefit. The 2016 ACC Expert Consensus statement on nonstatins did not include niacin in their treatment algorithms.
- Ezetimibe is the only available cholesterol absorption inhibitor and effectively lowers LDL-C either as a monotherapy or as a combination therapy with a statin.

I. Introduction

The five classes of nonstatin medications discussed in this chapter are omega-3 fatty acids (FAs), fibric acid derivatives, bile acid sequestrants (BASs), niacin, and cholesterol absorption inhibitors. Although statins are considered first-line therapy for lipid modification for the prevention and treatment of atherosclerotic vascular disease (ASCVD), nonstatin medications are used to supplement or augment the statin therapy in patients with severe hypercholesterolemia or mixed dyslipidemia.[1] Nonstatin medications may also be used as an alternative therapy for patients who do not tolerate statins.[1]

Although evidence for reducing or preventing cardiovascular events and/or deaths with nonstatin medications has been inconsistent or not been as strong as those with statins, lipid-modifying effects of nonstatin therapy are well documented. Nonstatin medications still play a key role in dyslipidemia management, and it is important to determine when and how to use these medications appropriately. The treatment of each nonstatin class is described in this chapter. The PCSK9 inhibitors, lomitapide, and mipomersen will be discussed in Chapter 12, "Familial Hypercholesterolemia."

II.   Omega-3 FAs (Fish Oils)

Omega-3 polyunsaturated FAs include eicosapentaenoic acid (EPA), docosahexaenoic acid (DHA), and α-linoleic acid (ALA). The metabolic precursor, ALA, is converted to EPA and further to DHA.[2] ALA is found in vegetable sources, and EPA and DHA enter the food chain through phytoplankton and are only present in marine organisms.[2] Omega-3 FAs are therefore commonly referred to as fish oil, and variable amounts of omega-3 FAs are contained in fish oil preparations in the forms of triglycerides (ie, esterified to a glycerol backbone), ethyl esters, or free fatty acids (ie, carboxylic acids).[2]

The omega-3 FA formulations approved by the United States (U.S.) Food and Drug Administration (FDA), omega-3-acid ethyl esters (Lovaza; generics available), omega-3-acid ethyl esters A (Omtryg), omega-3-carboxylic acids (Epanova), and icosapent ethyl (Vascepa), are listed in Table 9.1. The principal constituents of these FDA-approved preparations are EPA and DHA, while the icosapent ethyl product purely contains EPA. These are indicated as an adjunct to diet to reduce triglyceride (TG) levels in adult patients with severe hypertriglyceridemia (>500 mg/dL).[3–6]

A. **Mechanism of action (MOA)** The mechanism of action of omega-3 FAs is not completely elucidated. However, the following five pathways had been proposed: (1) decreased lipogenesis by inhibiting the conversion of acetyl-coenzyme A to FAs; (2) increased β-oxidation; (3) inhibition of phosphatidic acid phosphatase, an enzyme catalyzing conversion of phosphatidic acid to diacylglycerol, and diacylglycerol acyltransferase, an enzyme catalyzing the final step in TG synthesis; (4) increased degeneration of apolipoprotein B; and (5) increased lipoprotein lipase activity, an enzyme catalyzing the conversion of very-low-density lipoprotein (VLDL) to low-density lipoprotein (LDL) particles.[3–8] These pathways result in reduced hepatic TG production and enhanced TG clearance (Fig. 9.1).[7,9]

Table 9.1. Prescription Omega-3 Fatty Acid Products			
Product	**Omega-3 Acid Ethyl Esters (Lovaza)**	**Omega-3 Acid Ethyl Esters A (Omtryg)**	**Omega-3 Carboxylic Acids (Epanova)**	**Icosapent Ethyl (Vascepa)**
Capsule size	1 g	1.2 g	1 g	1 g
EPA and DHA contents	EPA ~0.465 g DHA ~0.375 g	EPA ~0.465 g DHA ~0.375 g	EPA 0.55 g DHA 0.2 g	EPA 1 g
Dosing	• 4 capsules daily • 2 capsules bid	• 4 capsules daily • 2 capsules bid	• 2 capsules daily • 4 capsules daily	• 4 capsules daily • 2 capsules bid
Administration	• Swallow capsules whole • Take with or without food	• Swallow capsules whole • Take with food	• Swallow capsules whole • Take with or without food	• Swallow capsules whole • Take with food
Generic availability	yes	no	no	no

EPA, eicosapentaenoic acid; DHA, docosahexaenoic acid; bid, twice daily.
Lovaza (omega-3-acid ethyl esters) Prescribing Information. Research Triangle Park, NC: GlaxoSmithKline; 2014.
Omtryg (omega-3-acid ethyl esters A) Prescribing Information. Arlington, VA: Trygg Pharma, Inc.; 2014.
Epanova (omega-3-carboxylic acids) Prescribing Information. Wilmington, DE: AstraZeneca Pharmaceuticals LP; 2014.
Vascepa (icosapent ethyl) Prescribing Information. Bedminster, NJ: Amarin Pharma Inc.; 2015.

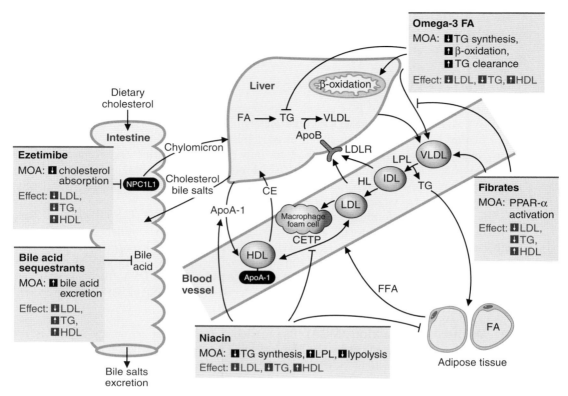

FIGURE 9.1: Mechanism of action for omega-3 fatty acids, fibrates, bile acid sequestrants, niacin, and cholesterol absorption inhibitors. ApoB, apolipoprotein B; CE, cholesteryl ester; CETP, cholesteryl ester transfer protein; FA, fatty acid; FFA, free fatty acid; HDL, high-density lipoprotein; HL, hepatic lipase; IDL, intermediate-density lipoprotein; LDL, low-density lipoprotein; MOA, mechanism of action; NPC1L1, Niemann-Pick C1-like 1 transporter; PPAR, peroxisome proliferator-activated receptor; TG, triglyceride; VLDL, very-low-density lipoprotein.

Omega-3 FAs are also proposed to modulate the activity of transcription factors, such as peroxisome proliferator-activated receptors (PPARs) and sterol regulatory element binding protein (SREBP)-1c, potentially affecting gene expressions involved in adipogenesis and glucose and lipid metabolism.[10] Other potential properties of omega-3 FAs include anti-inflammatory, antithrombotic, and antiarrhythmic effects.[10] Additionally, potential effects on lowering blood pressure and improving endothelial function are also reported with omega-3 FAs.[10]

B. Dosage and administration Table 9.1 summarizes dosages and administration instructions for each FDA-approved product. Omega-3 FAs may be administered either once or twice daily, based on patient's response and tolerability. Pill burden typically becomes high with administration of omega-3 FAs. Especially when over-the-counter fish oil supplements are selected, depending on available formulations, more than 10 capsules may be needed to acquire equivalent amounts of EPA and DHA with prescription products. Capsule sizes vary among products (most capsules are large), and it is good to check whether patients can readily swallow these capsules. Some patients may freeze or refrigerate supplemental products to minimize gastrointestinal adverse effects such as nausea, belching, and a fishy aftertaste or smell. One concern of refrigerating or freezing fish oil supplements is it has not been demonstrated that the absorption remains the same. The FDA-approved products are recommended to be stored at room temperature and should not be frozen.[3–6]

C. **Pharmacokinetics** For omega-3 FAs administered as ethyl esters, dose-dependent increases in serum EPA concentrations were observed. In contrast, increases in DHA concentrations were less pronounced and not dose dependent.[3,4] Omega-3 carboxylic acids were reported to have better bioavailability than ethyl ester forms in healthy volunteer studies.[11,12] According to data from MARINE, ANCHOR, EVOLVE, and ESPRIT, the plasma concentrations of EPA from icosapent ethyl appeared to be comparable to the total plasma concentrations of EPA plus DHA from omega-3-carboxylic acids after long-term administration.[7] Fish oil preparations available as nutritional supplements are not subject to FDA regulations concerning bioavailability, and it is advisable to use products that are externally tested and certified.

D. **Drug interactions** No significant drug-drug interactions have been reported. Prescribing information of omega-3 FA products lists potential interaction with anticoagulants due to previously noted prolongation of bleeding time.[3–6] However, the prolongation usually remains within normal limits.[3–6] Increased risk of clinically significant bleeding episodes is not reported with use of omega-3 FAs in combination with a medication affecting coagulation.[13] If patients are on warfarin or antiplatelet agents, more frequent monitoring may be advised, but omega-3 FAs can still be used.

E. **Contraindications and precautions** The prescription products are derived from fish sources and should be used with caution if patients are allergic to fish and/or shellfish.[3–6] Despite speculated antiarrhythmic effect, more frequent recurrences of symptomatic atrial fibrillation or flutter happened among patients with paroxysmal or persistent atrial fibrillation, especially within the first 2-3 months of treatment initiation, during a clinical trial of omega-3 acid ethyl esters (Lovaza and Omtryg).[3,4]

F. **Efficacy**
   1. **Triglyceride lowering** Effects of omega-3 acid ethyl esters on lipid parameters were investigated in patients with very high (≥500 and <2000 mg/dL) TG levels (Table 9.2).[14,15] Similarly, EVOLVE and MARINE studies were conducted for omega-3 carboxylic acids and icosapent ethyl, respectively (Table 9.2).[16,17] COMBOS (omega-3 acid ethyl esters), ESPRIT (omega-3 carboxylic acids), and ANCHOR (icosapent ethyl) examined the effect in combination with statin therapy among patients with high (≥200 and <500 mg/dL) TG levels (Table 9.2).[18–20] Both EPA and DHA have established TG-lowering effect.[21]

   2. **Non-HDL-C, LDL-C, and HDL-C effects** Although DHA raises LDL-C, EPA is suggested to reduce or only slightly increase LDL-C[21]; however, non-HDL-C and apolipoprotein B are slightly reduced with all agents.[21]
      DHA, but not EPA, is associated with increases in high-density lipoprotein cholesterol (HDL-C).[21]

   3. **Overall lipid effects** As the overall effect, omega-3 FAs are associated with ~30% reductions in TG, minimal elevation in HDL-C, modest elevation in LDL-C, and 8%-14% reductions in non-HDL-C.[22]

   4. **Antiarrhythmic effects** Regarding potential antiarrhythmic effect, the administration of omega-3 FAs was suggested to be protective against atrial fibrillation if patients have structural heart disease such as heart failure, but omega-3 FAs are not

Table 9.2.   Effects of Prescription Omega-3 Fatty Acid Products on Lipid Parameters (Percent Changes from Baseline)

	TG	LDL-C	HDL-C	Total-C	Non-HDL-C	VLDL-C	ApoB
Omega-3 acid ethyl esters (Lovaza)[a]	−45%	+45%	+9%	−10%	−14%	−42%	NA
with statin[b]	−30%	+0.7%	+3%	−5%	−9%	−28%	−4%
Omega-3 acid ethyl esters A (Omtryg)[a]	−25%	+20%	0%	−8%	−9%	−21%	NA
Omega-3 carboxylic acids (Epanova)[a]	−31%	+26%	+5%	−6%	−8%	−35%	+6%
with statin[b]	−21%	+1%	+3%	−4%	−7%	−22%	−2%
Icosapent ethyl (Vascepa)[a]	−27%	−5%	−4%	−7%	−8%	−20%	−4%
with statin[b]	−18%	+2%	−1%	−3%	−5%	−12%	−2%

NA, not available.

[a]Data were based on patients with very high (≥500 and <2000 mg/dL) TG levels at baseline.

[b]Data with statin therapy were based on patients with high (≥200 and <500 mg/dL) TG levels at baseline.

(Data from *Omtryg (omega-3-acid ethyl esters A) Prescribing Information*. Arlington, VA: Trygg Pharma, Inc.; 2014;

Harris WS, et al. Safety and efficacy of Omacor in severe hypertriglyceridemia. *J Cardiovasc Risk*. 1997;4(5-6):385–391;

Pownall HJ, et al. Correlation of serum triglyceride and its reduction by omega-3 fatty acids with lipid transfer activity and the neutral lipid compositions of high-density and low-density lipoproteins. *Atherosclerosis*. 1999;143(2):285–297;

Kastelein JJ, et al. Omega-3 free fatty acids for the treatment of severe hypertriglyceridemia: the EpanoVa fOr Lowering Very high triglyceridEs (EVOLVE) trial. *J Clin Lipidol*. 2014;8(1):94–106;

Bays HE, et al. Icosapent ethyl, a pure EPA omega-3 fatty acid: effects on lipoprotein particle concentration and size in patients with very high triglyceride levels (the MARINE study). *J Clin Lipidol*. 2012;6(6):565–572;

Davidson MH, et al. A novel omega-3 free fatty acid formulation has dramatically improved bioavailability during a low-fat diet compared with omega-3-acid ethyl esters: the ECLIPSE (Epanova compared to Lovaza in a pharmacokinetic single-dose evaluation) study. *J Clin Lipidol*. 2012;6(6):573-584;

Maki KC, et al. A highly bioavailable omega-3 free fatty acid formulation improves the cardiovascular risk profile in high-risk, statin-treated patients with residual hypertriglyceridemia (the ESPRIT trial). *Clin Ther*. 2013;35(9):1400.e1-3-1411.e1-3;

Ballantyne CM, et al. Efficacy and safety of eicosapentaenoic acid ethyl ester (AMR101) therapy in statin-treated patients with persistent high triglycerides (from the ANCHOR study). *Am J Cardiol*. 2012;110(7):984-992.)

likely helpful for lone atrial fibrillation.[9,23] Evidence is not sufficient to support use of omega-3 FAs for the antiarrhythmic effect nor should they be used for the treatment of atrial fibrillation or flutter.

5. **Blood pressure** Regarding potential effect on blood pressure, omega-3 FAs were shown to lower both systolic and diastolic blood pressure in a dose-dependent manner.[9,24] When omega-3 FAs were administered at a dose of ≥3 g/d, modest reductions of 0.66 mm Hg systolic and 0.35 mm Hg diastolic blood pressure were observed per g of omega-3 FAs.[9,24]

6. **Cardiovascular morbidity and mortality**
   a. According to a recent systematic review, the majority of earlier randomized controlled trials investigating the use of omega-3 FAs showed a reduction in cardiovascular risk or events.[25] However, some concerns of these earlier studies were inadequate designs, and more recent randomized controlled trials were not able to replicate the reduction in cardiovascular risk or event rates.[25] A meta-analysis of both randomized controlled trials and prospective cohort studies indicated that EPA + DHA may be associated with reducing CHD risk, with a greater benefit observed among those at higher risk in the randomized controlled trials (Alexander DD, et al. Mayo Clin Proc. 2017;92:15-29).
   b. Although the role of omega-3 FAs is well established in reducing TG levels, especially among patients with hypertriglyceridemia, it is an ongoing discussion whether omega-3 FA therapy provides direct benefit in preventing cardiovascular events and deaths.

G. **Adverse drug reactions (ADRs)** As a class, omega-3 prescription products have a favorable safety profile and generally well tolerated.[7] The most commonly reported ADRs are eructation (burping or belching), dyspepsia, and taste perversion with omega-3 acid ethyl esters (Lovaza and Omtryg); diarrhea, nausea, abdominal pain/discomfort, and eructation with omega-3 carboxylic acids (Epanova); and arthralgia with icosapent ethyl (Vascepa).[3-6] The EPA-only product (Vascepa) did not have increased incidence of gastrointestinal ADRs.[6]

The prescribing information recommends to monitor alanine aminotransferase (ALT) and aspartate aminotransferase (AST) levels periodically in patients with hepatic impairment.[3-6] While some experimental studies indicate improvement of insulin sensitivity, multiple meta-analyses showed no significant effect of omega-3 FA supplementation on fasting glucose or HgbH1c in patients with diabetes.[10] Among studies reporting increase in fasting plasma glucose, the observed increase was about 3 mg/dL for every 1 g/d omega-3 FA use.[10] Although evidence is not entirely conclusive, no major harmful or beneficial effect is expected on development of diabetes.[10]

III. Fibric Acid Derivatives (Fibrates)

Fibric acid derivatives presently available for clinical use are fenofibrate (available under various brands: Antara, Fenoglide, Lipofen, Tricor, Lofibra, Triglide), fenofibric acid (Fibricor, Trilipix), and gemfibrozil (Lopid) (Table 9.3). These medications are also available as generic

Table 9.3. Formulations of Fibric Acid Derivatives

Generic Name	Brand Name	Strengths/Forms	Administration
Fenofibrate (generic available)	*Nonmicronized*		
	Fenoglide	40, 120 mg tablet	With food Swallow tables whole
	Lipofen	50, 150 mg capsule (Lidose)	With food Swallow capsules whole
	Lofibra	54, 160 mg tablet	With food
	Triglide	50, 160 mg tablet (IDD-P)	With or without food Swallow tablets whole
	Nanocrystal (nonmicronized)		
	Tricor	48, 145 mg tablet	With or without food Swallow tablets whole
	Micronized		
	Antara	30, 90 mg capsule	With or without food Swallow capsules whole
	Lofibra	67, 134, 200 mg capsule	With food
Fenofibric acid (generic available)	Fibricor	35, 105 mg tablet	With or without food Swallow tablets whole
	Trilipix	45, 145 mg tablet	With or without food Swallow tablets whole
Gemfibrozil (generic available)	Lopid	600 mg tablet	30 min before meals

Data from *Fenoglide (fenofibrate) Prescribing Information*. San Diego, CA: Santarus, Inc.; 2012;
Lipofen (fenofibrate) Prescribing Information. Montgomery, AL: Kowa Pharmaceuticals America, Inc.; 2013;
Triglide (fenofibrate) Prescribing Information. Florham Park, NJ: Shionogi Inc.; 2015;
Antara (fenofibrate) Prescribing Information. Baltimore, MD: Lupin Pharma; 2015;
Lofibra (fenofibrate) Prescribing Information. Sellersville, PA: Gate Pharmaceuticals; 2010;
Tricor (fenofibrate) Prescribing Information. North Chicago, IL: AbbVie, Inc.; 2013;
Fibricor (fenofibric acid) Prescribing Information. Philadelphia, PA: Mutual Pharmaceutical Company, Inc.; 2014;
Trilipix (fenofibric acid) Prescribing Information. North Chicago, IL: AbbVie Inc.; 2015;
Lopid (gemfibrozil) Prescribing Information. New York, NY: Parke-Davis; 2014;
Ling H, Tuoma JT, Hilleman D. A review of currently available fenofibrate and fenofibric acid formulations. *Cardiol Res*. 2013;4(2):47-55.

products. Clofibrate was withdrawn from the market, and ciprofibrate and bezafibrate are not available in the United States.[25]

There are two FDA-approved indications for fibrates as an adjunctive therapy to diet: (1) to reduce elevated LDL-C, total-C, TG, and apolipoprotein B (apoB) and to increase HDL-C in primary hypercholesterolemia or mixed dyslipidemia and (2) to reduce TG in severe hypertriglyceridemia.[26–34] Only gemfibrozil carries an indication to prevent pancreatitis in patients whose TG level is >2000 mg/dL.[1] The primary role of fibrates for clinical use is to lower TG levels.

A. Mechanism of action The pharmacological effect of fibrates is mediated by PPAR-α activation, which reduces synthesis of apolipoprotein C-III, an inhibitor of lipoprotein lipase, and enhances lipoprotein lipase activity (Fig. 9.1).[26–34] The results are increased lipolysis and elimination of TG-rich particles.[26–34] The decrease in TG also alters the size and composition of LDL from small, dense articles to large buoyant particles, which are less atherogenic due to greater affinity to cholesterol receptors for better catabolism.[26–34] Synthesis of VLDL apolipoprotein B-100 is diminished in patients with hypertriglyceridemia.[1] The PPAR-α activation additionally leads to increased production of apolipoproteins A-I and A-II, major protein components of HDL, though this effect on HDL appears to be heterogeneous among fibrates.[1,26–35]

B. Dosage and administration

1. **Dosing** The standard doses of fenofibrate and fenofibric acid are 43-160 mg administered once daily, depending on strengths available for a selected product (Table 9.3). Gemfibrozil 600 mg is administered twice daily 30 minutes prior to morning and evening meals.[34]

2. **Titration** Titration of doses with fenofibrate or fenofibric acid is not necessary; the highest-strength tablet or capsule of selected product can be initiated for primary hypercholesterolemia or mixed dyslipidemia.[26–33] Fenofibrate or fenofibric acid may be initiated at lower strengths for the indication of hypertriglyceridemia.[26–33] The lower-strength therapy can be titrated up at 1- to 2-month intervals, based on patient's response.

3. **Use in renal impairment** If patients have mild-moderate renal impairment with creatinine clearance (CrCl) of 31-80 mL/min, initiating fenofibrate or fenofibric acid at lower strengths is recommended.[26–33] If patients have severe renal impairment or are on dialysis, fibrates should be avoided.[26–34] Both the National Lipid Association and the National Kidney Foundation recommend against the use of fenofibrate or fenofibric acid if CrCl is <15 mL/min.[36,37] Gemfibrozil is the preferred fibrate for patients with chronic kidney failure or with previous kidney transplant.[36,37] The National Lipid Association recommends adjusting the dosing frequency of gemfibrozil 600 mg from twice daily to once daily if CrCl is 15-59 mL/min and avoiding the use if CrCl is <15 mL/min.[36] Certain fenofibrate products (Fenoglide, Lipofen, Lofibra) should be administered with meals for better absorption (Table 9.3).

C. Pharmacokinetics

1. Fenofibrate is highly lipophilic and virtually insoluble in water, making this compound poorly absorbable.[38] Fenofibrate products are formulated in many different ways, including nonmicronized (Fenoglide, Lipofen, Lofibra, Triglide), micronized (Antara, Lofibra), and nanocrystal (Tricor) forms.[38]

2. The micronized formulations have smaller particle size than the nonmicronized formulations, and the nanoparticle formulations further reduced particle size to improve solubility and bioavailability.[38] Microcoating of micronized particles with hydrophilic polyvinylpyrrolidone (Lofibra) increased dissolution rates for greater bioavailability.[30,38] Insoluble drug delivery microparticle (IDD-P) tablets (Triglide) use phospholipid surface-modifying agent to prevent reaggregation of the micropar-ticles.[28,38] Lidose drug delivery technology (Lipofen) utilizes a lipid excipient mixture to enhance bioavailability.[27,38]

Fenofibrate is a prodrug, and the active metabolite, fenofibric acid, is also avail-able, being most hydrophilic with the highest bioavailability.[32,33,38] Differently formulated fenofibrates and fenofibric acids are not equivalent on a milligram-to-milligram basis, and appropriate dose needs to be prescribed if patients are switch-ing products.[38] After fenofibrate and gemfibrozil undergo extensive metabolism by glucuronidation and by oxidation and glucuronidation, respectively, the metabo-lites are eliminated renally.[26-34]

D. Drug interactions

1. Most clinically significant interactions of fibrates are reported with statins, repa-glinide, colchicine, warfarin, and bile acid–binding resins.[26-34]

2. Due to the risk of myopathy and rhabdomyolysis, which likely results from inhibited glucuronidation of statins, gemfibrozil should be avoided in a combination with a statin and is specifically contraindicated with simvastatin.[1,34,36] If a combination therapy of a statin and a fibrate is necessary, fenofibrate is the preferred fibrate; a fenofibrate dose not exceeding 48 mg should be initiated with caution, while the statin dose remains below the maximal dose.[36]

3. Coadministration of repaglinide and gemfibrozil is also contraindicated due to the risk of severe hypoglycemia from increased exposure to repaglinide.[34] Chronic use of colchicine at therapeutic doses with a fibrate may potentiate development of myopa-thy; fibrates should be cautiously used especially in geriatric patients and patients with renal impairment, who are considered at a higher risk.[26-34]

4. When a fibrate is concomitantly used with warfarin, prolongation of prothrombin time/international normalized ratio (PT/INR) is reported.[26-34] Warfarin dose may need to be reduced, and PT/INR should be frequently monitored until the level is stabilized.[26-34] Fenofibrate or fenofibric acid should be administered at least 1 hour before or 4-6 hours after a BAS to maintain absorption.[26-33] Gemfibrozil should be given at least 2 hours apart from colestipol to keep desired gemfibrozil exposure.[34]

5. Fibrates may increase risk of cholelithiasis by concurrent ezetimibe therapy as a result of increased cholesterol excretion into the bile.[36,39] However, cases of gallblad-der disease and cholecystectomies are uncommon.[36,39] If cholelithiasis is suspected, gallbladder studies are indicated.[36,39] In addition, alternative therapy should be used in this case.[36,39] If a fibrate needs to be combined with ezetimibe, fenofibrate is the recommended fibrate due to insufficient data with other fibrates.[36,39]

E. Contraindications and precautions Gemfibrozil is contraindicated in patients with (1) hepatic or severe renal dysfunction, including primary biliary cirrhosis, (2) preexisting gallbladder disease, (3) hypersensitivity to gemfibrozil, or (4) concomitant repaglinide or simvastatin therapy.[34]

Fenofibrates and fenofibric acids are contraindicated in patients with (1) gallblad-der disease; (2) hypersensitivity to fenofibrate or fenofibric acid; (3) active liver disease, including primary biliary cirrhosis or unexplained persistent abnormalities in liver function tests; or (4) severe renal impairment (or patients on dialysis).[26–33] Although fibrates are classified as pregnancy category C, nursing mothers should avoid fenofibrate or fenofibric acid as this is considered a contraindication.[26–33]

F. Efficacy

1. **Lipids** Previously reported effects of fibric acid derivatives on lipid parameters are shown in Table 9.4. Fibrates have a demonstrated effect on lowering TG levels (–36%) and moderately increasing HCL-C levels (+10%); mild reduction in LDL-C (–8%) is also observed.[22] A meta-analysis showed mean reductions in LDL particles (–10%), non-HDL-C (–14%), and apoB (–6%).[41]

2. **Cardiovascular morbidity and mortality in randomized clinical trials**
   a. The 5-year primary prevention Helsinki Heart Study (HHS) showed gemfibrozil was associated with 34% relative reduction in the incidence of coronary heart disease.[42] The most profound effect was achieved in obese patients and patients with high TG or low HDL-C levels.[25,43] The secondary prevention Veterans Affairs HDL Intervention Trial (VA-HIT) showed 22% relative risk reduction in nonfatal myocardial infarction or death from coronary heart disease with gemfibrozil monotherapy.[44] The patients who benefited the most in this study were those with type 2 diabetes.[25,44]
   b. Following these gemfibrozil trials, fenofibrate has been primarily studied in patients with type 2 diabetes.[1] The Fenofibrate Intervention and Event Lowering in Diabetes (FIELD) study failed to show reduction in primary composite outcome of coronary events after treating diabetic patients with fenofibrate for 5 years, while the protocol allowed other lipid-lowering therapies to be started during the study.[45] Although the study did not meet the primary end point, significant reductions in secondary outcomes, such as nonfatal myocardial infarction and cardiovascular events, were shown.[45]
   c. The best results in the cardiovascular outcome were observed among patients younger than 65 years of age and in patients with TG levels of ≥200 mg/dL.[25,45] The Action to Control Cardiovascular Risk in Diabetes (ACCORD) trial did not demonstrate significant reductions in the primary composite outcome of nonfatal myocardial infarction, nonfatal stroke, or fatal cardiovascular events or the secondary outcomes with simvastatin-fenofibrate combination therapy, compared to simvastatin therapy alone.[46]

3. **Cardiovascular morbidity and mortality in reviews and meta-analyses** According to systematic reviews and meta-analyses, fibrate monotherapy was consistently associated with reductions in major cardiovascular events and nonfatal myocardial infarction but not with all-cause mortality.[25,47–54] Although earlier trials showed improvement in clinical outcomes with fibrate monotherapy, more recent trials evaluating a fibrate-statin combination therapy did not provide compelling evidence of benefit.[25]

Table 9.4.	Effects of Fibric Acid Derivatives on Lipid Parameters (Percent Changes from Baseline)			
Drug	TG	LDL-C	HDL-C	Total-C
Fenofibrate/fenofibric acid	−23% to −54%	−31% to +45%	+9% to +23%	−9% to −22%
Gemfibrozil	−20% to −60%	−30% to +30%	+10% to +30%	−2% to −16%

(Adapted from Ito MK. Dyslipidemias. In: Chisholm-Burns MA, et al., eds. *Pharmacotherapy Principles and Practice*. New York, NY: McGraw Hill; 2016.)

Based on a review of subgroup analyses of patient populations who benefited in terms of cardiovascular events, reasonable candidates for a fibrate-statin combination therapy are patients with metabolic syndrome, type 2 diabetes, or severely elevated TG and low HDL-C levels.[25]

G. Adverse drug reactions

1. **Hepatic** The most common ADRs listed under prescribing information are abnormal liver tests, increased ALT, increased AST, increased creatinine kinase (CK), and rhinitis.[26–34]

2. **Muscle associated** The most serious ADR associated with fibrates is myopathy.[22] The incidence of myopathy is known to increase with a fibrate-statin combination therapy, and fibrate monotherapy itself confers a 5.5-fold higher risk than a statin monotherapy.[22,36,55,56] Failure to discontinue the fibrate therapy despite muscle symptoms may lead to rhabdomyolysis even though this is rare.[22,36] Patients with diabetes, renal failure, or hypothyroidism and the elderly may be at an increased risk of myotoxicity.[36] Gemfibrozil has higher incidences of muscle symptoms than fenofibrate, so fenofibrate is considered the fibrate of choice when a combination therapy with a statin is desired.[22,36] A general recommendation is to check a baseline CK level before initiating a second lipid-lowering therapy and to use the lowest dose of a statin or fibrate.[36]

3. **Renal** Elevations of creatinine levels are also well-known ADR of fibrates.[22,36]
   However, these increases in creatinine are reversible, and decreases in glomerular filtration rate are not observed, suggesting an absence of intrinsic renal damage.[22,36] Gemfibrozil seems to have less effect on creatinine than fenofibrate.[36] Prior to initiating a fibrate, baseline serum creatinine should be obtained; if renal function is mild to moderately impaired, gemfibrozil (if patient is not on a statin) or a lower-strength fenofibrate should be considered with periodic monitoring of renal function.[36]

4. **Cholelithiasis** Infrequent incidence of cholelithiasis is also reported with fibrates; if cholelithiasis is suspected while a patient is on a fibrate, gallbladder studies, including ultrasound, is warranted.[36]

5. **Thromboembolic** A small and relatively uncommon increase in venothromboembolic events is another ADR, and elevations in homocysteine levels are suspected to be associated.[22,36] Routine monitoring of plasma homocysteine levels is not necessary as it is not clearly understood how the elevations in homocysteine levels are clinically relevant.[36]
   Overall, fibrates are well tolerated, and the rate of discontinuation was similar to that with placebo.[22,48]

IV.   **Bile Acid Sequestrants**

BASs are the oldest class of cholesterol medications; cholestyramine (Prevalite, Questran), colestipol (Colestid), and colesevelam (Welchol) are used in clinical practice (Table 9.5).[57–61] These products are as a powder for oral suspension, with colestipol and colesevelam also formulated as tablets. Cholestyramine and colestipol are available as generic products.

The indication of BASs is to treat primary hypercholesterolemia as a monotherapy or in combination with a statin.[1] The clinical use of cholestyramine and colestipol is limited due to poor palatability and gastrointestinal tolerance.[62] However, absence of systemic absorption is an advantageous characteristic, and BAS can be safely used in pregnant women and

Table 9.5.	Formulations of BAS			
Generic Name	Brand Name	Formulation	Ingredient Amount per Formulation	Dosage and Administration
Cholestyramine (generic available)	Prevalite Questran Questran Light	Powder for suspension Powder for suspension Powder for suspension	4 g per 5.5 g powder 4 g per 9 g powder 4 g per 5 g powder	• Start at 1 packet once or twice daily. • Titrate to 1-2 packets twice daily at intervals of ≥4 wk. • Max: 6 packets/day
Colestipol (generic available)	Colestid lavored Colestid Colestid	Powder for suspension Powder for suspension (orange flavor) Tablet	5 g per packet 5 g per packet 1 g per tablet	• Start at 1 packet once or twice daily. • Titrate to 1-6 packets once daily or in divided doses at 1- to 2-mo intervals. • Max: 6 packets/day • Start at 2 tablets once or twice daily. • Titrate dose by the increments of 2 tablets once or twice daily at 1- to 2-mo intervals. • Max: 16 tablets/day • Swallow tablets whole. • Take with liquid.
Colesevelam (generic unavailable)	Welchol Welchol	Powder for suspension Tablet	3.75 g packet 1.875 g packet 625 mg	• One 3.75-g packet once daily or one 1.875-g packet twice daily • Mix the packet with 4-8 ounces of water, fruit juice, or diet soft drinks. • Take with a meal. • 6 tablets once daily or 3 tablets twice daily • Take with a meal and liquid.

Data from *Prevalite (cholestyramine) Prescribing Information*. Maple Grove, MN: Upsher-Smith Laboratories, Inc.; 2015;
Questran (cholestyramine) Prescribing Information. Spring Valley, NY: Par Pharmaceutical Companies, Inc.; 2013;
Colestid (colestipol hydrochloride for oral suspension) Prescribing Information. New York, NY: Pharmacia & Upjohn Company; 2014;
Colestid (micronized colestipol hydrochloride tablets) Prescribing Information. New York, NY: Pharmacia & Upjohn Company; 2014;
Welchol (colesevelam) Prescribing Information. Parsippany, NJ: Daiichi Sankyo, Inc.; 2014.

children.[62] Colesevelam has improved gastrointestinal tolerability and specifically carries FDA-approved indications for treating boys and postmenarchal girls who are 10- to 17-year old with heterozygous familial hypercholesterolemia and for improving glycemic control in adults with type 2 diabetes mellitus.[61] Colestimide or colestilan is another BAS but not available in the United States.[63]

A. **Mechanisms of action** BASs bind to cholesterol-rich bile salts in the small intestine and block their enterohepatic recirculation to the liver, increasing fecal excretion of bile acids (Fig. 9.1).[1] This effect upregulates 7α-dehydroxylase, which catalyzes the rate-limiting step of bile acid production, leading to increased flux of intrahepatic cholesterol to synthesize more bile acids.[21] This further reduces intrahepatic cholesterol and upregulates LDL receptor activity, resulting in removal of LDL, intermediate-density lipoprotein (IDL), and VLDL from the systemic circulation.[21] The efficacy of BASs may decline as hepatocytes compensate by increasing cholesterol synthesis with long-term use, signifying a use of another lipid-lowering agent in combination.[21]

With regard to BASs' glycemic effect, various mechanisms have been proposed. Farnesoid X receptors (FXRs) are expressed in the liver and intestine to modulate gene transcription.[10] FXR not only is involved in biosynthesis of bile acids and metabolism of cholesterols but also acts as a glucose sensor in gluconeogenesis, glucagon synthesis, and adipose tissue functionality.[10,63,64] The FXR is inhibited as part of the negative feedback regulation by bile acids.[63] However, BAS makes the bile acid less available and deactivates the inhibition of the FXR.[63] This deactivation of FXR inhibition provides positive metabolic effects.[10,63] Additionally, bile acids bind and activate G protein–coupled receptor, TGR5, which is expressed in the enterohepatic axis, brown adipose tissue, and skeletal muscle.[10,64] The activation of TGR5 induces the hormone, glucagonlike peptide-1, playing a role in insulin production and insulin sensitivity.[10,63] Corresponding to how bile acids participate in energy homeostasis, use of a BAS may positively influence glycemic control in diabetic patients.

B. **Dosage and administration** The formulation of BASs is summarized with dosage and administration instructions in Table 9.5. The oral powder for suspension always need to be mixed with water or other fluid and should not be taken in dry form to avoid accidental inhalation or esophageal distress.[59,61] Cholestyramine oral powder should be mixed with 2-3 ounces of liquid or alternatively can be mixed with applesauce, crushed pineapple, soups, or pulpy fruits.[62] Due to tablet size, oral suspension may be preferred if a patient has difficulty swallowing the tablets. Additionally, it is advisable to swallow one tablet at a time. No dose adjustments are necessary for impaired renal function since BASs are not systemically absorbed.[57–61]

C. **Pharmacokinetics** Cholestyramine and colestipol are insoluble, high molecular weight basic anion exchange polymers and are not absorbed systemically.[57–60] Colesevelam is also an insoluble nondigestible positively charged resin but has a more gelatinous consistency than cholestyramine in the intestinal tract, improving tolerability of this drug.[65] BASs are fecally eliminated as a complex bound with bile acids.[57–61]

D. **Drug interactions** Cholestyramine and colestipol can bind to concomitant oral medications and may delay or reduce the absorption.[57–60] BASs may also disrupt exposure to drugs that undergo enterohepatic circulation due to their bile acid binding effect.[57–61] Other oral medications, including other lipid-lowering agents, should be taken ≥1-hour before or ≥4-hour after taking cholestyramine or colestipol.[57–60] Colesevelam has a unique structure, polyallylamine cross-linked with epichlorohydrin and alkylated groups, which augments interactions with bile salt and reduces potential interactions with other drugs.[65] Owing to the less binding interactions, colesevelam may be taken with other oral medications except those with a narrow therapeutic index.[61] If coadministered drug has a narrow therapeutic index, it is prudent to take the medication ≥4 hours prior to cholestyramine or alternatively to monitor the drug levels.[61]

Drugs known to interact with colesevelam and have decreased exposure are cyclosporine, glimepiride, glipizide, glyburide, olmesartan, and oral contraceptives containing ethinyl diol and norethindrone.[61] Drugs known to interact with colesevelam and to have increased exposure are metformin extended release.[61] Postmarketing reports added interaction of colesevelam with phenytoin (decreased phenytoin levels), warfarin (lowered INR), and thyroid hormone replacement therapy (elevated thyroid-stimulating hormone levels).[61] Phenytoin and thyroid hormone replacement should be administered 4 hours prior to colesevelam, and INR should be monitored more frequently during colesevelam initiation.[61] Colesevelam had no drug-drug interaction with lovastatin and fenofibrate.[61]

E. **Contraindications and precautions**

1. BASs may increase TG levels, so these agents are preferentially initiated at TG level ≤200 mg/dL and need to be avoided at TG level >500 mg/dL.[57–61] Increased TG is particularly noted with colesevelam when this is administered with insulin or sulfonylureas, and this may precipitate as acute pancreatitis.[61] Cholestyramine

is contraindicated in patients with complete biliary obstruction.[57,58] Colesevelam is contraindicated in patients with a history of bowel obstruction or history of hypertriglyceridemia-induced pancreatitis.[61]

2. BASs interfere with fat digestion and absorption and may decrease absorption of fat-soluble vitamins (vitamins A, D, E, and K), iron, folic acid, and magnesium; use caution in patients susceptible to these deficiencies, and supplementation may be considered with long-term use of a BAS.[57-61,66]

3. The oral powder for suspension, except Colestid (tasteless formulation), contains aspartame and therefore phenylalanine; caution should be exercised especially for patients with phenylketonuria.[57-59,61]

F. Efficacy

1. **Lipids** The effects of colesevelam on lipid parameters are summarized in Table 9.6. BASs are known to lower LDL-C moderately (approximately –5% to –30%) in a dose-dependent manner.[1] BAS also mildly increases HDL-C and may increase TG.[57-61] A meta-analysis of BASs showed –9% reduction in LCL particles, –16% reduction in non-HDL-C, and –13% reduction in apoB.[41] According to a review by Agency for Healthcare Research and Quality, combination of a BAS and a statin provided additional 14% reduction of LDL-C.[67] The review also identified that a combination of a low-potency statin and a BAS is more effective than mild-potency statin alone to decrease LDL-C levels.[67] This finding supports the use of a BAS in patients who cannot tolerate dose escalation of statins.

2. **Glucose and HbA1c** Colesevelam was studied to evaluate the effect on HbA1c and fasting plasma glucose levels when added to other existing antidiabetic therapy in patients with type 2 diabetes. The observed reductions in HbA1c from baseline were –0.4% (placebo +0.2%) with metformin, –0.34% (placebo –0.02%) with pioglitazone, –0.3% (placebo +0.2%) with sulfonylurea, and –0.4% (placebo +0.1%) with insulin.[61] The reductions in fasting plasma glucose levels were –3 mg/dL (placebo +11 mg/dL) with metformin, –4.8 mg/dL (placebo +9.9 mg/dL) with pioglitazone, –4 mg/dL (placebo +10 mg/dL) with sulfonylurea, and +2 mg/dL (placebo +16 mg/dL) with insulin.[61]

3. **Cardiovascular events** Despite the documented LDL-C reduction and the metabolic effect, evidence of BASs from randomized controlled trials evaluating cardiovascular outcomes is scarce. In the Lipid Research Clinics Coronary Primary Prevention Trial (LRC-CPPT), 19% risk reduction was observed in the incidence of nonfatal myocardial infarction and death related to coronary heart disease after a

Table 9.6.	Effects of a Colesevelam on Lipid Parameters (Percent Changes from Baseline)					
Therapy	TG	LDL-C	HDL-C	Total-C	Non-HDL-C	ApoB
Colesevelam	+10%	−15%	+3%	−7%	−10%	−12%
Colesevelam + atorvastatin 10 mg	−1%	−48%	+11%	−31%	−40%	−38%
Colesevelam + simvastatin 10 mg	−12%	−42%	+10%	−28%	−37%	−33%
Colesevelam + fenofibrate 160 mg	+6%	−10%	0%	−6%	−8%	−7%

The dosage of colesevelam is 3.8 g (6 tablets).
(Data from *Welchol (colesevelam) Prescribing Information*. Parsippany, NJ: Daiichi Sankyo, Inc.; 2014.)

7-year follow-up of men treated with cholestyramine 24 g/d.[25,68] A study evaluating use of colestipol (5 g 3 times daily) also reported significant decrease in deaths related to coronary heart disease among men, where 20%-30% of participants had a history of atherosclerotic heart disease at the study entry.[25,69] Although BASs were shown to improve cardiovascular outcomes as monotherapy, it is yet unclear whether reduction of LDL-C directly translates to improvement in cardiovascular mortality by a use of a BAS and statin combination therapy.[25]

G. **Adverse drug reactions** The most common ADR of this class is constipation. Predisposing factors for constipation are high dose of BAS and increased age (>60-year old).[57-61] BASs may also worsen preexisting constipation. The dosage of BAS should be gradually increased to prevent development of fecal impaction. Patients should take a BAS with plenty of fluid, and increasing fiber intake is encouraged to alleviate constipation. Use of a stool softener may be needed occasionally. Most constipation cases are mild and transient, but some patients may require a temporary dose reduction or discontinuation of therapy.[57-61] BAS-induced constipation may aggravate hemorrhoids.[57-61]

Besides constipation, other common ADRs are abdominal discomfort, flatulence, nausea, vomiting, and dyspepsia.[57-61] Compared to cholestyramine and colestipol, colesevelam are better tolerated.[65] In terms of the metabolic effect, BASs are not associated with increased risk of hypoglycemia or weight gain.[10]

V.   Niacin

Niacin is water-soluble vitamin B_3; nicotinic acid and nicotinamide are both called niacin, but only nicotinic acid has lipid-modifying effects.[70] Three formulations of niacin marketed to this date are immediate release (IR), sustained release (SR), and extended release (ER).[70] Whereas many over-the-counter niacin supplements have not been officially reviewed by the FDA for the treatment of dyslipidemia, one niacin IR (Niacor) and one niacin ER (Niaspan) products have received an FDA approval (Table 9.7). The niacin ER was available as fixed-dose combination products with lovastatin (Advicor) and simvastatin (Simcor); however, the FDA withdrew approval for these due to safety issues (Table 9.7). A combination product of niacin with laropiprant, a strong antagonist of the prostaglandin D2 receptor, is available in Europe but was not approved by the FDA due to safety concerns.[71] Over-the-counter "no-flush niacin" is also marketed, but the active ingredient is often inositol hexaniacinate, not nicotinic acid.[70] While this "no-flush niacin" or "flush-free niacin" product technically contains niacin, the amount of free or bioavailable niacin is not sufficient to modify lipid levels effectively.[70] In clinical practice, niacin ER is the formulation most preferentially used.

Niacin-containing products available by prescription are indicated for primary hyperlipidemia, mixed dyslipidemia, and hypertriglyceridemia.[72-75] Niacin raises HDL-C levels and is the only currently available agent consistently shown to elevate HDL-C levels[70]; however at present, HDL-C is not a target for therapy. Niacin ER also carries indications to lower risk of recurrent nonfatal myocardial infarction in patients with a history of myocardial infarction and hyperlipidemia.[73] In addition, combination of niacin ER and a BAS is indicated to slow progression or promote regression of atherosclerotic disease in patients with a history of coronary artery disease and hyperlipidemia.[73]

Given the information from recent randomized clinical trials (discussed below), the indications, safety, and efficacy for use of niacin preparations have been questioned. In the 2016 ACC Expert Consensus Decision Pathway on the Role of Non-Statin Therapies for LDL-Cholesterol Lowering in the Management of Atherosclerotic Cardiovascular Disease Risk (JACC Vol. 68, No. 1. 2016 p. 92-125), niacin is not included in any of the treatment

Table 9.7.   FDA-Approved Niacin Products

Generic Name	Brand Name	Formulation	Strength (mg)	Dosage and Administration	Generic Availability
Niacin	Niacor	IR tablet	500	• Start at ½ tablet (250 mg) once daily following the evening meal. • Increase dose every 4-7 d up to 1500-2000 mg/d and maintain this dosage at least for 2 mo. • If necessary, further increase the dose at 2-4 wk intervals to 1000 mg 3 times daily. • Maintenance dose: 1000-2000 mg 2-3 times daily	Yes
Niacin	Niaspan	ER tablet	500, 750, and 1000	• Start at 500 mg once daily. • Do NOT increase dose by >500 mg in any 4-wk period. • Maintenance dose: 1000-2000 mg once daily • Take at bedtime with a low-fat snack. • Swallow each tablet whole.	Yes
Niacin/ lovastatin	Advicor	ER (niacin) tablet	500/20, 750/20, 1000/20, and 1000/40	• Niacin dose must be titrated (as Niaspan). • Maintenance dose: 500/20-2000/40 mg once daily • Take at bedtime with a low-fat snack. • Swallow each tablet whole.	No
Niacin/ simvastatin	Simcor	ER (niacin) tablet	500/20, 500/40, 750/20, 1000/20, and 1000/40	• Niacin dose must be titrated (as Niaspan). • Maintenance dose: 500/20-2000/40 mg once daily • Take at bedtime with a low-fat snack. • Swallow each tablet whole.	No

Data from *Niacor (niacin) Prescribing Information*. Minneapolis, MN: Upsher-Smith Laboratories, Inc.; 2000; *Niaspan (niacin extended-release) Prescribing Information*. North Chicago, IL: AbbVie Inc.; 2015; *Advicor (niacin extended-release/lovastatin) Prescribing Information*. North Chicago, IL: AbbVie Inc.; 2013; *Simcor (niacin extended-release/simvastatin) Prescribing Information*. North Chicago, IL: AbbVie Inc.; 2013.

algorithms. Information on niacin is presented here as to help the practitioner to determine when this class of medications may be helpful.

A. **Mechanism of action** Niacin has been proposed to act on several pathways to exert various lipid-modifying effects (Fig. 9.1). One proposed mechanism is inhibition of adenosine triphosphate synthase β-chain expression, which decreases catabolic rate of HDL and increases the half-life.[70] Another mechanism is increased level and production rate of apoA-I, which functions in HDL assembly and in reverse cholesterol transport, without affecting apoA-II known to have deleterious effect on cardiovascular health.[76,77] Niacin also decreases hepatic cholesteryl ester transfer protein (CETP) expression and the activity.[70] CETP is a protein catalyzing 1:1 exchange of cholesteryl ester in HDL for TG in VLDL, IDL, and LDL, and the CETP inhibition increases HDL levels.[76] Besides these mechanisms raising HDL, niacin inhibits diacylglycerol O-acyltransferase 2, an enzyme essential for TG synthesis, decreasing the availability of TG for subsequent lipoprotein production.[70] Increased degradation of apoB, a key component of VLDL, LDL, and lipoprotein(a), is similarly reported with niacin, resulting in decreased synthesis of these apoB-containing lipoproteins.[70,71] Niacin may activate the G protein–coupled hydroxy-carboxylic acid receptor 2, also termed GPR-109A, in adipose tissue.[70,76] This GPR-109A inhibition is considered to suppress the free fatty acid flux from the adipose tissue to the liver, reducing VLDL production.[70,76]

In addition to the ability to increase the level of HDL and to reduce atherogenic lipoprotein levels, various pleiotropic effects of niacin have also been studied. One well-documented pleiotropic effect of niacin is anti-inflammatory property, which may be independent of changes in plasma lipids.[76] Antioxidant property and improved endothelial vasorelaxation are also reported with niacin.[70,76]

B. Dosage and administration FDA-approved niacin products are summarized with the information on dosage and administration in Table 9.7.

1. **Dose** A minimum dose of 1 g/d is required for the LDL-modifying effect, while the greatest efficacy for both LDL-C and triglycerides lowering is seen at 2 g/d.[21]

2. **Administration** Taking niacin with low-fat meal or snack is recommended to reduce the risk of gastrointestinal upset and to slow the absorption, which may also help reduce severity of flushing, one of the most bothersome ADRs of niacin.[73] More specifically, niacin IR is recommended to be best taken in the middle of a meal instead of just before or after a meal.[78] Although niacin ER has better tolerability in terms of flushing, it is recommended to administer niacin at bedtime and to use non-enteric-coated aspirin 325 mg, ibuprofen 200 mg, or other nonsteroidal anti-inflammatory drug 30 minutes prior to taking the niacin to minimize the flushing by inhibiting the prostaglandin synthesis.[62,78] It is advisable to time alcohol, hot or spicy foods/beverages, and hot baths/showers sufficiently before or after niacin administration to prevent worsening of flushing.[78] If niacin is discontinued for an extended period (≥3 days), dose needs to be titrated upward again from the lowest dose to safely reinstitute the therapy.[72–75,78] If a patient is switching from niacin IR to niacin ER, the lowest dose of niacin ER should be initiated, followed by gradual dose titration.[73]

C. Pharmacokinetics The concentrations of niacin in systemic circulation are dose dependent but can be highly variable owing to the extensive and saturable first-pass metabolism.[73] Niacin is metabolized via two pathways. In the first conjugation pathway, niacin is conjugated with glycine and forms nicotinuric acid.[73] When the nicotinuric acid concentration increases, this causes vasodilation, leading to flushing.[71] In the second amidation pathway, niacin forms nicotinamide and pyrimidine products after redox reactions.[70,71]

The conjugation pathway is a low-affinity high-capacity pathway, whereas the amidation pathway is a high-affinity low-capacity pathway.[71] Therefore, niacin IR can quickly saturate the amination pathway and more readily undergoes the conjugation pathway, causing significant flushing.

In contrast, niacin SR is more extensively metabolized by the amidation pathway. Niacin slowly released over 12 hours does not saturate the amidation pathway and accumulates hepatotoxic metabolites, causing a higher incidence of dose-related hepatotoxicity.[62,70] In terms of dissolution rate, niacin ER falls between the IR and SR formulations, providing a better safety profile than niacin IR and niacin SR.[70] Both niacin and metabolites are excreted renally.[73]

D. Drug interactions Niacin has few drug interactions. Due to binding effect of BASs, niacin ER should be separated from cholestyramine or colestipol by at least 4-6 hours.[62,73] If niacin at a dose >1 g/d is to be combined with a statin, caution is necessary due to case reports of myopathy/rhabdomyolysis.[73]

Clinical evidence and postmarketing surveillance studies do not support a common occurrence of muscle symptoms from niacin either alone or in combination with a statin.[70,78] Higher-risk patient populations for the myotoxicity are elderly patients and patients with diabetes, renal failure, or uncontrolled hypothyroidism, and these patients should be monitored carefully for any signs and symptoms of muscle pain, tenderness, or weakness.[73]

Small dose-related reductions in platelet count and small increases in prothrombin time are reported with niacin though niacin can be safely used in patients receiving warfarin.[73,78] Platelet counts and prothrombin time may be monitored closely if niacin is coadministered with an anticoagulant.[73]

E. Contraindications and precautions

1. **Liver** Niacin is extensively metabolized by the liver and is contraindicated in patients with active liver disease, including unexplained persistent elevations in hepatic transaminase levels.[73] With a past history of jaundice, hepatobiliary disease, or peptic ulcer disease or with substantial alcohol consumption, patients should be monitored closely for hepatotoxicity.[73] It is recommended to obtain serum transaminase levels prior to treatment initiation, every 6-12 weeks during the first year, and periodically thereafter.[73]

2. **Renal** Since the major route of elimination is renal excretion, niacin should be used with caution in patients with renal impairment.[73] Niacin needs to be cautiously administered in patients with unstable angina or in the acute phase of a myocardial infarction especially if another vasoactive drug is used, such as nitrates, calcium channel blockers, or adrenergic blocking agents.[73]

3. **Gout and phosphorous** Uric acid level may become elevated due to competitive inhibition of tubular secretion by niacin.[73] Caution is needed for patients predisposed to gout by measuring a uric acid level at baseline and periodically thereafter.[73,78] Small dose-dependent reductions in phosphorus levels have been reported with niacin; periodic monitoring of phosphorus levels is not necessary unless patients are at risk for hypophosphatemia.[73,78]

F. Efficacy

1. **Lipid lowering** The dose-dependent effect of niacin on lipid parameters is summarized in Table 9.8. In a systematic review, niacin decreased LDL-P by 14%, non-HDL-C by 14%, and apoB by 15% for patients who received 0.5-3 g niacin.[41] Gender effect exists in response to niacin, and women tend to respond slightly better than men.[73] Overall, niacin can substantially lower LDL-C, TG, apoB, and lipoprotein(a) levels while favorably changing LDL particle size and number.[70,76] Niacin is considered the most potent agent to raise HDL-C although HDL-C again is not a target for therapy.[70,76]

Table 9.8. Effects of Niacin ER on Lipid Parameters in a Dose Escalation Study (Percent Changes from Baseline)

Dose	TG	LDL-C	HDL-C	Total-C	ApoB
500 mg	−5%	−3%	+10%	−2%	−2%
1000 mg	−11%	−9%	+15%	−5%	−7%
1500 mg	−28%	−14%	+22%	−11%	−15%
2000 mg	−35%	−17%	+26%	−12%	−16%

Data from *Niaspan (niacin extended-release) Prescribing Information*. North Chicago, IL: AbbVie Inc.; 2015.

2. **Morbidity and mortality**

   a. The first study, which investigated how niacin would affect mortality, was the coronary drug project (CDP). After 6.5 years of follow-up, niacin IR (up to 3 g/d) decreased the risk of stroke by 24%, myocardial infarction by 26%, and coronary revascularization by 67% among men with prior history of myocardial infarction.[79] Although no significant reduction in mortality was observed at this 6.5-year follow-up, a post hoc analysis after 15 years of follow-up demonstrated reduction in total mortality by 11% in the niacin group, compared to the placebo group.[79,80]

   b. The initial study, which examined the effect of niacin combined with a statin, was the HDL Atherosclerosis Treatment Study (HATS) conducted among patients with coronary heart disease. In this study, the incidence of major clinical events, including death, myocardial infarction, stroke, and revascularization, was significantly reduced in the niacin plus simvastatin group by 90% after 38 months.[81]

   c. One limitation of the HATS was a lack of statin-only arm, and the Arterial Biology for the Investigation of the Treatment Effects of Reducing Cholesterol (ARBITER) trials were conducted to evaluate the effect of adding niacin ER in addition to existing statin therapy on carotid intima-media thickness.[82–84] Among patients with coronary heart disease and receiving a statin, the addition of niacin ER 1 g daily showed no progression of carotid intima-media thickness at 12 months (ARBITER-2), followed by regression after additional 12 months in the open-label extension (ARBITER-3).[82,83] In the ARBITER-6, patients were randomized to receive either niacin ER with target dose of 2 g daily or ezetimibe 10 mg daily, in combination with a preexisting statin, and this study was prematurely terminated due to adjudicated benefit of niacin ER.[84]

   d. On the contrary, the Atherothrombosis Intervention in Metabolic Syndrome with Low HDL/High Triglycerides: Impact on Global Health Outcomes (AIM-HIGH) trial was stopped early after a mean follow-up of 3 years due to a lack of benefit in the niacin group.[85] In the AIM-HIGH, patients (85% men, 92% white) with established cardiovascular disease were randomized to receive niacin ER with a dose titration to 1500 mg/d or 2000 mg/d or placebo, which contained niacin IR 50 mg. For patients in the AIM-HIGH, LDL-C levels were optimally controlled by simvastatin with or without ezetimibe, and despite favorable changes in HDL-C, TG, and LDL-C, no significant reduction in major cardiovascular events was observed with the niacin therapy.[85]

   e. The results of the AIM-HIGH suggested that raising HDL-C levels may not result in additional reduction in cardiovascular events if LDL-C levels are at an optimal level by a use of a statin.[70] This was supported by a post hoc analysis of the Justification for the Use of Statins in Primary Prevention: An Intervention Trial Evaluating Rosuvastatin (JUPITER) trial, where HDL-C level was not a predictive factor of residual vascular risk once LDL-C levels were lowered by the statin therapy.[86] The finding of the AIM-HIGH did not terminate Heart Protection Study 2: Treatment of the HDL to Reduce the Incidence of Vascular Events (HPS2-THRIVE) study, which had a more diverse patient cohort. In the HPS2-THRIVE, niacin ER plus laropiprant was added to simvastatin for patients with a history of cardiovascular disease. Aligning with the results of the AIM-HIGH, the HPS2-THRIVE did not demonstrate a significant reduction in the incidence of major vascular events after 3.9 years of follow-up by the addition of niacin to simvastatin.[87]

Although early study of niacin IR achieved better cardiovascular outcomes, adding niacin to moderate-to-intensive statin therapy was not proven to reduce cardiovascular events in patients with established coronary heart disease. Without proven mortality benefits, indication of niacin as an add-on therapy to a statin remains unclear at this moment.

G. Adverse drug reactions

1. One of the most well-known ADR of niacin is flushing, which may adversely affect adherence to this therapy. It is important to educate patients on certain preventive measures (refer to the Dosage and Administration section above) and to let patients know that flushing typically starts to diminish by the fourth week of therapy as tachyphylaxis develops with continued use.[88] After 1 year of consistent use, most patients experience no flushing at all.[78] Niacin-induced flushing can be distinguished from hot flush in menopausal women by the absence of diaphoresis.[78]

2. Flushing is more common with niacin IR, while hepatotoxicity is associated more with niacin SR.[70] Due to the higher risk of hepatotoxicity, niacin SR is rarely used and is not currently available by prescription in the United States.[70] Niacin ER has not been significantly associated with hepatotoxicity and has a lower incidence of flushing than niacin IR, making the ER formulation most preferable.[70]

3. Besides flushing, other common ADRs (incidence > 5%) are diarrhea, nausea, vomiting, increased cough, and pruritus though diarrhea, nausea, and vomiting are uncommon at a dose <2000 mg/d.[73,78]

4. Niacin may increase fasting blood glucose, and dose-dependent increase in glucose intolerance is reported in diabetic patients.[73] Increase in glucose levels can be transient and reversible with continued therapy.[10,89] However, the increased insulin resistance could also lead to an increased incidence of new-onset diabetes mellitus.[70] The concern of hyperglycemia was mostly originated from early studies, where much higher doses of niacin were used than recommended today.[62,78] Fasting glucose levels should be periodically monitored in all patients, particularly in patients with diabetes mellitus, during initiation of niacin and dose titration.[70,73] The glucose dysregulation may be less prominent with the ER formulation, lower dosages, and gradual titration.[10]

   Although changes in fasting plasma glucose and HbA1c levels are not likely large (increase of 4%-5% in fasting glucose and of ≤0.3% in HbA1c), diet and/or antidiabetic therapy may need to be adjusted to maintain optimal glycemic control.[62,73,89]

VI. Cholesterol Absorption Inhibitor

The only cholesterol absorption inhibitor currently available in the United States is ezetimibe (Zetia) (Table 9.9). Ezetimibe is also formulated as a fixed-dose combination with simvastatin (Vytorin) and with atorvastatin (Liptruzet) (Table 9.9). Ezetimibe is indicated as an adjunct to diet to[39] (1) reduce elevated total-C, LDL-C, apoB, and non-HDL-C in primary hyperlipidemia (with or without a statin) or in mixed hyperlipidemia (with or without fenofibrate), (2) reduce elevated total-C and LDL-C in homozygous familial hypercholesterolemia (with atorvastatin or simvastatin), and (3) reduce elevated sitosterol and campesterol in patients with homozygous sitosterolemia (phytosterolemia).

Table 9.9.   Ezetimibe Products

Generic Name	Brand Name	Strength and Form	Dosage and Administration	Generic Availability
Ezetimibe	Zetia	10 mg tablet	• 10 mg (1 tablet) once daily • Take with or without food.	Yes
Ezetimibe/atorvastatin	Liptruzet	10/10, 10/20, 10/40, 10/80 mg tablet	• Start at 10/10 or 10/20 mg/day. • Start at 10/40 mg/d if requiring >55% reduction in LDL-C.	No
Ezetimibe/simvastatin	Vytorin	10/10, 10/20, 10/40, 10/80 mg tablet	• Start at 10/10 or 10/20 mg/day. • Do not use 10/80 mg dose unless patients have been taking this strength chronically (≥12 mo) with no evidence of muscle toxicity. • 10/40 mg dose should not be titrated to 10/80 mg.	No

Data from *Zetia (ezetimibe) Prescribing Information*. Whitehouse Station, NJ: Merck & Co., Inc.; 2013;
Liptruzet (ezetimibe and atorvastatin) Prescribing Information. Whitehouse Station, NJ: Merck & Co., Inc.; 2014;
Vytorin (ezetimibe and simvastatin) Prescribing Information. Whitehouse Station, NJ: Merck & Co., Inc.; 2015.

A. **Mechanism of action** Ezetimibe was originally developed as a potential inhibitor of intracellular acyl-coenzyme A cholesterol acyltransferase.[92] However, the development actually led to identification of ezetimibe as a cholesterol absorption inhibitor.

The molecular target of ezetimibe is the sterol transporter called Niemann-Pick C1-like 1 (NPC1L1) located at the brush border of the small intestine (Fig. 9.1).[39,92] The NPC1L1 transporter is involved in the intestinal uptake of cholesterol and phytosterols, and the binding of ezetimibe inhibits this transporter, leading to decreased delivery of intestinal cholesterol to the liver.[39,92] This reduction in cholesterol delivery results in upregulation of hepatic LDL receptors to take up LDL particles from the circulation.[1] This MOA is considered to be complementary to that of statins and of fenofibrate, supporting use of combination therapy.[39]

B. **Dosage and administration** Ezetimibe is given once daily at a dose of 10 mg with or without food, and no dose titration is necessary (Table 9.9).

C. **Pharmacokinetics** After absorption, ezetimibe is extensively conjugated to a pharmacologically active phenolic glucuronide, ezetimibe-glucuronide, which is highly bound (>90%) to human plasma proteins.[39] Ezetimibe undergoes enterohepatic recycling prior to biliary and renal excretion, which is the major route of elimination for ezetimibe and ezetimibe-glucuronide, respectively.[39]

D. **Drug interactions** Clinically significant drug interactions are reported with cholestyramine, colestipol, warfarin, cyclosporine, and fibrates.[39,62] Ezetimibe needs to be taken ≥2 hours prior to or ≥4 hours after administration of cholestyramine or colestipol to maintain adequate exposure to ezetimibe.[39,62]

If ezetimibe is initiated in patients receiving warfarin, additional INR monitoring is advised due to postmarketing reports indicating potential elevation of INR.[39,62] When cyclosporine and ezetimibe are coadministered, caution is necessary due to increased exposure to both medications, especially in patients with severe renal insufficiency.[39] Cyclosporine concentrations should be monitored closely when ezetimibe is administered with cyclosporine. Fibrates may increase cholesterol excretion into the bile, which may result in cholelithiasis with ezetimibe.[39] In a case of suspected cholelithiasis, gallbladder studies are indicated, and alternative lipid-modifying therapy should be considered.[39] Due to insufficient data with other fibrates, fenofibrate is the only fibrate recommended with concomitant ezetimibe.[39]

E. **Contraindications and precautions** The only contraindication specific to ezetimibe is hypersensitivity to product components; contraindications of a statin or fenofibrate apply when a combination therapy is used.[39] Ezetimibe is not recommended in patients with moderate to severe hepatic impairment due to unknown effects of increased exposure to the drug.[39] If simvastatin and ezetimibe combination therapy is used in patients with moderate to severe renal impairment (estimated glomerular filtration rate <60 mL/min/1.73 m^2), the dose of simvastatin should not exceed 20 mg.[39]

F. **Efficacy**

1. **Lipids** The effects of ezetimibe on lipid parameters are summarized in Table 9.10. Ezetimibe provides moderate reduction in LDL-C, TG, and non–HDL-C and small increase in HDL-C. The maximal response, in terms of lipid-modifying effect, is generally achieved within 2 weeks and maintained during continued therapy.[39]

2. **Morbidity and mortality**
   a. Evidence on the vascular effects of ezetimibe on atherosclerosis progression has not been entirely consistent. While the Stop Atherosclerosis in Native Diabetics Study (SANDS) and the Vytorin on Carotid Intima-Media Thickness and Overall Arterial Rigidity (VYCTOR) study showed atherosclerosis regression, negative outcomes are reported by the Ezetimibe and Simvastatin in Hypercholesterolemic Enhances Atherosclerosis Regression (ENHANCE) trial and the ARBITER-6.[93–96]
   b. The first study investigating the effect of ezetimibe on major cardiovascular events was Simvastatin and Ezetimibe in Aortic Stenosis (SEAS) trial. In the SEAS, no significant benefit was demonstrated in reducing the primary outcome of major cardiovascular events when patients with mild-to-moderate aortic stenosis were treated for 4 years with ezetimibe/simvastatin 10/40 mg, despite achievement of LDL-C reduction.[97] The Study of Heart and Renal Protection (SHARP) trial examined the clinical outcome benefit of ezetimibe/simvastatin 10/20 mg in patients with chronic kidney disease.[98] After 5 years of therapy, 17% reduction was demonstrated in major atherosclerotic events, and the risk reduction was proportional to magnitude of LDL-C reduction.[98]
   c. One of the largest trials investigating the incremental benefit of adding a non-statin treatment to a statin was the Improved Reduction of Outcomes: Vytorin

Table 9.10.   Effects of Ezetimibe on Lipid Parameters (Percent Changes from Baseline)

Treatment	TG	LDL-C	HDL-C	Total-C	Non-HDL-C	ApoB
Ezetimibe	−8%	−18%	+1%	−13%	−16%	−16%
Ezetimibe + ongoing statin	−14%	−25%	+3%	−17%	−23%	−19%
Ezetimibe + fenofibrate	−44%	−20%	+19%	−22%	−30%	−26%

Data from *Zetia (ezetimibe) Prescribing Information*. Whitehouse Station, NJ: Merck & Co., Inc.; 2013.

Efficacy International Trial (IMPROVE-IT). In the IMPROVE-IT, ezetimibe/ simvastatin 10/40 mg and simvastatin 40 mg monotherapy were compared in patients with acute coronary syndrome.[99] After 6 years of therapy, 2% reduction was shown in the composite primary outcome of cardiovascular death, nonfatal myocardial infarction, coronary revascularization, nonfatal stroke, or unstable angina necessitating rehospitalization.[99] While the IMPROVE-IT revalidated that the goal of achieving low LDL-C levels is clinically relevant, the interpretation of the study is slightly challenging. The risk reduction achieved by the addition of ezetimibe was relatively small, and the used statin was moderate-intensity even though the current guideline recommends high-intensity statins in this patient population.

Ezetimibe was shown to be effective in lowering LDL-C as a monotherapy or as a combination therapy with a statin. The evidence on the atherosclerosis progression and major clinical outcomes has been mixed. However, the finding from the IMPROVE-IT supports the use of ezetimibe in patients with acute coronary syndrome. Ezetimibe as an add-on therapy can be a beneficial treatment option when further LDL-C reduction is desired in case patient is not tolerating a high-intensity statin.

G. **Adverse drug reactions** Ezetimibe is well tolerated with minimal adverse reactions.[62,100] Reported with ezetimibe monotherapy (incidence ≥ 2%) include upper respiratory infection, diarrhea, arthralgia, sinusitis, and pain in extremity.[39] Although small increase in the incidence of hepatic aminotransferase elevations is reported with combination therapy of ezetimibe and a statin, this increase may not be significant, compared to statin therapy alone.[62,100] Baseline liver tests should be obtained when ezetimibe is added to an ongoing statin for a monitoring purpose.[39] The combination therapy of ezetimibe and a statin also does not appear to increase incidence of elevated creatinine kinase levels or myositis, compared to statin monotherapy.[100] However, ezetimibe and any statin or fenofibrate should be immediately discontinued if myopathy is diagnosed or suspected.[39]

VII. Place in Therapy for Nonstatin Medications

1. While statin therapy is considered the first line, nonstatin medications play an important role in cholesterol management. In order to select appropriate therapy for patients, clinicians need to know the unique properties of these medications and available evidence for lowering risks of ASCVD and mortality.

2. According to the 2013 American College of Cardiology (ACC)/American Heart Association Guideline, "clinicians treating high-risk patients who have a less than-anticipated response to statins, who are unable to tolerate a less-than recommended intensity of a statin, or who are completely statin intolerant, may consider the addition of a nonstatin cholesterol lowering therapy."[101] To follow up this recommendation, the ACC published expert consensus in 2016 on the use of nonstatins. According to this consensus, add-on nonstatin therapy may be considered in four major statin benefit groups identified in the 2013 guideline: (1) ≥21-year-old patients with clinical ASCVD, (2) ≥21-year-old patients with LDL-C ≥190 mg/dL, (3) 40- to 75-year-old patients with diabetes and LDL-C 70-189 mg/dL, and (4) 40- to 75-year-old patients with LDL-C 70-189 mg/dL and 10-year ASCVD risk ≥7.5% estimated by the Pooled Cohort Equations (Table 9.11).[101,102]

Table 9.11.   Consideration of an Add-on Nonstatin Medication According to the 2016 ACC Consensus

Major Statin Benefit Group	Subcategory of the Group	Statin Use	Criteria for Consideration of Adding Nonstatin Medication with Maximally Tolerated Statin	Treatment Options
1. ≥21-year-old patients with clinical ASCVD	**A.** Without comorbidities	Secondary prevention	• <50% LDL-C reduction • LDL-C ≥100 mg/dL	• Consider ezetimibe first • BAS may be considered first if ezetimibe intolerant and TG <300 mg/dL • Consider adding or replacing with PCSK9 inhibitor second
	B. With comorbidities	Secondary prevention	• <50% LDL-C reduction • LDL-C ≥70 mg/dL • Non-HDL-C ≥100 mg/dL	
	C. Baseline LDL-C ≥190 mg/dL	Secondary prevention	• <50% LDL-C reduction or • LDL-C ≥70 mg/dL	
2. ≥21-year-old patients with LDL-C ≥190 mg/dL (without ASCVD)		Primary prevention	• <50% LDL-C reduction • LDL-C ≥100 mg/dL	• Consider ezetimibe or PCSK9 inhibitor. • BAS may be considered first if ezetimibe intolerant and TG <300 mg/dL • BAS is a second line
3. 40- to 75-year-old patients with LDL-C 70-189 mg/dL and diabetes (without ASCVD)		Primary prevention	• <50% LDL-C reduction • LDL-C ≥100 mg/dL • Non-HDL-C ≥130 mg/dL	• Consider ezetimibe • BAS may be considered first if ezetimibe intolerant and TG <300 mg/dL • BAS is a second line
4. 40- to 75-year-old patients with LDL-C 70-189 mg/dL and 10-y ASCVD risk ≥7.5% (without ASCVD or diabetes)		Primary prevention	• <50% LDL-C reduction • LDL-C ≥100 mg/dL	

Adapted from Lloyd-Jones DM, et al. 2016 ACC expert consensus decision pathway on the role of nonstatin therapies for LDL-cholesterol lowering in the management of atherosclerotic cardiovascular disease risk: a report of the American College of Cardiology Task Force on Clinical Expert Consensus Documents. *J Am Coll Cardiol.* 2016;68:92-125.

3. Evaluation before adding another therapy includes (1) therapy adherence, (2) lifestyle modification, (3) intensity of statin therapy, (4) statin intolerance, (5) control of other risk factors, and (6) referral to a lipid specialist and a registered dietician nutritionist.[102] Criteria, which may prompt consideration of adding a nonstatin medication, are listed in Table 9.11.

4. The 2016 ACC consensus points out that before adding the second agent, clinician-patient discussion should take place to consider (1) potential for additional ASCVD risk reduction, (2) potential for adverse events or drug interactions, and (3) patient's preference.[102]

5. Ezetimibe is recommended in all four groups as a first line with maximally tolerant statin (Table 9.11).[102] BAS is considered second line but may be considered first if a patient is ezetimibe intolerant and TG <300 mg/dL (Table 9.11).[102] Currently, niacin does not have a clear indication for a routine use as an add-on therapy due to lack of evidence proving efficacy outweighing the potential harms.[102] Omega-3 FAs and fibrates are not addressed in the 2016 ACC consensus because these are the agents primarily used in hypertriglyceridemia. It is essential to understand the primary action and unique properties of each nonstatin therapy, so that clinicians can select the most effective and safe treatment for the individual patient and for his/her therapy goal.

References

1. Gotto AM Jr, Moon JE. Pharmacotherapies for lipid modification: beyond the statins. *Nat Rev Cardiol.* 2013;10(10):560-570.
2. De Caterina R. n-3 fatty acids in cardiovascular disease. *N Engl J Med.* 2011;364(25):2439-2450.
3. *Lovaza (omega-3-acid ethyl esters) Prescribing Information.* Research Triangle Park, NC: GlaxoSimithKline; 2014.
4. *Omtryg (omega-3-acid ethyl esters A) Prescribing Information.* Arlington, VA: Trygg Pharma, Inc.; 2014.
5. *Epanova (omega-3-carboxylic acids) Prescribing Information.* Wilmington, DE: AstraZeneca Pharmaceuticals LP; 2014.
6. *Vascepa (icosapent ethyl) Prescribing Information.* Bedminster, NJ: Amarin Pharma Inc.; 2015.
7. Weintraub HS. Overview of prescription omega-3 fatty acid products for hypertriglyceridemia. *Postgrad Med.* 2014;126(7):7-18.
8. Bays HE, et al. Prescription omega-3 fatty acids and their lipid effects: physiologic mechanisms of action and clinical implications. *Expert Rev Cardiovasc Ther.* 2008;6(3):391-409.
9. Christou GA, et al. Confronting the residual cardiovascular risk beyond statins: the role of fibrates, omega-3 fatty acids, or niacin, in diabetic patients. *Curr Pharm Des.* 2014;20(22):3675-3688.
10. Zafrir B, Jain M. Lipid-lowering therapies, glucose control and incident diabetes: evidence, mechanisms and clinical implications. *Cardiovasc Drugs Ther.* 2014;28(4):361-377.
11. Offman E, et al. Steady-state bioavailability of prescription omega-3 on a low-fat diet is significantly improved with a free fatty acid formulation compared with an ethyl ester formulation: the ECLIPSE II study. *Vasc Health Risk Manag.* 2013;9:563-573.
12. Davidson MH, et al. A novel omega-3 free fatty acid formulation has dramatically improved bioavailability during a low-fat diet compared with omega-3-acid ethyl esters: the ECLIPSE (Epanova compared to Lovaza in a pharmacokinetic single-dose evaluation) study. *J Clin Lipidol.* 2012;6(6):573-584.
13. Wachira JK, Larson MK, Harris WS. n-3 Fatty acids affect haemostasis but do not increase the risk of bleeding: clinical observations and mechanistic insights. *Br J Nutr.* 2014;111(9):1652-1662.
14. Harris WS, et al. Safety and efficacy of Omacor in severe hypertriglyceridemia. *J Cardiovasc Risk.* 1997;4(5-6):385-391.
15. Pownall HJ, et al. Correlation of serum triglyceride and its reduction by omega-3 fatty acids with lipid transfer activity and the neutral lipid compositions of high-density and low-density lipoproteins. *Atherosclerosis.* 1999;143(2):285-297.
16. Kastelein JJ, et al. Omega-3 free fatty acids for the treatment of severe hypertriglyceridemia: the EpanoVa fOr Lowering Very high triglyceridEs (EVOLVE) trial. *J Clin Lipidol.* 2014;8(1):94-106.
17. Bays HE, et al. Icosapent ethyl, a pure EPA omega-3 fatty acid: effects on lipoprotein particle concentration and size in patients with very high triglyceride levels (the MARINE study). *J Clin Lipidol.* 2012;6(6):565-572.
18. Davidson MH, et al. Efficacy and tolerability of adding prescription omega-3 fatty acids 4 g/d to simvastatin 40 mg/d in hypertriglyceridemic patients: an 8-week, randomized, double-blind, placebo-controlled study. *Clin Ther.* 2007;29(7):1354-1367.
19. Maki KC, et al. A highly bioavailable omega-3 free fatty acid formulation improves the cardiovascular risk profile in high-risk, statin-treated patients with residual hypertriglyceridemia (the ESPRIT trial). *Clin Ther.* 2013;35(9):1400.e1-3-1411.e1-3.
20. Ballantyne CM, et al. Efficacy and safety of eicosapentaenoic acid ethyl ester (AMR101) therapy in statin-treated patients with persistent high triglycerides (from the ANCHOR study). *Am J Cardiol.* 2012;110(7):984-992.
21. Tiwari V, Khokhar M. Mechanism of action of anti-hypercholesterolemia drugs and their resistance. *Eur J Pharmacol.* 2014;741:156-170.
22. Ito MK. Long-chain omega-3 fatty acids, fibrates and niacin as therapeutic options in the treatment of hypertriglyceridemia: a review of the literature. *Atherosclerosis.* 2015;242(2):647-656.
23. Sakabe M, et al. Omega-3 polyunsaturated fatty acids prevent atrial fibrillation associated with heart failure but not atrial tachycardia remodeling. *Circulation.* 2007;116(19):2101-2109.
24. Geleijnse JM, et al. Blood pressure response to fish oil supplementation: metaregression analysis of randomized trials. *J Hypertens.* 2002;20(8):1493-1499.
25. Sando KR, Knight M. Nonstatin therapies for management of dyslipidemia: a review. *Clin Ther.* 2015;37(10):2153-2179.
26. *Fenoglide (fenofibrate) Prescribing Information.* San Diego, CA: Santarus, Inc.; 2012.
27. *Lipofen (fenofibrate) Prescribing Information.* Montgomery, AL: Kowa Pharmaceuticals America, Inc.; 2013.
28. *Triglide (fenofibrate) Prescribing Information.* Florham Park, NJ: Shionogi Inc.; 2015.
29. *Antara (fenofibrate) Prescribing Information.* Baltimore, MD: Lupin Pharma; 2015.
30. *Lofibra (fenofibrate) Prescribing Information.* Sellersville, PA: Gate Pharmaceuticals; 2010.
31. *Tricor (fenofibrate) Prescribing Information.* North Chicago, IL: AbbVie, Inc.; 2013.
32. *Fibricor (fenofibric acid) Prescribing Information.* Philadelphia, PA: Mutual Pharmaceutical Company, Inc.; 2014.
33. *Trilipix (fenofibric acid) Prescribing Information.* North Chicago, IL: AbbVie Inc.; 2015.

34. *Lopid (gemfibrozil) Prescribing Information.* New York, NY: Parke-Davis; 2014.
35. Wierzbicki AS, Viljoen A. Fibrates and niacin: is there a place for them in clinical practice? *Expert Opin Pharmacother.* 2014;15(18):2673-2680.
36. Davidson MH, et al. Safety considerations with fibrate therapy. *Am J Cardiol.* 2007;99(6A):3C-18C.
37. Kasiske B, et al. Clinical practice guidelines for managing dyslipidemias in kidney transplant patients: a report from the Managing Dyslipidemias in Chronic Kidney Disease Work Group of the National Kidney Foundation Kidney Disease Outcomes Quality Initiative. *Am J Transplant.* 2004;4(suppl 7):13-53.
38. Ling H, Tuoma JT, Hilleman D. A review of currently available fenofibrate and fenofibric acid formulations. *Cardiol Res.* 2013;4(2):47-55.
39. *Zetia (ezetimibe) Prescribing Information.* Whitehouse Station, NJ: Merck & Co., Inc.; 2013.
40. Ito MK. Dyslipidemias. In: Chisholm-Burns MA, et al., eds. *Pharmacotherapy Principles and Practice.* New York, NY: McGraw Hill; 2016.
41. Rosenson RS, Underberg JA. Systematic review: evaluating the effect of lipid-lowering therapy on lipoprotein and lipid values. *Cardiovasc Drugs Ther.* 2013;27(5):465-479.
42. Frick MH, et al. Helsinki Heart Study: primary-prevention trial with gemfibrozil in middle-aged men with dyslipidemia. Safety of treatment, changes in risk factors, and incidence of coronary heart disease. *N Engl J Med.* 1987;317(20):1237-1245.
43. Tenkanen L, Manttari M, Manninen V. Some coronary risk-factors related to the insulin-resistance syndrome and treatment with gemfibrozil—experience from the Helsinki Heart-Study. *Circulation.* 1995;92(7):1779-1785.
44. Rubins HB, et al. Gemfibrozil for the secondary prevention of coronary heart disease in men with low levels of high-density lipoprotein cholesterol. Veterans affairs high-density lipoprotein cholesterol intervention trial study group. *N Engl J Med.* 1999;341(6):410-418.
45. Keech A, et al. Effects of long-term fenofibrate therapy on cardiovascular events in 9795 people with type 2 diabetes mellitus (the FIELD study): randomised controlled trial. *Lancet.* 2005;366(9500):1849-1861.
46. Ginsberg HN, et al. Effects of combination lipid therapy in type 2 diabetes mellitus. *N Engl J Med.* 2010;362(17):1563-1574.
47. Jun M, et al. Effects of fibrates on cardiovascular outcomes: a systematic review and meta-analysis. *Lancet.* 2010;375(9729):1875-1884.
48. Birjmohun RS, et al. Efficacy and safety of high-density lipoprotein cholesterol-increasing compounds: a meta-analysis of randomized controlled trials. *J Am Coll Cardiol.* 2005;45(2):185-197.
49. Allemann S, et al. Fibrates in the prevention of cardiovascular disease in patients with type 2 diabetes mellitus: meta-analysis of randomised controlled trials. *Curr Med Res Opin.* 2006;22(3):617-623.
50. Abourbih S, et al. Effect of fibrates on lipid profiles and cardiovascular outcomes: a systematic review. *Am J Med.* 2009;122(10):962.e1-968.e1.
51. Keene D, et al. Effect on cardiovascular risk of high density lipoprotein targeted drug treatments niacin, fibrates, and CETP inhibitors: meta-analysis of randomised controlled trials including 117,411 patients. *BMJ.* 2014;349:g4379.
52. Gudzune KA, et al. Effectiveness of combination therapy with statin and another lipid-modifying agent compared with intensified statin monotherapy: a systematic review. *Ann Intern Med.* 2014;160(7):468-476.
53. Studer M, et al. Effect of different antilipidemic agents and diets on mortality: a systematic review. *Arch Intern Med.* 2005;165(7):725-730.
54. Saha SA, Arora RR. Fibrates in the prevention of cardiovascular disease in patients with type 2 diabetes mellitus—a pooled meta-analysis of randomized placebo-controlled clinical trials. *Int J Cardiol.* 2010;141(2):157-166.
55. Gaist D, et al. Lipid-lowering drugs and risk of myopathy: a population-based follow-up study. *Epidemiology.* 2001;12(5):565-569.
56. Graham DJ, et al. Incidence of hospitalized rhabdomyolysis in patients treated with lipid-lowering drugs. *JAMA.* 2004;292(21):2585-2590.
57. *Prevalite (cholestyramine) Prescribing Information.* Maple Grove, MN: Upsher-Smith Laboratories, Inc.; 2015.
58. *Questran (cholestyramine) Prescribing Information.* Spring Valley, NY: Par Pharmaceutical Companies, Inc.; 2013.
59. *Colestid (colestipol hydrochloride for oral suspension) Prescribing Information.* New York, NY: Pharmacia & Upjohn Company; 2014.
60. *Colestid (micronized colestipol hydrochloride tablets) Prescribing Information.* New York, NY: Pharmacia & Upjohn Company; 2014.
61. *Welchol (colesevelam) Prescribing Information.* Parsippany, NJ: Daiichi Sankyo, Inc.; 2014.
62. Wiggins BS. Pharmacology of lipid-lowering medications. In: Wiggins BS, Saseen JJ, eds. *Pharmacist's Guide to Lipid Management.* Lenexa, KS: American College of Clinical Pharmacy; 2014:80-121.
63. Goyal P, et al. Cardiometabolic impact of non-statin lipid lowering therapies. *Curr Atheroscler Rep.* 2014;16(2):390.
64. Hansen M, Sonne DP, Knop FK. Bile acid sequestrants: glucose-lowering mechanisms and efficacy in type 2 diabetes. *Curr Diab Rep.* 2014;14(5):482.
65. Scaldaferri F, et al. Use and indications of cholestyramine and bile acid sequestrants. *Intern Emerg Med.* 2013;8(3):205-210.

66. Ewang-Emukowhate M, Wierzbicki AS. Lipid-lowering agents. *J Cardiovasc Pharmacol Ther.* 2013;18(5): 401-411.
67. Monroe AK, et al. Combination therapy versus intensification of statin monotherapy: an update. *Rockville (MD).* 2014.
68. Rifkind BM. The Lipid Research Clinics Coronary Primary Prevention Trial Results. 2. The relationship of reduction in incidence of coronary heart-disease to cholesterol lowering. *JAMA.* 1984;251(3):365-374.
69. Dorr AE, et al. Colestipol hydrochloride in hypercholesterolemic patients—effect on serum cholesterol and mortality. *J Chronic Dis.* 1978;31(1):5-14.
70. Creider JC, Hegele RA, Joy TR. Niacin: another look at an underutilized lipid-lowering medication. *Nat Rev Endocrinol.* 2012;8(9):517-528.
71. Cooper DL, et al. Effects of formulation design on niacin therapeutics: mechanism of action, metabolism, and drug delivery. *Int J Pharm.* 2015;490(1-2):55-64.
72. *Niacor (niacin) Prescribing Information.* Minneapolis, MN: Upsher-Smith Laboratories, Inc.; 2000.
73. *Niaspan (niacin extended-release) Prescribing Information.* North Chicago, IL: AbbVie Inc.; 2015.
74. *Advicor (niacin extended-release/lovastatin) Prescribing Information.* North Chicago, IL: AbbVie Inc.; 2013.
75. *Simcor (niacin extended-release/simvastatin) Prescribing Information.* North Chicago, IL: AbbVie Inc.; 2013.
76. Boden WE, Sidhu MS, Toth PP. The therapeutic role of niacin in dyslipidemia management. *J Cardiovasc Pharmacol Ther.* 2014;19(2):141-158.
77. Castellani LW, Lusis AJ. ApoA-II versus ApoA-I: two for one is not always a good deal. *Arterioscler Thromb Vasc Biol.* 2001;21(12):1870-1872.
78. Guyton JR, Bays HE. Safety considerations with niacin therapy. *Am J Cardiol.* 2007;99(6a):22c-31c.
79. Clofibrate and niacin in coronary heart disease. *JAMA.* 1975;231(4):360-381.
80. Canner PL, et al. Fifteen year mortality in Coronary Drug Project patients: long-term benefit with niacin. *J Am Coll Cardiol.* 1986;8(6):1245-1255.
81. Brown BG, et al. Simvastatin and niacin, antioxidant vitamins, or the combination for the prevention of coronary disease. *N Engl J Med.* 2001;345(22):1583-1592.
82. Taylor AJ, et al. Arterial Biology for the Investigation of the Treatment Effects of Reducing Cholesterol (ARBITER) 2: a double-blind, placebo-controlled study of extended-release niacin on atherosclerosis progression in secondary prevention patients treated with statins. *Circulation.* 2004;110(23):3512-3517.
83. Taylor AJ, Lee HJ, Sullenberger LE. The effect of 24 months of combination statin and extended-release niacin on carotid intima-media thickness: ARBITER 3. *Curr Med Res Opin.* 2006;22(11):2243-2250.
84. Taylor AJ, et al. Extended-release niacin or ezetimibe and carotid intima-media thickness. *N Engl J Med.* 2009;361(22):2113-2122.
85. Boden WE, et al. Niacin in patients with low HDL cholesterol levels receiving intensive statin therapy. *N Engl J Med.* 2011;365(24):2255-2267.
86. Ridker PM, et al. HDL cholesterol and residual risk of first cardiovascular events after treatment with potent statin therapy: an analysis from the JUPITER trial. *Lancet.* 2010;376(9738):333-339.
87. Landray MJ, et al. Effects of extended-release niacin with laropiprant in high-risk patients. *N Engl J Med.* 2014;371(3):203-212.
88. Stern RH, et al. Tolerance to nicotinic acid flushing. *Clin Pharmacol Ther.* 1991;50(1):66-70.
89. Goldberg RB, Jacobson TA. Effects of niacin on glucose control in patients with dyslipidemia. *Mayo Clin Proc.* 2008;83(4):470-478.
90. *Liptruzet (ezetimibe and atorvastatin) Prescribing Information.* Whitehouse Station, NJ: Merck & Co., Inc.; 2014.
91. *Vytorin (ezetimibe and simvastatin) Prescribing Information.* Whitehouse Station, NJ: Merck & Co., Inc.; 2015.
92. Gryn SE, Hegele RA. Ezetimibe plus simvastatin for the treatment of hypercholesterolemia. *Expert Opin Pharmacother.* 2015;16(8):1255-1262.
93. Howard BV, et al. Effect of lower targets for blood pressure and LDL cholesterol on atherosclerosis in diabetes: the SANDS randomized trial. *JAMA.* 2008;299(14):1678-1689.
94. Meaney A, et al. The VYtorin on Carotid intima-media thickness and overall arterial rigidity (VYCTOR) study. *J Clin Pharmacol.* 2009;49(7):838-847.
95. Kastelein JJP, et al. Simvastatin with or without ezetimibe in familial hypercholesterolemia. *N Engl J Med.* 2008;358(14):1431-1443.
96. Kastelein JJ, Bots ML. Statin therapy with ezetimibe or niacin in high-risk patients. *N Engl J Med.* 2009;361(12):2180-2183.
97. Rossebo AB, et al. Intensive lipid lowering with simvastatin and ezetimibe in aortic stenosis. *N Engl J Med.* 2008;359(13):1343-1356.
98. Baigent C, et al. The effects of lowering LDL cholesterol with simvastatin plus ezetimibe in patients with chronic kidney disease (Study of Heart and Renal Protection): a randomised placebo-controlled trial. *Lancet.* 2011;377(9784):2181-2192.
99. Cannon CP, et al. Ezetimibe added to statin therapy after acute coronary syndromes. *N Engl J Med.* 2015;372(25):2387-2397.

100. Phan BA, Dayspring TD, Toth PP. Ezetimibe therapy: mechanism of action and clinical update. *Vasc Health Risk Manag.* 2012;8:415-427.
101. Stone NJ, et al. 2013 ACC/AHA guideline on the treatment of blood cholesterol to reduce atherosclerotic cardiovascular risk in adults: a report of the American College of Cardiology/American Heart Association Task Force on Practice Guidelines. *J Am Coll Cardiol.* 2014;63(25 Pt B):2889-2934.
102. Lloyd-Jones DM, et al. 2016 ACC expert consensus decision pathway on the role of non-statin therapies for LDL-cholesterol lowering in the management of atherosclerotic cardiovascular disease risk: a report of the American College of Cardiology Task Force on Clinical Expert Consensus Documents. *J Am Coll Cardiol* 2016;68:92-125.

CHAPTER 10

Hypertriglyceridemia

Ashley Buffomante and Kavita Sharma

Key Points

- Up until recently, triglycerides have historically been an underemphasized risk factor for cardiovascular disease.

- While treatments for hyperlipidemia have been mostly targeted at LDL levels, guidelines do recommend using non-HDL levels (which include triglycerides) as target for therapy.

- The mainstay of treatment for all patients with elevated triglycerides includes aggressive dietary and lifestyle counseling and modifications.

- There are genetic conditions that lead to hypertriglyceridemia.

- Statins continue to be first line for mild to moderately elevated triglycerides, as these medications have the most data for cardiovascular disease risk reduction.

- For those with moderately to severely elevated triglycerides, fibrates and omega-3 fatty acids should be used.

- Patients with severely elevated triglycerides are at risk for complications including acute pancreatitis and may need to be treated with additional medications.

- There are several novel therapeutics in clinical trials that are designed to specifically target triglyceride synthesis/metabolism that may be alternative options for patients with severe and familial forms of hypertriglyceridemia.

I.   Overview of Triglycerides

Triglycerides are molecules formed by the esterification of a glycerol molecule and three fatty acids and are an important source of energy for the human body. The fatty acid components can be released from the triglyceride molecule when necessary and used to generate energy via oxidation in the Krebs cycle. However, elevated plasma levels of triglycerides have been associated with several pathologic conditions including cardiovascular disease (CVD), pancreatitis, and nonalcoholic fatty liver disease (NAFLD).

II.   Overview of Metabolism

In order to understand the various mechanisms that can result in hypertriglyceridemia, an understanding of the basic pathways involved in triglyceride metabolism is important (see Fig. 10.1).

A. Dietary triglycerides Dietary triglycerides are transported from the gastrointestinal tract in the form of lipoprotein molecules known as chylomicrons. Chylomicrons are made up of triglycerides, cholesterol esters, phospholipids, and various apolipoproteins.

B. Hepatic synthesis In addition to the dietary supply of lipids, the liver is also able to produce its own triglyceride-containing lipoproteins. This process occurs to ensure adequate availability of lipids in the plasma at all times regardless of dietary intake.

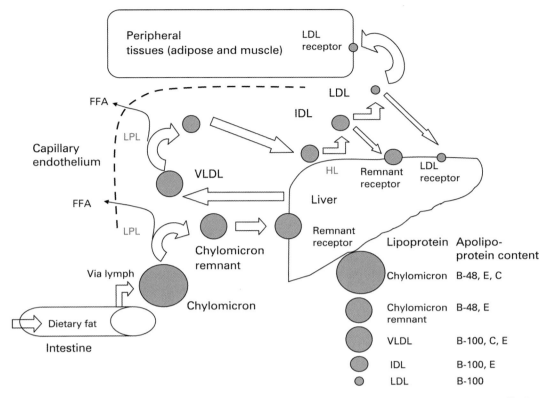

FIGURE 10.1: Pathways in triglyceride metabolism. (Reprinted with permission from Ferns G, Keti V, Griffin B. Investigation and management of hypertriglyceridaemia. *J Clin Pathol.* 2008;61:1174-1183.)

Instead of chylomicrons, the liver produces a lipoprotein known as very-low-density lipoprotein (VLDL). Both chylomicrons and VLDL are high in concentration of triglycerides; however, chylomicrons contain the apolipoprotein B48 (Apo-B48), whereas VLDL contains the apolipoprotein B100 (Apo-B100).

C. **Utilization of triglycerides for energy** In the plasma, free fatty acids can be liberated from the triglyceride molecule by the action of an enzyme known as lipoprotein lipase (LPL). The free fatty acids can then be taken up by skeletal muscle for metabolism or adipose tissue for storage or can be transported back to the liver for reprocessing into VLDL.

D. **Regulation of metabolism** The activity of LPL is regulated by two apolipoproteins, C-II and C-III (Apo-CII and Apo-CIII, respectively). Apo-CII activates the function of LPL, whereas Apo-CIII inhibits its function. Genetic defects resulting in loss of function mutations in the LPL enzyme or the Apo-CII lipoproteins are responsible for certain inherited forms of hypertriglyceridemia as triglyceride molecules are unable to be cleared from the blood.[1]

E. **Relationship among other lipoproteins** During metabolism, VLDL can exchange some of its triglycerides for cholesterol esters found in high-density lipoprotein (HDL) particles by way of an enzyme called cholesterol ester transfer protein (CETP) to become an intermediate-density lipoprotein (IDL). The IDL particle can undergo additional hydrolysis by LPL and becomes a low-density lipoprotein (LDL). Similar metabolic processes occur in the chylomicrons transferring triglycerides from the gastrointestinal tract.

F. **Pathogenesis in human disease** To be discussed in greater detail in subsequent sections, the Apo-B lipoproteins are important in the pathogenesis of hypertriglyceridemia as they have been directly implicated in atherogenesis and cardiovascular disease.[2] The synthesis of VLDL in the liver is dependent upon the availability of free fatty acids and Apo-B100 particles. Therefore, certain conditions (ie, genetic defects, insulin resistance) that increase the availability of these building blocks can result in hypertriglyceridemic states. The intermediate hydrolyzed triglyceride products, sometimes referred to as triglyceride remnants, have also been implicated in atherogenesis.[3] The enzyme hepatic triglyceride lipase (HTGL) aids in removal of the triglyceride remnants from the blood. Defects in the gene encoding this enzyme can result in hypertriglyceridemia and premature cardiovascular disease.

III. Overview of Hypertriglyceridemia

The most recent National Cholesterol Education Program (NCEP) guidelines define a normal fasting triglyceride value as <150 mg/dL. Triglycerides in the 150-199 range are considered borderline high, 200-499 mg/dL are considered high, and >500 mg/dL are considered very high.[4] Unlike the other lipoproteins measured on a basic lipid panel (LDL, HDL), triglyceride values are highly influenced by dietary intake the day preceding the test and can vary greatly from day to day in a particular individual based on what they have eaten. Some advocate for the use of nonfasting triglyceride levels as a screening for hypertriglyceridemia as most people spend a minority of the day in a fasting state, and this value may underestimate the degree of hypertriglyceridemia.[5] In addition, this would add to ease in screening. In patients without hypertriglyceridemia, TG levels in the nonfasting state should be <200 mg/dL.

A. **Epidemiology** About one-third of American adults have triglyceride values greater than normal. In the United States, hypertriglyceridemia is more common in men compared with women and in Mexican Americans compared with other ethnic groups and increases in prevalence according to age up until about age 70, where prevalence then begins to decrease again. Over the last several decades, mean triglyceride levels have been increasing (and especially so in the younger populations) and mirrors the increasing rates of obesity, diabetes, and cardiovascular disease.[5]

B. **Association between hypertriglyceridemia and disease** To be discussed in greater detail later in the chapter, hypertriglyceridemia is intimately associated with the metabolic syndrome and atherogenic dyslipidemia (high LDL and low HDL). There is a well-established link between elevated triglycerides and cardiovascular disease; however, it has been controversial whether triglycerides themselves have a direct role in atherogenesis or if elevated triglyceride levels just serve as a marker for increased cardiovascular risk given their association with conditions such as obesity or type II diabetes mellitus.[6]

C. **Clinical features of hypertriglyceridemia** Unless very severe, most cases of hypertriglyceridemia present asymptomatically. Patients may have clinical findings suggestive of the metabolic syndrome, which include abdominal obesity, hypertension, and insulin resistance (which can manifest as acanthosis nigricans, a dark pigmentation of the skin found on the back of the neck or in the axilla). Physical exam findings specific to hypertriglyceridemia are usually absent unless triglyceride levels are >1000-2000 mg/dL.

1. *Eruptive xanthomas*, which are small, reddish to yellowish papules typically found on the extensor surfaces of the arms and legs, as well as the lower back and buttocks, can be seen in severe hypertriglyceridemia. Histopathologically, eruptive xanthomas are characterized by high concentrations of lipid-laden macrophages.

2. *Lipemia retinalis.* Although rare, at very high levels of triglycerides (>4000 mg/dL), ocular manifestations of hypertriglyceridemia, such as lipemia retinalis, may occur. Lipemia retinalis is a result of lipid infiltration of the retinal vessels and can be seen as a whitish discoloration on funduscopic exam. Normalization of the serum triglycerides usually results in reversal of lipemia retinalis.

IV. Genetic Causes of Elevated Triglycerides

It is often difficult to distinguish genetic forms of hypertriglyceridemia from the hypertriglyceridemia associated with obesity and the metabolic syndrome. Genetic causes of hypertriglyceridemia should be suspected in cases of severely elevated triglycerides (>500 mg/dL), in those with minimal risk factors (younger age, normal body weight, healthy diet), or in those with multiple family members presenting with elevated triglycerides. Table 10.1 outlines the genetic forms of hypertriglyceridemia.

A. **Familial combined hyperlipidemia** Familial combined hyperlipidemia (FCHL) is the most common genetic cause of dyslipidemia, with estimated prevalence of around 1%-2% in the general population. Features of this disorder include elevated cholesterol levels, triglycerides, or both. Often times, genetically predisposed individuals will have normal serum triglyceride levels early in adulthood, but if they acquire a "second hit" (obesity, metabolic syndrome, oral contraceptive use), more severe hypertriglyceridemia can occur.

1. **Genetics** There is no one single gene associated with FCHL; in fact, there have been at least 35 genes identified that have been associated with familial combined hyperlipidemia. The common mechanisms among the various genetic abnormalities are defects

Table 10.1.	Genetic Causes of Hypertriglyceridemia	
Familial combined hyperlipidemia (FCHL)	Very common disorder (1%-2% of population), genetically diverse and diagnosis is made clinically based on family history	Moderately elevated cholesterol and triglycerides (200-1000 mg/dL), elevated Apo-B levels
Familial hypertriglyceridemia	Most common genetic cause of elevated triglycerides. Genetically diverse disorder that results in VLDL overproduction or reduced VLDL metabolism	Moderately elevated triglycerides (200-1000 mg/dL), Apo-B levels are not elevated
Dysbetalipoproteinemia (familial type III)	Autosomal recessive, defect in Apo E II that results in elevated triglycerides	Moderately elevated triglycerides (200-1000 mg/dL)
Heterozygous LPL deficiency	Relatively rare	Moderate elevations in serum triglycerides (200-1000 mg/dL)
Homozygous LPL deficiency	Autosomal recessive	Results in significant elevations in circulating chylomicrons (TG > 1000 mg/dL). Can be associated with lipemia retinalis, eruptive xanthomas, hepatosplenomegaly, and pancreatitis
Apo CII deficiency	Autosomal recessive	Results in significant elevations of circulating chylomicrons (TG > 1000 mg/dL)

that result in elevated levels of Apo-B100 (by either increased synthesis or impaired clearance) and an increased amount of small dense LDL particles. As discussed previously, the presence of Apo-B100 directly correlates with the number of VLDL particles secreted by the liver and Apo-B100 particles themselves have been implicated in atherosclerosis. Subsequently, the presence of many VLDL particles in the circulation promotes formation of atherogenic small, dense LDL particles.

2. **Diagnosis** There is no specific testing available that can detect the disorder, so detailed family history taking is key in establishing the diagnosis. As there is a well-defined relationship between FHCL and premature cardiovascular disease, it is important to recognize the disorder early so that family members can be screened and treated appropriately. The presumptive diagnosis can be made by findings of elevated triglycerides, cholesterol, and/or Apo-B levels in the patient and at least one first-degree relative.

B. **Familial hypertriglyceridemia** Familial hypertriglyceridemia (FHTG) is also a polygenic disorder characterized by elevations in plasma triglycerides (usually modest, with values ranging from 200 to 500 mg/dL), with relatively normal LDL levels. Marked elevations in serum triglycerides often occur in conjunction with heavy alcohol use, medications (estrogens), pregnancy, or other exacerbating factors and therefore does not usually present until adulthood.

1. **Genetics** Genetic studies in familial hypertriglyceridemia have been able to identify some specific genetic defects involved in this disorder; however, there are likely others as well. The most common mutation seems to be a heterozygous loss of function mutation of lipoprotein lipase (LPL), which is typically inherited in an autosomal recessive fashion. This is in contrast with the homozygous loss of function mutations in the LPL enzyme, which leads to severe fasting hypertriglyceridemia (>1000 mg/dL) as seen in the familial hyperchylomicronemia syndromes.

2. **Diagnosis** Familial hypertriglyceridemia is a known risk factor for premature coronary artery disease. Previously, it was believed that familial hypertriglyceridemia did not confer the same increased risk of CAD as did familial combined hyperlipidemia; however, recent analysis shows that the risks of premature CAD are about equal in each disorder.[7] Both disorders are also strongly associated with the metabolic syndrome. As there is no readily available testing for FHTG, the diagnosis is clinical and based strongly on family history.

C. **Hyperchylomicronemia syndromes** There are several genetic conditions that lead to markedly elevated levels of chylomicrons in the bloodstream. These disorders often manifest by acute pancreatitis, abdominal pain, or lipemia retinalis, due to the excess amount of chylomicrons and usually present in childhood. There have also been case reports about severe multiorgan dysfunction due to hyperchylomicronemia related to the resultant hyperviscosity of the blood.

1. **Genetics** The familial hyperchylomicronemia syndrome is associated with an autosomal recessive loss of function mutation in the gene encoding the enzyme lipoprotein lipase (LPL), which is used for metabolism and clearance of chylomicrons and VLDL particles from the bloodstream. There are other disorders, such as familial apolipoprotein CII deficiency, that present similarly. As mentioned previously, apolipoprotein CII is a regulatory enzyme that activates the function of LPL. Thus, in states of apolipoprotein-CII deficiency, there are reduced amounts of functioning LPL and impaired clearance of chylomicrons and VLDL from the serum.

2. **Diagnosis** Like the other genetic disorders, the diagnosis of familial hyperchylomi-cronemia syndrome is usually clinical and based on family history as well. Genetic testing for LPL gene mutations can be performed.

V. **Association of Triglycerides and Cardiovascular Disease Risk**

The association between elevated triglycerides and increased cardiovascular disease is well established; however, there has been much debate whether the triglycerides directly promote cardiovascular disease or if they are indirect markers for increased cardiovascular risk. For instance, hypertriglyceridemia is intimately associated with other conditions that are known risk factors for cardiovascular disease, including diabetes, low HDL levels, and high LDL levels.

A. **Association with cardiovascular disease** There are, however, more data now to suggest that triglycerides may be an independent risk factor for cardiovascular disease. In one large study, elevated triglycerides were associated with increased risk of coronary artery disease even after controlling for traditional risk factors such as HDL and LDL.[8–10]

B. **Chylomicron remnants** There is some evidence that the intermediate breakdown products of triglyceride metabolism, referred to as triglyceride remnants, may be directly involved in atherosclerosis. Although large VLDL and chylomicrons are likely too large to cross the arterial wall, the triglyceride remnant particles have been found to be present in coronary atherosclerotic plaques. Remnant particles that contain high levels of Apo-CIII tend to be smaller and more atherogenic. These remnant particles have been demonstrated to promote inflammation, cause endothelial dysfunction, inhibit vasodilation, and stimulate platelet aggregation. Similar to LDL and IDL particles, triglyceride remnants are rich in atherogenic Apo-B100.[11,12]

C. **Formation of LDL** In addition to directly promoting atherosclerosis, high circulating levels of VLDL activate cholesterol ester transfer protein (CETP) and aid in the formation of small, dense LDL particles, which also play an important role in atherogenesis. Small, dense LDL particles are thought to promote atherogenesis by their susceptibility to oxidation and small size, which eases their transport across the arterial lining. These same metabolic processes cause reductions in HDL levels, which also can lead to increased cardiovascular risk.

VI. **Atherogenic Dyslipidemia and Metabolic Syndrome**

The atherogenic lipoproteins are all the Apo-B–containing lipoproteins including LDL, IDL, VLDL, and chylomicrons. Together, these make up the so-called "non-HDL" lipoproteins. Data from the Lipid Research Clinics Program suggest that levels of non-HDL cholesterol (which includes LDL, IDL, VLDL, and chylomicrons), as compared with LDL levels alone, were a stronger predictor of cardiovascular disease.[13,14]

A. **The metabolic syndrome** Hypertriglyceridemia is strongly associated with the metabolic syndrome. The metabolic syndrome is defined by having three of the following features: abdominal obesity (a waist circumference of 40 in or above in males, 35 in or above in females), triglycerides of ≥150 mg/dL, low HDL levels (<40 mg/dL for men or <50 mg/dL in women), elevated blood pressure (>130/85), and a fasting plasma glucose of ≥100 mg/dL.

B. Effects of insulin resistance A key association between the metabolic syndrome and dyslipidemia is related to insulin resistance. Insulin resistance causes elevations in triglycerides by several mechanisms. First, there is increased systemic lipolysis, which results in larger amounts of free fatty acids delivered to the liver and therefore increased VLDL secretion. Insulin has also been shown to aid in degradation of Apo-B100 so therefore in states of insulin resistance, there is more Apo-B100 available for VLDL synthesis.

VII. Role of Lifestyle Modifications for Treatment

All patients with elevated triglycerides should be counseled about lifestyle modifications, regardless of whether the patient is placed on pharmacologic therapy. The mainstay of treatment is encouraging weight loss, certain dietary changes, and physical activity. These nonpharmacologic therapies can lower triglyceride levels between 20% and 50%. Table 10.2 outlines the key components of lifestyle therapy.

A. Weight loss Weight loss of even just 5%-10% of total body weight has been shown to reduce triglyceride levels of up to 20%. While both visceral and subcutaneous abdominal adiposity are associated with hypertriglyceridemia, there is a much stronger correlation between abnormal lipid profiles and the visceral form of obesity. Although there are likely multiple mechanisms by which weight loss lowers triglycerides, one major pathway is improvement in insulin sensitivity.

B. Effects of sugar and other refined carbohydrates Diets high in refined carbohydrates or added sugars, such as in processed foods and soft drinks, are also highly associated with hypertriglyceridemia. The American Heart Association recommends that no more than 60% of total calories in the diet come from carbohydrates and no more than 5%-10% of total calories from added sugars.[5,15] With regard to added sugar, this comes out to be around 9 teaspoons per day, which is roughly the equivalent of the sugar content in one 12 oz can of soda. Currently, it is estimated that the average American is consuming around 20 teaspoons of added sugar per day, and this continues to be on the rise. The 2015 guidelines were the first year in which there was a recommended limit on sugar consumption as more information is coming out with regard to sugar consumption and risks for obesity and cardiovascular disease.[4]

C. The effects of fructose Many processed foods also contain high levels of fructose, in the form of high fructose corn syrup or sucrose, both of which contain roughly 50% fructose and 50% glucose. Although there has previously been controversy over the effects of consuming high amounts of dietary fructose, several studies have confirmed a stronger adverse effect of fructose (at levels >50 g/d) on plasma triglyceride levels than with equivalent amounts of glucose.

Table 10.2. Key Components of Lifestyle Modification for Reducing Triglycerides	
Lifestyle Modifications for Reducing Triglycerides	
Weight loss	Weight loss of 5%-10% of total body weight can reduce triglycerides up to 20%.
Limit carbohydrate intake	Limit carbohydrate intake to <60% of total calories; limit added sugar intake to 5%-10% of total calories; avoid high intake of fructose (high fructose corn syrup) or highly processed foods.
Encourage a "Mediterranean-like" diet	Encourage intake of fresh fruits, vegetables, legumes, whole grains.
Limit alcohol use	Limit alcohol intake to <1 drink per day for women and <2 drinks per day for men.

D. **The "Mediterranean-style" diet** Diets similar to the "Mediterranean-style" diet, which is rich in whole grains, legumes, fruits, vegetables, and mono- and poly-unsaturated fatty acids, are associated with improved triglyceride levels and should be encouraged in all patients. These diets worked better to lower triglyceride levels than those that were extremely low in fat.

E. **Alcohol** Heavy alcohol consumption has also been shown to adversely affect triglyceride levels. Although moderate alcohol consumption (defined as one drink per day for women and two drinks per day for men) has been associated with a decreased risk of cardiovascular disease, consumption above this amount is strongly associated with hypertriglyceridemia. Alcohol is known to inhibit lipoprotein lipase, the enzyme responsible for hydrolysis of chylomicrons and VLDL particles. These effects of alcohol on triglyceride levels are likely amplified by the high carbohydrate content of alcohol as well as the propensity to consume higher calorie containing foods after heavy drinking.

VIII. Secondary Causes of Hypertriglyceridemia

A search for secondary causes of hypertriglyceridemia (Table 10.3) should be sought in all patients. In addition to the lifestyle factors mentioned in the previous section (diets high in saturated fat and refined carbohydrates, sedentary lifestyle, alcohol use), certain medications and disease states can cause or exacerbate hypertriglyceridemia.

A. **Medications** Common medications implicated include exogenous hormones (oral estrogens, selective estrogen receptor modulators), glucocorticoids, atypical antipsychotics, antiretroviral medications, immunosuppressive medication (cyclosporine, sirolimus), thiazide diuretics, and beta-blockers.

B. **Diabetes mellitus** As mentioned in previously, hypertriglyceridemia is also intimately linked with insulin resistance; therefore, all patients should be screened for diabetes. Improved glucose control can result in marked improvements in serum triglycerides.

C. **Thyroid disorders** Elevated triglycerides are also commonly seen in patients with hypothyroidism. Thus, all patients should be screened for thyroid disorders as well. Treatment with thyroid replacement results in improvement of the lipid profile.

Table 10.3. **Secondary Causes of Hypertriglyceridemia**	
Lifestyle Factors	**Renal Disease**
• Excessive alcohol use • Diets high in saturated fat or refined carbohydrates • Obesity	• Nephrotic syndrome • Chronic kidney disease
Medications	**Endocrine Abnormalities**

• Immunosuppressants (tacrolimus, cyclosporine, rapamune, steroids)
• Estrogen therapy (oral contraceptives, estrogen replacement, selective estrogen receptor modifiers [SERMs])
• Beta-blockers
• Protease inhibitors
• Thiazide diuretics
• *Antipsychotic medications*
  - Bile acid resins
  - Alpha interferon
  - Sertraline
	• Hypothyroidism
	• Uncontrolled diabetes
	• Pregnancy

	Lipodystrophy
	HIV associated Genetic lipodystrophy Autoimmune

D. Chronic kidney disease (CKD) Chronic kidney disease (CKD) is also commonly associated with hypertriglyceridemia. Several studies suggest that the activity of LPL is reduced in chronic kidney disease, thereby inhibiting hydrolysis of VLDL and chylomicron particles. In uremic states, the ratio of Apo-CIII (an inhibitor of LPL) to Apo-CII (an activator of LPL) increases, thus also reducing the amount of functioning LPL. Similarly, CKD is also associated with insulin resistance, and thus, triglycerides can be elevated via this pathway as well.[16]

IX.   Pharmacologic Treatment

In all patients, treatment of hypertriglyceridemia includes counseling on intensive lifestyle modifications along with medications (Table 10.4). The 2004 Adult Treatment Panel (ATP) III guidelines recommend treatment of triglycerides at levels >500 mg/dL as this is the range in which the complications such as pancreatitis are more likely to occur.[17] The 2013 ACC/AHA guidelines do not specifically give recommendations regarding treatment of triglycerides but emphasize using statins for overall cardiovascular risk reduction. Both the National Lipid Association (NLA) and the International Atherosclerosis Society recommend using both LDL and non-HDL as targets for therapy for cardiovascular disease risk reduction in this population. In fact, although the NLA recommendations target both non-HDL and LDL, they list non-HDL first to emphasize its importance, as non-HDL encompasses triglyceride levels while LDL does not.[14] Chapter 6 outlines the step-by-step plan for diagnosis and management of elevated LDL-C, non-HDL-C, and triglycerides. Chapters 9 and 10 provide in-depth discussion on lipid-lowering medications.

A. Statins

1. **Indications** Typically, for mild to moderate hypertriglyceridemia, the HMG-CoA reductase inhibitors (statins) are first-line therapy after lifestyle changes. In severe hypertriglyceridemia (>500 mg/dL), fibrates and fish oil are preferred therapy, but there are other medications including niacin, ezetimibe, and some newer novel agents that may be utilized as well.

2. **Cardiovascular risk reduction** Although usually first line, statins are not the most efficacious at lowering triglycerides; however, they do have the most data for cardiovascular risk factor reduction. Statins can reduce triglyceride levels from 20% to 40%. Statins are thought to reduce triglycerides by reducing VLDL synthesis and up-regulating the LDL receptor on cells, which facilitates clearance of triglyceride remnants from the plasma.

Table 10.4.	Medications to Treat Hypertriglyceridemia	
Drug	**Reduction in Triglycerides**	**Mechanism of Action**
Fibrates	30%-50%	Activates peroxisome proliferator-activated receptor-α (PPAR-α), increases beta-oxidation of fatty acids, enhances the function of LPL, reduces Apo-CIII levels
Niacin	20%-50%	Inhibits diacylglycerol acyltransferase-2
Omega-3	20%-50%	Inhibits VLDL secretion and increases VLDL clearance
Statins	10%-30%	Reduces synthesis of VLDL, increases LDL receptors on cells, which aids in clearance of triglyceride remnants
Ezetimibe	5%-10%	Reduces absorption of dietary cholesterol from gastrointestinal tract

B. Fibrates

1. **Mechanism and risks** Fibrates work by activating peroxisome proliferator-activated receptor-α (PPAR-α) that increases beta-oxidation of fatty acids, which decreases the amount of fatty acids available for VLDL synthesis. Fibrates also enhance LPL function and reduce Apo-CIII levels, which promote metabolism of triglycerides in the plasma. Fibrates can lower triglyceride levels from 20% to 70%. There is increased risk of rhabdomyolysis when used in combination with statins. Fenofibrate has less risk for rhabdomyolysis when combined with statins compared with other fibrates such as gemfibrozil and therefore is recommended when combination therapy is indicated.

2. **Cardiovascular risk reduction** Results from a large meta-analysis of 45 058 patients showed that fibrate therapy resulted in a 10% risk reduction for major cardiovascular events (95% CI 0-12, p < .048) and a 13% risk reduction in coronary heart disease (95% CI 7-19, p < .0001) compared with placebo.[18] However, results from the ACCORD-LIPID study showed no improvement in cardiovascular disease mortality or nonfatal MI when fibrates are added to statin therapy in type II diabetics.[19]

C. Fish oils

1. **Mechanism** Fish oils that contain n-3 polyunsaturated fatty acids (PUFAs), such as docosahexanoic acid (DHA) and eicosapentaenoic acid (EPA), can reduce triglycerides. The n-3 PUFAs work by inhibiting VLDL secretion and increasing VLDL clearance. Typically, high doses (2-4 g/d) are required for optimal triglyceride reduction. Fish oils are generally well tolerated and can be combined with either statins or fibrates for patients with severe hypertriglyceridemia. The PUFAs also have been shown to improve endothelial function, decrease platelet aggregation, and improve vasodilatation, which may be protective against cardiovascular disease.

2. **Newer agents** The FDA recently approved a newer formulation of fish oil, Epanova (omega-3-carboxylic acids), which has been shown to have superior bioavailability compared with older preparations and can be taken with or without meals. The STRENGTH trial is currently under way that is investigating the risk of developing cardiovascular disease in patients on statins plus Epanova vs statin therapy alone.[20] Vascepa (icosapent ethyl), which is an EPA-only product, is another prescription formulation that has been shown to have superior effects on the lipid profile compared with combined EPA and DHA products.[21]

D. Niacin

1. **Mechanisms** Niacin has also been used successfully to reduce triglyceride levels. Although the mechanism is not entirely clear, it appears that at high doses Niacin works by inhibiting the enzyme diacylglycerol acyltransferase-2, which is found in hepatocytes and is necessary for triglyceride synthesis.

2. **Dosing** Niacin is generally titrated up starting with 500 mg of a sustained-release (SR) formulation and titrated up to 2000 mg daily.[22] Serum triglyceride levels can be reduced by up to 50% with higher doses.

3. **Risks and side effects** The SR niacin has been associated with more hepatotoxicity than the immediate release (IR) formulations are is therefore not recommended for routine use.[23] Another major side effect of niacin is flushing; this can be reduced by taking aspirin (325 mg dose is needed) prior to administration of the niacin. In addition, avoidance of alcohol use or spicy foods can alleviate the flushing. Niacin has

been shown to reduce the risk of cardiovascular disease when used by itself; however, results from the AIM-HIGH trial have shown no additional mortality benefit when added to statin therapy.[24] The use of niacin in treatment of dyslipidemia has lessened due to side effects and overall efficacy. See Chapters 10 and 12 for further discussion about use of niacin.

E. **Ezetimibe** Ezetimibe is a triglyceride-lowering agent that reduces the absorption of dietary cholesterol from the gastrointestinal tract, with lower efficacy when compared to other agents. Ezetimibe can lower triglycerides by 5%-10%; however, they are more effective in lowering LDL levels, which they lower about 20%. This medication is useful as an adjunct to statin therapy in individuals who have not reached their LDL or non-HDL goals on maximal doses of statins.

F. **Drugs in development**

1. Apo-CIII synthesis inhibitors. A newer class of triglyceride-lowering therapy is in development, an agent known as Volanesorsen (previously ISIS 304801), which is an antisense oligonucleotide that inhibits the synthesis of apolipoprotein C-III by binding the Apo-CIII mRNA and causing degradation rather than protein translation. This drug was created based on the observation that those individuals with low levels of Apo-CIII (as with loss of function genetic mutations) had lower triglyceride levels and a reduced risk of cardiovascular disease. Apo-CIII is responsible for inhibiton of LPL function and also acts to increase VLDL secretion in the liver; therefore, reduction in the amount of Apo-CIII should effectively reduce plasma triglyceride levels. Early studies have shown up to a 56%-86% reduction in triglyceride levels in patients with familial hyperchylomicronemia syndromes.

2. **Apo-B synthesis inhibitors** There is another similar type of drug, known as Mipomersen, which works by inhibiting translation of Apo-B mRNA. The result is decreased production of the atherogenic Apo-B–containing lipoproteins including LDL, IDL, and VLDL. Although currently used for its LDL-reducing properties (as in familial hypercholesterolemia), studies have shown around a 36% reduction in plasma triglyceride levels when compared with placebo.

3. **Gene therapy** In Europe, gene therapy has been successfully used for patients with hyperchylomicronemia syndromes resulting from LPL deficiency. The gene that encodes the LPL protein can be transmitted effectively to humans using a viral vector (an adeno-associated virus). Major limitations to this therapy include loss of effectiveness by around 18-24 months, presumably due to patient antibody formation against the viral vector. Concurrent immunosuppressive therapies to suppress antibody formation have also been unsuccessful.[25,26]

G. **MTP inhibitors** Lomitapide, a microsomal triglyceride transfer protein (MTP) inhibitor, is also available and FDA approved for homozygous familial hypercholesterolemia. In addition to LDL-lowering properties, trials have shown up to a 45% reduction in plasma triglyceride levels.[25,27]

X. Conclusion

In conclusion, hypertriglyceridemia often results from genetics, lifestyle, medications or a combination of these factors. At very high levels, hypertriglyceridemia can result in pancreatitis and other physical exam findings such as eruptive xanthomas. At moderately elevated levels, there is an association with increased cardiovascular disease risk. Trials are ongoing to assess whether the addition of triglyceride-lowering medications to a statin will lower CVD risk. In addition, there are ongoing trials related to Apo-CIII inhibition. However, the mainstay of management of hypertriglyceridemia is with optimal diet and exercise habits.

References

1. Chait A, Subramanian S, Brunzell J. *Genetic Disorders of Triglyceride Metabolism.* Endotext [Internet]. 2015 Jun 12. Available at: http://www-ncbi-nlm-nih-gov.proxy.lib.ohio-state.edu/books/NBK326743/

2. Olofsson SO, Boren J. Apolipoprotein B: a clinically important apolipoprotein which assembles atherogenic lipoproteins and promotes the development of atherosclerosis. *J Intern Med.* 2005;258(5):395-410.

3. Talayero BG, Sacks FM. The role of triglycerides in atherosclerosis. *Curr Cardiol Rep.* 2011;13(6):544-552.

4. U.S. Department of Health and Human Services and U.S. Department of Agriculture. *2015–2020 Dietary Guidelines for Americans.* 8th ed. December 2015. Available at: http://health.gov/dietaryguidelines/2015/guidelines/

5. Miller M, Stone NJ, Ballantyne C, et al.; on behalf of the American Heart Association Clinical Lipidology, Thrombosis, and Prevention Committee of the Council on Nutrition, Physical Activity, and Metabolism, Council on Arteriosclerosis, thrombosis and Vascular Biology, Council on Cardiovascular Nursing, and Council on the Kidney in Cardiovascular disease. Triglycerides and cardiovascular disease: a scientific statement from the American Heart Association. *Circulation.* 2011;123:2292-2333.

6. Austin MA. Epidemiology of hypertriglyceridemia and cardiovascular disease. *Am J Cardiol.* 1999;83(9B):13F-16F.

7. Hopkins PN, Heiss G, Ellison RC, et al. Coronary artery disease risk in familial combined hyperlipidemia and familial hypertriglyceridemia: a case-control comparison from the National Heart, Lung, and Blood Institute Family Heart Study. *Circulation.* 2003;108:519-523.

8. Tenembaum A, Klempfner R, Fisman EZ. Hypertriglyceridemia: a too long unfairly neglected cardiovascular risk factor. *Cardiovasc Diabetol.* 2014;13:159.

9. Cullen P. Evidence that triglycerides are an independent coronary heart disease risk factor. *Am J Cardiol.* 2000;86(9):943-949.

10. Hokanson JE, Austin MA. Plasma triglyceride level is a risk factor for cardiovascular disease independent of high density lipoprotein level: a meta-analysis of population-based prospective studies. *J Cardiovasc Risk.* 1996;3:213-219.

11. Carmena R, Duriez P, Fruchart JC. Atherosclerosis: evolving biology and clinical implications: atherogenic lipoprotein particles in atherosclerosis. *Circulation.* 2004;109:2-7.

12. Hodis HN. Triglyceride-rich lipoprotein remnant particles and risk of atherosclerosis. *Circulation.* 1999;99:2852-2854.

13. Cui Y, Blumenthal RS, Flaws JA, et al. Non-high-density lipoprotein cholesterol level as a predictor of cardiovascular disease mortality. *Arch Intern Med.* 2001;161:1413-1419.

14. Jacobson TA, Ito MK, Maki KC, et al. National Lipid Association recommendations for patient-centered management of dyslipidemia: part 1-executive summary. *J Clin Lipidol.* 2014;8:473-488.

15. U.S. Department of Health and Human Services. *Dietary Guidelines for Americans.* 6th ed. Available at: http://www.healtierus.gov. Accessed March 25, 2016; 2005.

16. Tsimihodimos V, Mitrogiani Z, Elisaf M. Dyslipidemia associated with chronic kidney disease. *Open Cardiovasc Med J.* 2011;5:41-48.

17. Grundy SM, Cleeman JI, Bairey Merz N, et al. Implications of recent clinical trials for the national cholesterol education program adult treatment Panel III Guidelines. *Circulation.* 2004;110:227-239.

18. Jun M, Foote C, Lv J, et al. Effects of fibrates on cardiovascular outcomes: a systematic review and meta-analysis. *Lancet.* 2010;375(9729):1875-1888.

19. The ACCORD Study Group. Effects of combination lipid therapy in type 2 diabetes mellitus. *N Engl J Med.* 2010;362:1563-1574.

20. AztraZeneca, Cleveland Clinic Coordinating Center for Clinical Research. Outcomes study to assess statin residual risk reduction with Epanova in high CV risk patients with hypertriglyceridemia. In: *Clinicaltrials.gov [Internet].* Available at: http://clinicaltrials.gov/show/NCT92194817. NLM Identifier: NCT02104717. Accessed March 25, 2016.

21. Hilleman DE, Malesker MA. Potential benefits of icosapent ethyl on the lipid profile: case studies. *Clin Med Insights Cardiol.* 2014;8:13-15.

22. Stone NJ, Robinson J, Lichtenstein AH, et al. 2013 ACC/AHA guideline on the treatment of blood cholesterol to reduce atherosclerotic cardiovascular risk in adults. *J Am Coll Cardiol.* 2013.

23. McKenney JM, Proctor JD, Harris S, Chinchili VM. A comparison of the efficacy and toxic effects of sustained vs immediate release niacin in hypercholesterolemic patients. *JAMA.* 1994;271(9):672-677.

24. The AIM-HIGH Investigators. Niacin in patients with low HDL cholesterol levels receiving intensive statin therapy. *N Engl J Med.* 2011;365:2255-2267.
25. Gryn SE, Hegele RA. Novel therapeutics in hypertriglyceridemia. *Curr Opin Lipidol.* 2015;26:484-491.
26. Stroes ES, Nieman MC, Meulenberg JJ, et al. Intramuscular administration of AAV1-lipoprotein lipase S447X lowers triglycerides in lipoprotein lipase-deficient patients. *Arterioscler Thromb Vasc Biol.* 2008;28:2303-2304.
27. Cuchel M, Meagher EA, du Toit Theron H, et al. Efficacy and safety of a microsomal triglyceride transfer protein inhibitor in patients with homozygous familial hypercholesterolemia: a single-arm, open-label, phase 3 study. *Lancet.* 2013;381:40-46.

CHAPTER 11

Safety and Tolerability of Lipid-Lowering Medications

Connie B. Newman and Jonathan A. Tobert

Key Points

- The safety and tolerability of statins have been established over three decades.

- The hallmark adverse effect of statins, myopathy (defined by FDA and in prescribing information as unexplained muscle pain or weakness accompanied by creatine kinase elevated above 10× ULN), occurs in <0.1% of patients. Rhabdomyolysis is a severe form of myopathy, in which creatine kinase is typically over 40 times the upper limit of normal with myoglobinuria, which can cause acute renal failure.

- Interactions with drugs that interfere with clearance of statins increase the risk of myopathy/rhabdomyolysis, and these interactions vary among statins.

- In patients with risk factors for diabetes, statins increase the risk of new-onset diabetes in a dose-related manner by 10%-20%. Statins reduce cardiovascular risk in patients with or without diabetes, and this outweighs the risk of new-onset diabetes by a large margin.

- In the United States, about 10% of patients stop taking statins because they report a variety of symptoms, most commonly muscle symptoms. However, in clinical trials, discontinuation of statin and that of placebo are consistently very similar. Furthermore, well-documented statin intolerance usually disappears under double-blind conditions. Statin intolerance is mainly the product of the nocebo effect, in which common background symptoms such as muscle aches are attributed to the statin.

- With the exception of niacin, other lipid-lowering agents appear to be generally safe, though data are more limited than with statins.

This chapter is intended as a general guide to the safety and tolerability (Box 11.1) of lipid-lowering drugs. For detailed information on individual agents, readers should consult the prescribing information.

I.   Overview: Benefit vs Risk for Lipid-Lowering Medications

A. Cardiovascular benefits of lipid-lowering drugs

1. **Statins** Lipid-lowering drugs are used to lower the risk of atherosclerotic disease, both in patients who have never suffered a myocardial infarction, stroke, or other manifestations of atherosclerotic disease and in those who have, to reduce the risk of further adverse cardiovascular outcomes. In the case of statins, the evidence for reduction of cardiovascular risk is derived from numerous randomized controlled trials (RCTs)[1] and is indisputable.

2. **Ezetimibe** In the case of ezetimibe, there is only one relevant RCT, but it showed a clear beneficial effect.[2]

3. **Other medications** For the other lipid-lowering drugs, the evidence for cardiovascular risk reduction is weaker or currently nonexistent. Because lipid-lowering medications are typically used for several decades if not a lifetime,

---

BOX 11.1 | Terminology

Adverse event: any untoward medical occurrence during use of a drug or placebo

- Adverse effect: an adverse event that is caused by a drug.
- A serious adverse event is life threatening, requires hospitalization, or disrupts normal functioning (eg, rhabdomyolysis). See full FDA definition

at http://www.fda.gov/Safety/MedWatch/HowTo Report/ucm053087.htm.

- A generally safe drug rarely causes serious adverse events.
- A well-tolerated drug has few adverse effects, serious or nonserious, and they are uncommon.

---

long-term safety is important; and because they are used not to relieve symptoms but to prevent cardiovascular events at some point in the future, tolerability is particularly important.

B. Evaluation of risk

1. **Randomized controlled trials** The best way to evaluate drug benefit, safety, and tolerability is the RCT.[3,4] Double-blind well-executed RCTs have the great advantage that the only variable (other than random error) affecting the results is allocation to the test treatment or the control. The main disadvantage of large RCTs is their high cost.

2. **Observational studies**
   a. Utility for rare adverse effects
      Observational studies can be useful to detect adverse effects that are too rare to be reliably apparent in RCTs, particularly when the background incidence is very low.[5] Prior to 2010, when simvastatin 80 mg was shown in an RCT to cause myopathy (unexplained muscle pain or weakness accompanied by creatine kinase >10× ULN), including rhabdomyolysis, much more frequently than simvastatin 20 mg,[6] there had been no statistically significant difference in RCTs in the incidence of this adverse effect, and its detection was thus essentially observational. In this case, observational data were reliable because idiopathic rhabdomyolysis is very rare, so that any case occurring during statin therapy without another known cause is very likely to be causally related to the statin. Observational data derived from postmarketing surveillance revealed that the risk of rhabdomyolysis with cerivastatin was much higher than with other statins, leading to its withdrawal from the market.[7]
   b. Disadvantages
      Because the comparisons made in observational studies are not randomized, all observational data are at risk of confounding.[5] Statistical adjustment can reduce the risk but not eliminate it. There are numerous examples of observational findings later refuted by RCTs. In cardiovascular medicine, among the best known is estrogen therapy to reduce CHD risk in postmenopausal women, which was supported by numerous epidemiological studies[8,9] and subsequently largely refuted by RCTs[10–12] that reported no overall cardiovascular benefit and possibly an increase in risk, especially for the combination of conjugated equine estrogen and medroxyprogesterone acetate in women without CHD. In addition, observational studies suggesting that vitamin E supplementation reduces the risk of cardiovascular events,[13] possibly because of antioxidant properties, were subsequently refuted by several RCTs.[13,14] Unless observational studies show very large differences in the groups compared, they should be interpreted cautiously.[5]

II. Proven Adverse Effects of Statins

A. Myopathy/rhabdomyolysis

This section deals with muscle adverse effects accompanied by marked increases in creatine kinase (CK), which are definitely caused by statins. Muscle symptoms without significant CK increases (ie, <3× ULN) are associated with statin therapy but rarely caused by statins. These are dealt with in Section 5, Statin Intolerance.

1. **Definitions**
   a. Myopathy
      Few drugs have toxic effects on skeletal muscle, but all statins occasionally cause myopathy. The terminology used to describe muscle adverse effects of statins varies among authors, clinical trials, and consensus groups.[15] **The original definition of statin-induced myopathy,[16] accepted by the FDA and specified in the prescribing information for all statins that provide a definition, is unexplained muscle pain or weakness accompanied by creatine kinase (CK) concentration >10 times the upper limit of normal; that is the terminology used here.** Muscle symptoms are bilateral and predominantly derive from the large muscles of the legs, back, and shoulders. Fortunately, the adverse effect is confined to skeletal muscle, and cardiomyopathy has never been associated with any statin.
   b. Rhabdomyolysis
      Rhabdomyolysis is a severe form of myopathy with CK > 40× ULN that may require hospitalization; muscle fiber necrosis results in myoglobinuria that can cause acute renal failure. Prompt recovery from myopathy/rhabdomyolysis typically occurs on cessation of therapy. However, there have been very rare cases in which treatment continued despite muscle symptoms and death occurred due to acute renal failure.

2. **Incidence** The incidence of myopathy/rhabdomyolysis increases with dose, but is <0.1% at the currently recommended doses of all statins, except for simvastatin 80 mg, for which the risk is unacceptably high at about 1%.[6] This dose is still marketed, but the prescribing information warns against its use except for patients who have taken 80 mg daily uneventfully for at least 12 months.

3. **Risk factors** Because of the rarity of the event for all doses of all statins except for simvastatin 80 mg, factors predisposing to myopathy/rhabdomyolysis are not well defined, but may include age, female sex, Chinese ancestry and possibly East Asian ancestry in general, and diabetes.

4. **Time of onset and mechanism** The risk of myopathy is greatest in the first year of therapy and after increasing statin dose or the addition of an interacting drug (see Box 11.3). The mechanism is usually a direct toxic effect (mechanism unknown) of the statin on skeletal muscle, but a very rare autoimmune necrotizing myopathy has also been described,[17] with an estimated incidence of 2-3 per 100 000 patients treated with statins. This condition should be suspected if CK remains elevated after stopping the statin and no other cause is found.

5. **Evaluation** Patients complaining of muscle symptoms during treatment with statins should be queried about unusual or strenuous exercise, which is a common cause and can produce substantial elevations of CK. Hypothyroidism and preexisting muscle disease should be ruled out, and the use of any drug known to interact with the statin in question should be explored. CK should be measured in any patient presenting with unexplained muscle symptoms.

6. **Creatine kinase with muscle symptoms** If >10 ULN (or >5× ULN in a vulnerable patient), the statin should be stopped immediately; if it is >40× ULN, and the patient is considered to be at risk of acute renal failure, hospitalization may be required. If >3× ULN but <10× ULN, and the symptoms are mild, the statin can be continued with another measurement in a few days to determine whether CK is rising or falling. If stable and <3× ULN, the statin can be continued. Stopping the statin in a patient with statin-induced myopathy is followed by prompt resolution of symptoms and a falling CK.

7. **Vigorous exercise** Patients who engage in vigorous athletic activities such as marathons may ask about possible effects of statins on exercise performance. It has long been known that statins produce a small (about 10%) increase in mean creatine kinase in clinical trials,[18] but this does not necessarily imply a deleterious effect on muscle, just as the small mean increases in hepatic transaminases produced by statins do not imply a deleterious effect on the liver. Limited evidence suggests that statins amplify the CK increases that commonly occur after prolonged vigorous exercise such as a marathon, but these are not randomized comparisons.[19] It is reasonable to suspend a statin a day or 2 before a marathon or other occasional strenuous exercise. Whether this will improve performance is unknown, as generally clinical trials investigating fitness or muscle performance have either not been double blind[20] or have yielded no significant differences between statin and placebo.[21,22] However, losing 2 days of treatment a week to avoid exposure during regular weekend exercise would compromise lipid-lowering efficacy and should be avoided.

B. **New-onset diabetes** RCTs have shown that statins increase the risk of new-onset diabetes in a dose-related manner by 10%-20%,[23-25] but this is observable only at the group level; it is not possible to identify specific patients in whom this adverse effect has occurred, just as it is not possible to identify specific patients in whom a myocardial infarction or stroke has been prevented. The mechanism is unclear at present, but it is believed that this adverse effect is attributable to patients with at least one risk factor for diabetes—impaired fasting glucose, metabolic syndrome, severe obesity, or raised HbA_{1c}—developing the disease earlier than they would have otherwise, rather than diabetes occurring unexpectedly in a patient with no major risk factors.[26,27] Statin therapy also may increase HbA_{1c} in patients with diabetes, but the average increase is very small, ~0.1%.[28] To establish a baseline, some practitioners measure HbA_{1c} before starting statin therapy in a patient with risk factors for diabetes. The increase in the risk of developing diabetes is outweighed by the major cardiovascular events prevented, even if the analysis is confined to patients with risk factors for diabetes and without clinically manifest atherosclerotic disease.[26,27] The same applies to the increase in HbA_{1c}.

C. **Hemorrhagic stroke** Although statins unquestionably reduce the risk of ischemic stroke, in some cardiovascular outcome studies, a trend toward an increase in the risk of hemorrhagic stroke in the statin group has been observed.[1] In SPARCL,[29] which compared atorvastatin 80 mg to placebo in patients with previous stroke/TIA, this increase was statistically significant, leading to a warning in the prescribing information. It is likely[1] but not certain[30] that other statins also increase the risk of hemorrhagic stroke. Hemorrhagic strokes account for only 10% of all strokes in Western countries and 20% in Asia.[31] The reduction in the risk of ischemic stroke outweighs any increase in the risk of hemorrhagic stroke, except in patients who have had a previous hemorrhagic stroke.

III.   Adverse Events of Statins Without Established Causality

A. **Common disorders** At one time or another, a variety of adverse events have been attributed to statins, including cataracts, sleep disturbances, cognitive dysfunction including memory loss, erectile dysfunction, and others. However, all of these are common conditions, so observational evidence is not compelling. RCTs have not shown a consistent difference between statin and placebo in the risk of any of these.[32–35]

B. **Cancer** A large meta-analysis provided no evidence that statins given for several years increase the risk of cancer.[36]

C. **Liver** Statins increase hepatic transaminases in a dose-related manner.[37] Liver function tests should be measured before starting statin treatment to rule out preexisting liver disease, but monitoring of liver function tests is no longer recommended because it is not effective in preventing serious liver injury. Clinical hepatitis is very rare in clinical trials with statins, and none have reported a significant difference vs placebo. A careful examination of Swedish national registry adverse event data, including an evaluation of causality in each case, suggests that the risk of serious statin-induced hepatotoxicity is about 0.001%.[38] This risk is too low to be detectable in clinical trials, even though some have randomized over 20 000 patients.[1] If serious hepatotoxicity occurs and no other cause is found, rechallenge with a statin is not recommended because of the risk of a further serious and possibly fatal reaction.[38]

D. **Congenital abnormalities** All statins are contraindicated during pregnancy. This is mainly because of theoretical concerns about fetal requirements for cholesterol, rather than good evidence for teratogenicity. Epidemiological studies of women exposed to statins during pregnancy have not provided evidence that statins can cause congenital abnormalities,[39] but they are not large enough to rule out moderate risks. In the event of inadvertent exposure during early pregnancy, the statin should be stopped immediately, but patients can be advised that the risk to the fetus is low.[39]

IV.   Drug Interactions

A. **CYP3A4-mediated interactions**

1. **Differences in metabolism among statins** Although the pharmacodynamic properties of statins (ie, their effects on lipids and lipoproteins) are qualitatively similar, their complex pharmacokinetic properties are not. The most important difference is that lovastatin, simvastatin, and atorvastatin are metabolized by CYP3A4, but the other four statins are not. These three statins are therefore vulnerable to interactions with CYP3A4 inhibitors, which increase HMG-CoA reductase inhibitory activity derived from the parent drug and/or active metabolites in plasma. This increases the risk of myopathy, including rhabdomyolysis. Lovastatin and simvastatin are subject to first-pass metabolism, and as a result, CYP3A4 inhibitors tend to produce larger increases in HMG-CoA reductase inhibitory activity with them than with atorvastatin.

2. **CYYP 3A4 inhibitors**

   a. Prescription drugs
       The CYP3A4 inhibitors producing the greatest increase in the risk of myopathy are those given in doses of several hundred milligrams, including the macrolide antibiotics, antifungal azoles, and HIV protease inhibitors.

   b. Grapefruit juice

In addition to prescription drugs, grapefruit juice contains bergamottin, which inhibits CYP3A4, and large quantities taken daily can produce a significant interaction. For example, one grapefruit or <250 mL grapefruit juice daily with breakfast is not likely to be enough to precipitate myopathy with simvastatin or lovastatin taken in the evening (as recommended),[40] but taken simultaneously, the interaction is greater and generally should be avoided.[41] Alternatively, as with other CYP3A4 interactions, atorvastatin is less susceptible and could be substituted for simvastatin or lovastatin in patients who consume >250 mL grapefruit juice regularly.[42]

B. OATP1B1 All statins are substrates for the organic anion transporter OATP1B1,[43] which conveys statins into the hepatocyte for excretion in bile. This is inhibited by cyclosporine and the fibrate gemfibrozil. Fenofibrate causes little if any interaction, and it is the fibrate of choice for coadministration with a statin. Although cyclosporine interacts with all statins, the interaction is least with fluvastatin, which may be the preferred statin in transplant patients taking cyclosporine, though other statins can be used at low doses.

C. Anticoagulants Several statins, including simvastatin, lovastatin, fluvastatin, and rosuvastatin, and possibly others, can modestly potentiate the anticoagulant activity of warfarin and other coumarin anticoagulants,[44,45] which should be taken into account when monitoring these patients.

D. Further information It is important that prescribers are familiar with statin drug interactions, especially for the statins they prescribe frequently or at high dosage. A full discussion is beyond the scope of this chapter, but further details can be found in the prescribing information for individual statins and in a recent comprehensive review.[46]

V. Statin Intolerance

A. The problem Statin therapy is a long-term endeavor, sometimes lifelong. As with any chronic therapy intended to prevent adverse outcomes rather than treat symptoms, adherence can be problematic.[47] Compounding the problem, in the United States and other English-speaking countries, about 10% of patients report adverse events during treatment with statins that lead to discontinuation (Box 11.2).[48,49] However, this rate is only 2% in Italy, Spain, Sweden, and Japan.[49] Cultural factors may play a part in this wide variation.[50]

BOX 11.2 Statin Intolerance Key Points

1. Statin intolerance is a common problem. In clinical practice, about 10% of U.S. patients experience adverse events that lead to cessation of therapy. About half of these have muscle symptoms without significantly elevated creatine kinase.

2. Statin intolerance does not usually occur under double-blind conditions, even in patients who have previously stopped taking statins because of intolerance, showing that the phenomenon is dependent on patients knowing they are taking a statin. This indicates that it is not caused by the statin (except in perhaps <1% of cases). The best explanation is a normal neuropsychological phenomenon, the nocebo effect.

3. Statin therapy can be restored by rechallenge, using the same statin at the same or a lower dose, or a different statin, in over 90% of patients with statin intolerance.

4. Minimizing the nocebo effect is important both when starting treatment with a statin and when attempting to restore statin treatment in a statin-intolerant patient (Box 11.5).

B. Muscle symptoms

1. **Incidence** About half of the adverse events that lead to statin discontinuation are muscle symptoms, typically pain or weakness.[50] These symptoms are usually not accompanied by significant elevations in creatine kinase or other objective changes.

2. **Randomized controlled outcome studies and meta-analyses** In large randomized placebo-controlled trials, the incidence of muscle symptoms is generally similar in the patient group allocated to the statin and the group allocated to placebo.[4,51] Meta-analyses of placebo-controlled studies have shown no difference between statin and placebo in the rates of muscle symptoms.[52,53]

3. **Studies of statin-intolerant patients** Furthermore, studies that have randomized patients with well-documented statin intolerance due to muscle symptoms to a statin or a control, either placebo[54] or an active comparator,[55] have found either no significant difference between statin and control[54,56,57] or a small difference,[58] and in the latter study, the data suggest self-unblinding by a minority of patients.[4,50] These findings indicate that the intolerance generally disappears under double-blind conditions and shows that in most cases the intolerance is not due to a toxic effect of statins.[4,50,51,59,60]

4. **High prevalence of muscle symptoms in middle-aged or elderly people** Muscle symptoms are subjective and common in untreated middle-aged or elderly patients. In the Heart Protection Study (HPS),[32] participants were directly questioned at every visit about muscle AEs (in addition to the standard general query for adverse events typically employed in clinical trials), and one-third reported these symptoms at least once in both the placebo and simvastatin groups. HPS illustrates the high prevalence of muscle symptoms in older people whether taking a statin or not.

C. Relationship of statin intolerance to the nocebo effect

1. **Influence of physician warnings and the media on expectations** The risk of myopathy and rhabdomyolysis is prominent in statin patient information leaflets, and clinicians warn patients to report muscle symptoms; furthermore, Internet searches bring up mainly misinformation about statin AEs, attributing causality without evidence. This is the fate of many advances in medicine, such as vaccination programs and fluoridation of water.[61] Therefore, some patients will expect to suffer these symptoms[62,63] and may associate background muscle AEs with their statin use. This phenomenon is the inverse of the placebo effect and is known as the nocebo effect.[62–64]

2. **What is the nocebo effect?** Just as an ineffective treatment may appear subjectively effective in an uncontrolled setting due to the placebo effect, an innocuous treatment may appear subjectively toxic due to the nocebo effect.[62,63] The placebo/nocebo effect reflects normal human neuropsychology and not drug efficacy/toxicity. Under double-blind randomized conditions, patients do not know what they are taking; the nocebo effect can increase the frequency of an adverse event in both groups, but cannot cause differences between the treatment and control groups.

D. Randomized controlled trials In recent years, various objections have been raised to the reassuring adverse effect profile demonstrated in cardiovascular outcome trials with statins, which include over 170 000 patients. Some have argued that the statin trials do not reflect clinical practice and therefore fail to reliably assess adverse effects.[65–67] Similar objections could be raised to many clinical trials of therapeutic agents of any kind.

Table 11.1.   Discontinuation due to Any Adverse Event in Randomized Double-Blind Placebo-Controlled Cardiovascular Outcome Trials of Statins in Patients with Advanced Disease[a]

Trial	N	Drug, Dose (mg)	Duration (Y)[b]	Patient Type	Age (Y)[b]	% Female	Discontinuation due to AEs (%)	
							Statin	Placebo
4S	4444	S 20-40	5.4	CHD	59	19	5.7	5.7
HPS	20 536	S 40	4.9	Mixed[c]	64	25	4.8	5.1
ALERT	2102	F 40-80	5.1	Renal transplant	50	34	14.8	16.3
4D	1255	A 20	4.0	Diabetes on dialysis	66	46	11.8	8.2
SPARCL	4731	A 80	4.9	Stroke/TIA[d]	63	40	17.5	14.5
CORONA	5011	R 10	2.7	Heart failure	73	24	9.6	12.1
GISSI-HF	4574	R 10	3.9	Heart failure	68	23	4.6	4.0
AURORA	2776	R 10	3.8	Hemodialysis	64	38	14.9[e]	16.8[e]
Total	**45 429**						**8.0**	**8.1**

[a]Trials are listed in order of publication date of the main results.
[b]Mean or median.
[c]65% CHD, 16% cerebrovascular disease, and 29% diabetes.
[d]69% stroke and 31% TIA.
[e]Included end point events.
Abbreviations: Y, years; AEs, adverse events; CHD, coronary heart disease; TIA, transient ischemic attack; S, simvastatin; F, fluvastatin; A, atorvastatin; R, rosuvastatin.
(Reprinted with permission from Tobert JA, Newman CB. Statin tolerability: in defence of placebo-controlled trials. *Eur J Prev Cardiol.* 2016;23(8):891-896.)

The present authors have investigated these objections and find them unfounded,[57] a view shared by a multinational group of experienced trialists and statisticians.[4] For example, the claim[67] that clinical trials underestimate AEs because they exclude participants more vulnerable to statin adverse effects, such as the elderly, women, and patients with renal failure or other complex medical histories, is not sustainable (Table 11.1). This table shows discontinuation rates due to any adverse event—a good measure of tolerability—in 8 large cardiovascular outcome trials comprising over 45 000 participants, many female and elderly, with complex medical histories including one or more of CHD, stroke, diabetes, chronic kidney disease, and heart failure. The discontinuation rates in patients allocated to statin and placebo were consistently similar, and withdrawal due to any adverse event in the 8 studies pooled was 8.0% and 8.1% in patients allocated to statin and placebo, respectively. Thus, there was no intolerance in these studies, not because of the characteristics of the participants, but because statins are well tolerated when treatment is blinded.

E. Evaluation of statin intolerance

1. **Dechallenge and rechallenge (Box 11.3)** Even though in most cases statin intolerance can be adequately explained by the nocebo effect, it remains a challenging clinical problem. Many patients and some clinicians are convinced that the intolerance has a pharmacological basis; in a typical scenario, a clinician prescribes a statin, the patient returns complaining of muscle symptoms with no obvious cause, the clinician or patient stop the statin and the symptoms resolve. The clinician would typically then rechallenge with the same or a different statin, which often succeeds, but sometimes symptoms recur. If so, this sequence of events convinces the patient and

---

BOX 11.3 | **Choices for Rechallenge, in Order of Preference**

1. **Same statin at same dose, or an equivalent dose of a different statin**, first choice because this does not sacrifice efficacy. For example, atorvastatin 20 mg could replace simvastatin 40 mg.
2. **Halve the dose of the same statin**. This will reduce the degree of LDL-C reduction by 6% on average from the original baseline. If this is well tolerated, the clinician may consider attempting to restore the original dose after a few months.
3. **Alternate-day dosing with a statin with a relatively long half-life**, such as rosuvastatin or atorvastatin, might be considered after 3 or 4 statins have been tried using daily dosing. Again, this will involve loss of efficacy, and restoring

daily treatment after a few months is worthwhile when possible.
4. **Addition of nonstatin LDL-C lowering medication**. If the maximum tolerated statin dose does not produce sufficient reduction of LDL cholesterol, another agent can be added, most commonly ezetimibe. This will produce an additional reduction in LDL cholesterol of about 20% from the on-statin level. Ezetimibe is a well-tolerated drug with cardiovascular outcome trial data showing a good long-term safety profile and a significant reduction in the risk of major cardiovascular events.[2] It is available as a generic product.

---

sometimes the clinician that the symptoms are caused by the statin. But this scenario is adequately explained by the nocebo effect and there is no reason to invoke drug toxicity.[50,57] However, even though the nocebo effect reflects normal human neuropsychology,[68] few patients will accept that their symptoms are psychosomatic, and this explanation is generally not therapeutic.

2. **Importance of restarting statin treatment** Devoting effort to restarting treatment with a statin is important, because stopping statins can be expected to increase the risk of cardiovascular events.[4,69] Furthermore, the only class of lipid-lowering agent capable of matching the efficacy of statins is the PCSK9 inhibitors, but as, these cost 50-100 times more than a generic statin. They may be used in addition to a statin in carefully selected cases, but should not be viewed as a statin substitute (Box 11.4).

F. Management of statin intolerance (Box 11.5)

1. **Physician-patient communication** As always, prevention is better than cure.[50] The prescribing information for all statins advises warning patients about the risk of myopathy/rhabdomyolysis and to promptly report unexplained muscle symptoms. Because warning patients about a potential subjective adverse event can substantially

---

BOX 11.4 | **Key Points: Nonstatin Therapies**

1. *Ezetimibe* has excellent safety and tolerability data and proven cardiovascular benefits and is available as a generic product. It is the medication of choice in most patients who require more LDL-C reduction than statins alone can provide.
2. Fenofibrate is generally well tolerated and much less likely than gemfibrozil to cause myopathy/rhabdomyolysis when given with a statin.
3. PCSK9 inhibitors, introduced in 2015, appear to be well tolerated.

4. Bile acid–binding resins (cholestyramine, colesevelam) and, to a lesser extent, omega-3 fatty acids commonly cause GI symptoms. Both are inconvenient to take, requiring multiple daily gram doses. Bile acid–binding resins decrease absorption of many medications.
5. Niacin is a toxic drug (at lipid-lowering doses) that should be used only by lipid specialists, if at all.

BOX 11.5 | **Minimizing the Nocebo Effect to Preempt and Manage Statin Intolerance**

1. When starting a statin, advise patients that:
   a. CV benefits and safety are proven over 30 years.
   b. Risk of rhabdomyolysis is <1 in a thousand.
   c. Aches and pains are very common in people *not* taking a statin.
   d. Statins as a common cause of muscle and other symptoms is a myth spread on the Internet.

2. Advise an intolerant patient that:
   a. Statin therapy can be restored in 9 out of 10 patients.

3. Stay positive—intolerance is a soluble problem.

---

increase the risk that it will be experienced,[62,70–72] the frequency of subjective adverse events can be strongly influenced by clinician-patient communication.[71] Therefore, it is important to inform the patient that myopathy/rhabdomyolysis occurs in <1 in 1000 patients and to put this very small risk in the context of the proven benefits of statins. Clinicians can also consider advising patients that statins rarely cause minor muscle symptoms and that information about statin adverse effects revealed by Internet searches is mostly incorrect.

2. **Ruling out other causes of muscle symptoms** If a patient stops the statin because of an adverse event, the first step is to rule out other explanations for the symptoms. If the symptoms are musculoskeletal as is commonly the case, unaccustomed, prolonged, or strenuous exercise may be the cause. Hypothyroidism is another cause of muscle symptoms, especially weakness, and diuretics can cause leg cramps. If the patient experienced similar symptoms before beginning statin treatment, this may suggest a different diagnosis, such as fibromyalgia.

3. **Communicating an optimistic outlook** Rechallenge is successful in about 90% of cases,[48] though not necessarily with the same statin or at the same dose. Patient expectations are critical.[62] Communicating an optimistic outlook[63,64] can reverse or reduce the effect of previous negative expectations.[61] Patients need to be aware that intolerance is a soluble problem that responds to therapy adjustments. It is also useful to remind the patient of the proven cardiovascular benefits of statins and to explore any ambivalence about the need to take a statin. Knowing the value of a treatment reduces the nocebo effect.[63]

VI. Adverse Effects of Nonstatin Therapies for Dyslipidemia

A. Ezetimibe

1. **Hepatic transaminases** Ezetimibe is well tolerated and has a good safety profile. Elevations in hepatic transaminases are rare and probably not causally related. Nevertheless, the prescribing information recommends against using ezetimibe in patients with moderate or severe liver disease.

2. **No evidence for cancer** Earlier concerns that ezetimibe might increase the risk of cancer,[73] based on limited interim clinical trial data, have not been borne out by the final data from these trials.[2,74]

3. **IMPROVE-IT trial** In the IMPROVE-IT trial in 18 000 patients with acute coronary syndrome followed for 6 years,[2] there were no differences between the ezetimibe/simvastatin group and the simvastatin group in any prespecified safety end points including myopathy and rhabdomyolysis, hepatic transaminases ≥3× ULN, gallbladder-related adverse events and cholecystectomy, and cancer.

4. **Cyclosporine** Ezetimibe increases plasma concentrations of cyclosporine, and therefore, cyclosporine concentrations should be monitored in patients taking ezetimibe.

B. Monoclonal antibodies to proprotein subtilisin kexin type 9 (PCSK9)

1. **Need for additional safety data** Evolocumab and alirocumab were approved in 2015. They appear to be generally well tolerated.[75,76]

2. **Serious adverse effects** The most serious adverse effects of PCSK9 monoclonal antibodies are severe hypersensitivity reactions, which are rare. Less severe allergic reactions include urticaria, nummular eczema, and hypersensitivity vasculitis.

3. **Injection site reactions** Injection site reactions (redness, pain, bruising) occurred in fewer than 10% of people in clinical trials.

4. **Potential neurocognitive adverse effects** There is some evidence that monoclonal antibodies to PCSK9 rarely cause neurocognitive adverse events such as amnesia, impaired memory, and confusion.[75,76] This is undergoing evaluation.

5. **Drug interactions** There are no known drug interactions to date.

6. **Safety at low levels of LDL-C** The combination of a statin and a PCSK9 inhibitor can drive LDL cholesterol down to very low levels, below 25 mg/dL. The evidence to date does not indicate any particular hazard attributable to very low LDL-C.[75,76]

   The main negative attribute of PCSK9 inhibitors is their high cost, which in the United States was more than $14 000 per year of treatment when launched in 2015, for both alirocumab and evolocumab.

   PCSK9 inhibitors are covered in detail in the chapter on PCSK9 inhibitors.

C. Fibrates

1. **Gemfibrozil**
   a. **Myopathy/rhabdomyolysis in combination with statins**
      Myopathy or rhabdomyolysis when gemfibrozil is given with a statin is the most serious safety concern and the main reason why gemfibrozil has been largely displaced by fenofibrate. The probable mechanism is inhibition of the organic anion transporter OATB1B1 inhibitor, reducing statin elimination in the bile.
   b. **Common adverse effects**
      Common adverse effects are gastrointestinal (dyspepsia, abdominal pain) and worsening of renal function in people with creatinine above 2.0 mg/dL.
   c. **Contraindications**
      Gemfibrozil is contraindicated in patients with liver disease or severe renal impairment. Repaglinide is contraindicated with gemfibrozil because of the risk of severe hypoglycemia.

2. **Fenofibrate**
   a. **Myopathy/rhabdomyolysis in combination with statins**
      The use of fenofibrate with a statin carries a much lower risk of myopathy/rhabdomyolysis than gemfibrozil plus a statin.[77]
   b. **LFTs and creatinine**
      Fenofibrate may cause increased liver function tests (3%-7% of patients) and can increase plasma creatinine. Both liver function tests and creatinine should be monitored.
   c. **Serious adverse events**
      Serious adverse events include cholelithiasis and possibly a small increased risk of pulmonary embolism.[78]

d. **Drug interactions**
Fenofibrate interacts with coumarin anticoagulants, immunosuppressants, bile acid binding resins, and colchicine. The dose of the coumarin anticoagulant should be adjusted to maintain the prothrombin time/INR at the desired level to avoid bleeding.

D. Bile acid–binding resins: Colestipol, cholestyramine, and colesevelam

1. **Constipation** The most common adverse reaction with bile acid–binding resins is constipation, which is probably due to binding of bile salts that normally would stimulate the colon. Constipation can be alleviated by gradual dose increments, increased fluid intake, fiber, and a stool softener.

2. **Other gastrointestinal adverse effects** Other less frequent gastrointestinal adverse effects include abdominal pain or cramping, bloating and flatulence, and transient elevations of liver function tests. Colesevelam may be better tolerated than the older medications, cholestyramine and colestipol.

3. **Decreased absorption of vitamins and medications** Bile acid–binding resins may decrease absorption of folic acid and fat-soluble vitamins (A, D, E, and K) as well as a variety of medications. Therefore, the interval between taking a bile acid–binding resin and any other medication should be as long as possible, preferably 2 to 4 hours before the bile acid resin or 4-6 hours afterward.

4. **Elevations in triglycerides** Bile acid–binding resins may cause modest increases in plasma triglycerides (10%-20%). They should not be used in patients with triglycerides above 500 mg/dL and should be discontinued in patients who develop triglycerides above 500 mg/dL or hypertriglyceridemia-related pancreatitis.

E. Omega-3 fatty acids (prescription): Omega-3 acid ethyl esters, omega-3 carboxylic acid, and icosapent ethyl

1. **Gastrointestinal adverse effects** Adverse effects are mostly related to the gastrointestinal tract and include eructation, taste perversion, diarrhea, nausea, abdominal pain, or discomfort.

2. **Potential hepatic effects** All omega-3 fatty acids should be used with caution in patients with hepatic disease, and ALT and AST levels should be monitored.

3. **Hypersensitivity to fish** Caution is also recommended when prescribing omega-3 fatty acids to people who are hypersensitive to fish; however, it is not known whether this increases the risk of allergic reactions.

4. **Increase in LDL-C** Omega-3 acid ethyl esters and omega-3 carboxylic acid may increase LDL-C levels.

5. **Bleeding** There is no conclusive evidence that prescription omega-3 fatty acids increase the risk of bleeding. Nevertheless, the prescribing information for each omega-3 fatty acid states that some studies have found prolonged bleeding time, but within the normal limits, and without clinically significant bleeding episodes. The manufacturers also recommend that patients on anticoagulants or antiplatelet agents should be carefully monitored when taking omega-3 fatty acids.

F. Niacin (lipid-lowering doses)

1. **Cutaneous and hepatic adverse effects** Prescription niacin has been used for 60 years to lower triglycerides, raise LDL-C, and increase HDL-C, despite a high incidence of cutaneous adverse effects including flushing and pruritus and occasional serious hepatotoxicity.

2. **Infection and bleeding** Recent RCTs show that niacin has other serious adverse effects, including infection and bleeding,[79–81] and it does not reduce cardiovascular events when given together with a statin.[80–82] As a result, prescription niacin is no longer available in most of Europe.[81]

3. **Benefits/risks** Although extended-release niacin is still marketed in the United States, in April 2016, the FDA withdrew the approval of the combination products containing niacin extended release (ER) with simvastatin or lovastatin because of the studies cited above demonstrating that the benefits no longer outweighed the risks (*Federal Register* vol. 81, No. 74, Monday April 18, 2016, Notices). Similarly, a recent Expert Consensus report from the American College of Cardiology concluded niacin does not add to the cardiovascular benefit of statins and may be harmful, and therefore niacin preparations should not be used together with statins.[83] Based on the results of the Coronary Drug Project and long-term follow-up of participants in this study,[84] which preceded the statin era, specialists may occasionally use niacin in the rare patient who cannot tolerate any statin at any dose.

References

1. Cholesterol Treatment Trialists' (CTT) Collaboration. Efficacy and safety of more intensive lowering of LDL cholesterol: a meta-analysis of data from 170,000 participants in 26 randomised trials. *Lancet.* 2010;376:1670-1681.
2. Cannon CP, Blazing MA, Giugliano RP, et al. Ezetimibe added to statin therapy after acute coronary syndromes. *N Engl J Med.* 2015;372(25):2387-2397.
3. Collins R, MacMahon S. Reliable assessment of the effects of treatment on mortality and major morbidity, I: clinical trials. *Lancet.* 2001;357(9253):373-380.
4. Collins R, Reith C, Emberson J, et al. Interpretation of the evidence for the efficacy and safety of statin therapy. *Lancet.* 2016;388(10059):2532-2561. http://dx.doi.org/10.1016/S0140-6736(16)31357-5.
5. MacMahon S, Collins R. Reliable assessment of the effects of treatment on mortality and major morbidity, II: observational studies. *Lancet.* 2001;357(9254):455-462.
6. Study of the Effectiveness of Additional Reductions in Cholesterol and Homocysteine (SEARCH) Collaborative Group. Intensive lowering of LDL cholesterol with 80 mg versus 20 mg simvastatin daily in 12,064 survivors of myocardial infarction: a double-blind randomised trial. *Lancet.* 2010;376:1658-1669.
7. Tobert JA. Lovastatin and beyond: the history of the HMG-CoA reductase inhibitors. *Nat Rev Drug Discov.* 2003;2(7):517-526.
8. Grady D, Rubin SM, Petitti DB, et al. Hormone therapy to prevent disease and prolong life in postmenopausal women. *Ann Intern Med.* 1992;117(12):1016-1037.
9. Grodstein F, Stampfer MJ, Manson JE, et al. Postmenopausal estrogen and progestin use and the risk of cardiovascular disease. *N Engl J Med.* 1996;335(7):453-461.
10. Hulley S, Grady D, Bush T, et al. Randomized trial of estrogen plus progestin for secondary prevention of coronary heart disease in postmenopausal women. Heart and Estrogen/progestin Replacement Study (HERS) Research Group. *JAMA.* 1998;280(7):605-613.
11. Writing Group for the Women's Health Initiative Investigators. Risks and benefits of estrogen plus progestin in healthy postmenopausal women: principal results From the Women's Health Initiative randomized controlled trial. *JAMA.* 2002;288(3):321-333.
12. Anderson GL, Limacher M, Assaf AR, et al. Effects of conjugated equine estrogen in postmenopausal women with hysterectomy: the Women's Health Initiative randomized controlled trial. *JAMA.* 2004;291(14):1701-1712.
13. Tatsioni A, Bonitsis NG, Ioannidis JP. Persistence of contradicted claims in the literature. *JAMA.* 2007;298(21):2517-2526.
14. Heart Protection Study Collaborative Group. MRC/BHF Heart Protection Study of antioxidant vitamin supplementation in 20,536 high-risk individuals: a randomised placebo-controlled trial. *Lancet.* 2002;360(9326):23-33.
15. Stroes ES, Thompson PD, Corsini A, et al. Statin-associated muscle symptoms: impact on statin therapy—European Atherosclerosis Society Consensus Panel Statement on Assessment, Aetiology and Management. *Eur Heart J.* 2015;36(17):1012-1022.
16. Tobert JA. Efficacy and long-term adverse effect pattern of lovastatin. *Am J Cardiol.* 1988;62(15):28j-34j.
17. Mammen AL. Statin-associated autoimmune myopathy. *N Engl J Med.* 2016;374(7):664-669.
18. Keech A, Collins R, MacMahon S, et al. Three-year follow-up of the Oxford Cholesterol Study: assessment of the efficacy and safety of simvastatin in preparation for a large mortality study. *Eur Heart J.* 1994;15(2):255-269.

19. Parker BA, Augeri AL, Capizzi JA, et al. Effect of statins on creatine kinase levels before and after a marathon run. *Am J Cardiol.* 2012;109(2):282-287.
20. Mikus CR, Boyle LJ, Borengasser SJ, et al. Simvastatin impairs exercise training adaptations. *J Am Coll Cardiol.* 2013;62(8):709-714.
21. Parker BA, Capizzi JA, Grimaldi AS, et al. Effect of statins on skeletal muscle function. *Circulation.* 2013;127(1):96-103.
22. Panza GA, Taylor BA, Dada MR, Thompson PD. Changes in muscle strength in individuals with statin-induced myopathy: a summary of 3 investigations. *J Clin Lipidol.* 2015;9(3):351-356.
23. Sattar N, Preiss D, Murray HM, et al. Statins and risk of incident diabetes: a collaborative meta-analysis of randomised statin trials. *Lancet.* 2010;375:735-742.
24. Preiss D, Seshasai SR, Welsh P, et al. Risk of incident diabetes with intensive-dose compared with moderate-dose statin therapy: a meta-analysis. *JAMA.* 2011;305(24):2556-2564.
25. Preiss D, Sattar N. Pharmacotherapy: statins and new-onset diabetes—the important questions. *Nat Rev Cardiol.* 2012;9(4):190-192.
26. Ridker PM, Pradhan A, MacFadyen JG, Libby P, Glynn RJ. Cardiovascular benefits and diabetes risks of statin therapy in primary prevention: an analysis from the JUPITER trial. *Lancet.* 2012;380(9841):565-571.
27. Robinson JG. Statins and diabetes risk: how real is it and what are the mechanisms? *Curr Opin Lipidol.* 2015;26(3):228-235.
28. Erqou S, Lee CC, Adler AI. Statins and glycaemic control in individuals with diabetes: a systematic review and meta-analysis. *Diabetologia.* 2014;57(12):2444-2452.
29. Amarenco P, Bogousslavsky J, Callahan A, et al. High-dose atorvastatin after stroke or transient ischemic attack. *N Engl J Med.* 2006;355(6):549-559.
30. Hackam DG, Woodward M, Newby LK, et al. Statins and intracerebral hemorrhage: collaborative systematic review and meta-analysis. *Circulation.* 2011;124:2233-2242.
31. O'Donnell MJ, Xavier D, Liu L, et al. Risk factors for ischaemic and intracerebral haemorrhagic stroke in 22 countries (the INTERSTROKE study): a case-control study. *Lancet.* 2010;376(9735):112-123.
32. Heart Protection Study Collaborative Group. MRC/BHF Heart Protection Study of cholesterol lowering with simvastatin in 20 536 high risk individuals: a randomised placebo-controlled trial. *Lancet.* 2002;360:7-22.
33. Pedersen TR, Berg K, Cook TJ, et al. Safety and tolerability of cholesterol lowering with simvastatin during 5 years in the Scandinavian Simvastatin Survival Study. *Arch Intern Med.* 1996;156:2085-2092.
34. Keech AC, Armitage JM, Wallendszus KR, et al. Absence of effects of prolonged simvastatin therapy on nocturnal sleep in a large randomized placebo-controlled study. Oxford Cholesterol Study Group. *Br J Clin Pharmacol.* 1996;42(4):483-490.
35. Kostis JB, Dobrzynski JM. The effect of statins on erectile dysfunction: a meta-analysis of randomized trials. *J Sex Med.* 2014;11(7):1626-1635.
36. Cholesterol Treatment Trialists' (CTT) Collaboration. Lack of effect of lowering LDL cholesterol on cancer: meta-analysis of individual data from 175,000 people in 27 randomised trials of statin therapy. *PLOS ONE.* 2012;7(1):e29849.
37. Dujovne CA, Chremos AN, Pool JL, et al. Expanded clinical evaluation of lovastatin (EXCEL) study results: IV. Additional perspectives on the tolerability of lovastatin. *Am J Med.* 1991;91(1b):25s-30s.
38. Björnsson E, Jacobsen EI, Kalaitzakis E. Hepatotoxicity associated with statins: reports of idiosyncratic liver injury post-marketing. *J Hepatol.* 2012;56(2):374-380.
39. Karalis DG, Hill AN, Clifton S, Wild RA. The risks of statin use in pregnancy: a systematic review. *J Clin Lipidol.* 2016;10(5):1081-1090. doi:10.1016/j.jacl.2016.07.002.
40. Rogers J, Zhao J, Liu L, et al. Grapefruit juice has minimal effects on plasma concentrations of lovastatin-derived 3-hydroxy-3-methylglutaryl coenzyme A reductase inhibitors. *Clin Pharmacol Ther.* 1999;66:358-366.
41. Lilja JJ, Neuvonen M, Neuvonen PJ. Effects of regular consumption of grapefruit juice on the pharmacokinetics of simvastatin. *Br J Clin Pharmacol.* 2004;58(1):56-60.
42. Reddy P, Ellington D, Zhu Y, et al. Serum concentrations and clinical effects of atorvastatin in patients taking grapefruit juice daily. *Br J Clin Pharmacol.* 2011;72(3):434-441.
43. Niemi M, Pasanen MK, Neuvonen PJ. Organic anion transporting polypeptide 1B1: a genetically polymorphic transporter of major importance for hepatic drug uptake. *Pharmacol Rev.* 2011;63(1):157-181.
44. Yu CY, Campbell SE, Zhu B, et al. Effect of pitavastatin vs. rosuvastatin on international normalized ratio in healthy volunteers on steady-state warfarin. *Curr Med Res Opin.* 2012;28(2):187-194.
45. Andrus MR. Oral anticoagulant drug interactions with statins: case report of fluvastatin and review of the literature. *Pharmacotherapy.* 2004;24(2):285-290.
46. Kellick KA, Bottorff M, Toth PP; The National Lipid Association's Safety Task F. A clinician's guide to statin drug-drug interactions. *J Clin Lipidol.* 2014;8(3 suppl):S30-S46.
47. Grundy SM. Statin discontinuation and intolerance: the challenge of lifelong therapy. *Ann Intern Med.* 2013;158(7):562-563.

48. Zhang H, Plutzky J, Skentzos S, et al. Discontinuation of statins in routine care settings: a cohort study. *Ann Intern Med.* 2013;158(7):526-534.
49. Hovingh GK, Gandra SR, McKendrick J, et al. Identification and management of patients with statin-associated symptoms in clinical practice: a clinician survey. *Atherosclerosis.* 2015;245:111-117.
50. Tobert JA, Newman CB. The nocebo effect in the context of statin intolerance. *J Clin Lipidol.* 2016;10(4):739-747.
51. Newman CB, Tobert JA. Statin intolerance: reconciling clinical trials and clinical experience. *JAMA.* 2015;313(10):1011-1012.
52. Kashani A, Phillips CO, Foody JM, et al. Risks associated with statin therapy: a systematic overview of randomized clinical trials. *Circulation.* 2006;114(25):2788-2797.
53. Ganga HV, Slim HB, Thompson PD. A systematic review of statin-induced muscle problems in clinical trials. *Am Heart J.* 2014;168(1):6-15.
54. Joy TR, Monjed A, Zou GY, Hegele RY, McDonald CG, Mahon JL. N-of-1 (single-patient) trials for statin-related myalgia. *Ann Intern Med.* 2014;160:301-310.
55. Moriarty PM, Thompson PD, Cannon CP, et al. Efficacy and safety of alirocumab vs ezetimibe in statin-intolerant patients, with a statin rechallenge arm: the ODYSSEY ALTERNATIVE randomized trial. *J Clin Lipidol.* 2015;9(6):758-769.
56. Newman CB, Tobert JA. Comment on the article by Moriarty et al. *J Clin Lipidol.* 2016;10(1):209-210.
57. Tobert JA, Newman CB. Statin tolerability: in defence of placebo-controlled trials. *Eur J Prev Cardiol.* 2016;23(8):891-896.
58. Nissen SE, Stroes E, Dent-Acosta RE, et al. Efficacy and tolerability of evolocumab vs ezetimibe in patients with muscle-related statin intolerance: the GAUSS-3 randomized clinical trial. *JAMA.* 2016;315(15):1580-1590.
59. Brown WV, Moriarty PM, McKenney JM. JCL roundtable: PCSK9 inhibitors in clinical practice. *J Clin Lipidol.* 2016;10(1):5-14.
60. Brown WV. From the editor: new drugs, old lessons. *J Clin Lipidol.* 2016;10(1):1-2.
61. Crichton F, Petrie KJ. Accentuate the positive: counteracting psychogenic responses to media health messages in the age of the Internet. *J Psychosom Res.* 2015;79(3):185-189.
62. Faasse K, Petrie KJ. The nocebo effect: patient expectations and medication side effects. *Postgrad Med J.* 2013;89(1055):540-546.
63. Bingel U. Avoiding nocebo effects to optimize treatment outcome. *JAMA.* 2014;312(7):693-694.
64. Häuser W, Hansen E, Enck P. Nocebo phenomena in medicine: their relevance in everyday clinical practice. *Dtsch Arztebl Int.* 2012;109(26):459-465.
65. Maningat P, Breslow JL. Needed: pragmatic clinical trials for statin-intolerant patients. *N Engl J Med.* 2011;365(24):2250-2251.
66. Fernandez G, Spatz ES, Jablecki C, Phillips PS. Statin myopathy: a common dilemma not reflected in clinical trials. *Cleve Clin J Med.* 2011;78(6):393-403.
67. Jacobson TA. NLA Task Force on Statin Safety—2014 update. *J Clin Lipidol.* 2014;8(3 suppl):S1-S4.
68. Tracey I. Getting the pain you expect: mechanisms of placebo, nocebo and reappraisal effects in humans. *Nat Med.* 2010;16(11):1277-1283.
69. Horton R. Offline: lessons from the controversy over statins. *Lancet.* 2016;388(10049):1040.
70. Mondaini N, Gontero P, Giubilei G, et al. Finasteride 5 mg and sexual side effects: how many of these are related to a nocebo phenomenon? *J Sex Med.* 2007;4(6):1708-1712.
71. Colloca L, Finniss D. Nocebo effects, patient-clinician communication, and therapeutic outcomes. *JAMA.* 2012;307(6):567-568.
72. Myers MG, Cairns JA, Singer J. The consent form as a possible cause of side effects. *Clin Pharmacol Ther.* 1987;42:250-253.
73. Nissen SE. Analyses of cancer data from three ezetimibe trials. *N Engl J Med.* 2009;360(1):86-87; author reply 87.
74. Baigent C, Landray MJ, Reith C, et al. The effects of lowering LDL cholesterol with simvastatin plus ezetimibe in patients with chronic kidney disease (Study of Heart and Renal Protection): a randomised placebo-controlled trial. *Lancet.* 2011;377(9784):2181-2192.
75. Robinson JG, Farnier M, Krempf M, et al. Efficacy and safety of alirocumab in reducing lipids and cardiovascular events. *N Engl J Med.* 2015;372(16):1489-1499.
76. Sabatine MS, Giugliano RP, Wiviott SD, et al. Efficacy and safety of evolocumab in reducing lipids and cardiovascular events. *N Engl J Med.* 2015;372(16):1500-1509.
77. Jones PH, Davidson MH. Reporting rate of rhabdomyolysis with fenofibrate + statin versus gemfibrozil + any statin. *Am J Cardiol.* 2005;95(1):120-122.
78. Keech A, Simes RJ, Barter P, et al. Effects of long-term fenofibrate therapy on cardiovascular events in 9795 people with type 2 diabetes mellitus (the FIELD study): randomised controlled trial. *Lancet.* 2005;366(9500):1849-1861.
79. Anderson TJ, Boden WE, Desvigne-Nickens P, et al. Safety profile of extended-release niacin in the AIM-HIGH trial. *N Engl J Med.* 2014;371(3):288-290.

80. Landray MJ, Haynes R, Hopewell JC, et al. Effects of extended-release niacin with laropiprant in high-risk patients. *N Engl J Med.* 2014;371(3):203-212.
81. Lloyd-Jones DM. Niacin and HDL cholesterol—time to face facts. *N Engl J Med.* 2014;371(3):271-273.
82. Aim-High Investigators. Niacin in patients with low HDL cholesterol levels receiving intensive statin therapy. *N Engl J Med.* 2011;365(24):2255-2267.
83. Lloyd-Jones DM, Morris PB, Ballantyne CM, et al. 2016 ACC expert consensus decision pathway on the role of non-statin therapies for LDL-cholesterol lowering in the management of atherosclerotic cardiovascular disease risk: a report of the American College of Cardiology Task Force on Clinical Expert Consensus Documents. *J Am Coll Cardiol.* 2016;68(1):92-125.
84. Canner PL, Berge KG, Wenger NK, et al. Fifteen year mortality in Coronary Drug Project patients: long-term benefit with niacin. *J Am Coll Cardiol.* 1986;8(6):1245-1255.

CHAPTER 12

Familial Hypercholesterolemia: Family Disease

Emanuel M. Ebin and Seth J. Baum

Key Points

- Familial hypercholesterolemia (FH) is a heterogeneous genetic disease.
- There are several aspects to identifying FH in a patient.
- Cascade (family) screening is essential.
- Management is focused on drug therapy although lifestyle modification still has a roll.
- Statins form the basis of treatment; however, in those with homozygous or severely elevated LDL-C, there are newer and more potent medications.

I.   Genetics

A. Historical background Brown and Goldstein are indisputably the fathers of familial hypercholesterolemia (FH). In 1972, they attributed the disorder to defective HMG-CoA reductase.[1] A year later, they recognized their miscalculation and determined that a genetic abnormality in receptors for LDL particles was at the root of FH.[2] Their presumption was that a mutation in the LDL receptor (LDLR) gene caused a malfunction in the liver's capacity to capture and degrade LDL particles circulating in the blood. The consequence of such a disorder was of course lifelong markedly elevated LDL levels (beginning in utero and resulting in the development of concomitant severe and premature atherosclerotic cardiovascular disease and even valvular and supravalvular stenosis in some cases).

B. Genetic causes of FH Studying a population of patients with premature atherosclerotic cardiovascular disease (ASCVD) and markedly elevated LDL levels, they calculated that the prevalence of FH was 1/500 in the heterozygous form (HeFH) and 1/1000000 in the homozygous form (HoFH).[3] (It is important to recognize that these two prevalence figures are inextricably bound to one another through the Hardy Weinberg Equilibrium Equation.) At the time of their discovery, Goldstein and Brown attributed a single mutation in the LDLR to all cases of FH. We have learned much since then, and more than 1700 LDLR mutations have already been discovered.[4,5] Additionally, mutations in other genes—and alterations of their downstream protein products—affecting the functionality of the LDL receptor (LDLR) are now recognized to also cause FH, for example, PCSK9 and apoB.[6-8] To better understand how multifarious mutations can cause a single disease, a quick review of the LDLR's role in lipid metabolism is called for.

C. The LDL receptor in FH Imagine the LDLR as a "Y-shaped" structure planted in the hepatocyte. Different ligands can bind the receptor at different sites on the exposed "Y": apoB, a large protein weaving in and out of the surface of atherogenic lipoprotein particles such as LDL, and PCSK9 at a different site. Under normal circumstances, LDL particles bind the LDLR to be internalized into the hepatocyte for degradation. Intracellular levels of cholesterol drive this process; less cholesterol means more internalization of LDL particles, while more intracellular cholesterol means less internalization. Anything disrupting the LDLR's ability to internalize and then destroy LDL particles will result in high blood levels of LDL-C. So if the LDLR itself is defective, or if something that interacts with the LDLR causes its functionality to be adversely disrupted (eg, PCSK9 and apoB), fewer LDL particles will be internalized and LDL-C levels can become severely elevated.[9]

D. **Nomenclature** Another post-Goldstein/Brown genetic development requiring explanation is the distinction among three types of HoFH. Recall that each gene has two alleles, one from the mother and the other from the father. Goldstein and Brown initially described HoFH as a condition in which an individual inherits a single and same mutation in the LDLR from each parent. This is now referred to as "simple HoFH."[10] It is, as you might intuit, a very rare event. While this can be confusing, the lexicon is pervasive in the literature, and therefore, our acquaintance with it is imperative.

Far more frequently, HoFH is the result of inheritance of two different pathogenic mutations in the same gene, the LDLR being most common. A person with this form of HoFH is referred to as a "compound heterozygote." Note that the term "heterozygote" is utilized here to describe a homozygote. Another common condition is when an individual inherits a mutation in one gene from the mother and a different gene from the father. As both mutations in this scenario adversely affect LDLR function, the person is born with FH. More specifically, they have HoFH, and even more specifically, they are a "double heterozygote." An example of such a circumstance would be inheriting a pathologic LDLR mutation from one parent, and a PCSK9 gain of function mutation from the other (PCSK9 is responsible for degrading the LDLR itself. Therefore, more PCSK9 means higher LDL-C levels).

II.   Epidemiology

A. **Prevalence** We mentioned early on that the presumed prevalence of FH was 1/500. This too has been refined in recent years. Based on large genetic studies from the Netherlands, Denmark, and the United States, we now know the prevalence of FH to be ~1/200[11] and consequently that of HoFH to be around 1/160 000.[12,13] Therefore, FH is more common than cystic fibrosis, neonatal hypothyroidism, and even type 1 diabetes mellitus. As typical clinical practices often comprise a few thousand patients or so, this translates into the fact that every practice cares for at least several FH patients.

Unfortunately, the diagnosis is typically unrecognized, leaving such individuals and their families undertreated and thereby more vulnerable to the consequences of lifelong LDL-C elevations. Our underappreciation of FH is so profound that one estimate went so far as to state that <1% of FH patients in the United States have been identified.[14] Consider this in the context of the fact that FH is an autosomal dominant disorder, meaning if you inherit a mutation, you have the disease. It also means that each child of an HeFH parent has a 50% likelihood of inheriting the disease. Thus, we have much work to do, which will be discussed in greater detail over the ensuing few pages.

B. **Clustering of FH in populations** Here's a quick caveat when it comes to prevalence statistics: they apply to the general population. Circumstances in which consanguinity is high (when individuals within a particular group tend to procreate predominantly within that group) produce even higher prevalence rates. Such groups have been dubbed founder populations. In the case of FH, French Canadians, South African Afrikaners, South African Ashkenazi Jews, Ashkenazi Jews in general, and Christian Lebanese are founder populations and can have an FH prevalence as high as 1/67.[15] So it is important to "know your audience" and be on the lookout for such individuals and their families in your practices.

C. Use of genetics in clinical care Finally, when it comes to the genetics of FH, there is a fairly heated debate as to whether or not genotyping should become the standard of care. It is so in smaller nations such as the Netherlands, but in the United States, experts in FH management have not adopted routine genotyping. The reason for this lies in the poor sensitivity of genetic testing. Studies have demonstrated that between 20% and even 70% of possible FH patients will have negative genetic tests.[16,17] The specificity of genotyping is on the contrary quite high; when pathogenic mutations are identified, the carrier definitely has FH. One circumstance in which few would argue against the merits of genotyping is in Cascade screening, also to be discussed in a future section of this chapter. Simply stated though, when a particular mutation is identified in one patient, it can be used to identify relatives who carry the same mutation and thus the disease as well.

III. Clinical Presentation

To assure that clinicians recognize patients with FH, the diagnosis must always be on the tips of our diagnostic tongues when we assess patients with high LDL levels.[18] Once the diagnosis becomes top of mind, evidence should be sought to confirm it. Remember though that the following clues are generalizations; variations occur and not all elements must be present to render the FH diagnosis. Such clues include:

A. A very high LDL (>95% for age/gender matched controls) with a typically normal TG and HDL. LDL particles are usually large, not small. Previously, very precise and high cut points in LDL-C existed in order to diagnose HeFH and HoFH. HoFH required an untreated LDL-C > 500 mg/dL and an LDL-C > 300 mg/dL when treated with lipid-lowering therapy (LLT).[19–21] The cut point for HeFH in an adult had similarly been >190 mg/dL. Recent studies in which genotyping has been performed revealed the fact that there is an unexpectedly large overlap of LDL-C among those with FH. To date, the lowest LDL-C in an untreated patient with HoFH is 170 mg/dL.[11] Thus, LDL-C levels have an enormous overlap between those with HeFH and HoFH. Still, there is no question that the higher the LDL-C, the more aggressive the vascular disease.

In the 2013 ACC/AHA Guidelines, FH is not a specific category meeting requirements for statin therapy. Instead, LDL-C ≥ 190 mg/dL is considered one of the four "ASCVD Statin Benefit Group."

B. Patients should have a family history of premature ASCVD, very high cholesterol, or both.

C. Premature ASCVD in a patient is a clue to FH. In fact, 20% of all MIs in people under age 45 are a consequence of FH.[22,23]

D. The expected response to lipid-lowering therapy is often blunted in these patients, their LDL falling less robustly than would normally be anticipated. This occurs because the common denominator for LDL lowering with standard medications such as statins, ezetimibe, and the bile acid sequestrants is an up-regulation of LDLRs. As these receptors are by definition defective, their up-regulation is less effective at internalizing LDL particles.[24–26]

E. Physical signs

1. **Skin** Physical signs can occur, but are not needed for the diagnosis of FH: extensor tendon xanthomas, typically affecting the Achilles or the hands; corneal arcus; and xanthelasma are manifestations of abnormal cholesterol deposition [Images]. A few clinical reminders are important here. With regard to corneal arcus, it does

not have to be circumferential. In fact, it often starts in the superior and inferior aspects of the cornea where the blood supply is greatest. Also, a corneal arcus in someone under 45 years old is pathognomonic for FH.[27] Regarding the Achilles tendon xanthomas, they do not have to be large and protuberant malformations. A simple thickening of the tendon is often all one palpates on examination. Thus, it is important to always examine the Achilles tendon when performing a physical exam. This way, you will recognize it when you feel one that is unusually thickened. It is important to recognize that because of the prevalent use of lipid lowering therapy, xanthomas are uncommon findings nowadays.

2. **Heart valves** Another physical finding that merits its own bullet point is valvular and supravalvular aortic stenosis. These two conditions can occur in the setting of HoFH.[28] Fortunately, they are quite rare. Still, such murmurs should always be considered when evaluating a patient with FH as both can be a major cause of death and disability in patients with HoFH.

F. **Lipoprotein (a)** Finally, another lab value requires special mention here. Lp(a) is a small lipoprotein particle that possesses two negative effects: it is highly atherogenic, and it is also prothrombotic. Elevated Lp(a) causes vascular disease independent of LDL levels,[29,30] but when combined with FH, it is particularly malignant.[31] Making matters worse, elevated Lp(a) is far more prevalent in the FH population than in the "normal" population (in which 20% of people have significant elevation). Thus, every FH patient—and probably every patient with a history of premature ASCVD—should have her Lp(a) assessed. Additionally, some believe that elevated Lp(a) alone can be a significant cause of FH.[31]

IV. Diagnosis and Cascade Screening

A. **Diagnosis of index case** Although most FH specialists in the United States diagnose FH on clinical grounds,[32] three systems are also available: Make Early Diagnosis to Prevent Early Death (MEDPED), The Dutch Lipid Clinic Network, and Simon Broome. Each has its own pros and cons, and none is essential to make the diagnosis. Still, it would be good to familiarize yourself with all three in case you wish to utilize them in clinical practice.

B. **Cascade screening** Once the diagnosis has been made in an individual patient, he/she is dubbed the proband, or the index case. As FH is an autosomal dominant disorder, and as early diagnosis and treatment can dramatically reduce the risk of future ASCVD events,[33] it is incumbent on clinicians to identify other members of the family in need of help. Screening relatives of the proband is called "cascade screening." In performing cascade screening, you work your way from first-degree relatives (parents, children, and siblings) outward all the way to third degree relatives. To identify FH in other members of the family, the three systems noted above can be utilized. Even simpler, when a first-degree relative of an FH patient has a total cholesterol or LDL-C > 95%, it is highly likely she too has FH.[34]

There are two methods of cascade screening, active and passive. In the United States, only passive screening is currently used. Passive screening employs the index case as the messenger to inform other family members and recommend further testing. As you might imagine, passive screening is fraught with challenges and is typically unsuccessful. In contradistinction, active cascade screening—a system in which clinicians rather than patients seek out affected family members—is extraordinarily effective. It was successfully performed in the Netherlands, a geographically far smaller country than the United States and also a nation with pockets of very high population density. Because of Netherlands' unique geographic and population characteristics (as well as a single national health care system), it was relatively easy for small groups of scientists/physicians to travel door to door to obtain cholesterol levels from relatives of the index cases. This active cascade screening system set the bar for the world, identifying nearly 75% of the Netherlands' FH population and adding 8 additional FH patients for every single index case identified.[11] Currently, the FH Foundation (www.thefhfoundation.org) is planning to initiate an active cascade screening system in the United States, the first of its kind.

V. Management

A. Identification of those with FH The most vital step in the management of FH is its identification. We cannot treat what we do not know, so it is essential for all clinicians to always keep FH on the tips of their differential diagnostic tongues. Using the criteria established above, the FH diagnosis can be rendered and therapy begun.[35]

B. LDL-C goals The mainstay of therapy in FH is to lower the LDL-C as much as possible. Different guidelines exist, providing various targets, but most would agree that getting the LDL-C < 70 mg/dL would be optimal.[36,37] Of course therapy is always matched with risk, so in the highest-risk FH patients, aggressive combination therapy should invariably be introduced. All patients with FH are considered high risk however, and for this reason, formal risk stratification with Framingham or other systems is never advised when guiding treatment in FH as it would not add anything.[37] Let's run through the management of a typical FH patient, one you are likely to see in your practice.

C. Therapeutic lifestyle changes First remember that Therapeutic Lifestyle Changes (TLC) is the foundation of all ASCVD prevention,[38] even in FH. FH patients will garner relatively less lipid advantage from TLC, but other beneficial cardiovascular consequences still require its emphasis. A healthful diet limited in saturated fats and simple sugars, daily aerobic exercise, avoidance of tobacco, maintenance of an optimal blood pressure and weight, and reduction of stress are all important.

D. Medications Concurrent with the establishment of TLC and the control of comorbidities, lipid-lowering medication should be initiated. Children with HeFH usually begin statin therapy at age 8, while those with HoFH begin treatment even younger (with lipoprotein apheresis) (see Chapter 15 for complete details on management in children). In the adult patient, current American Heart Association recommendations (2015) advise use of maximum intensity statins at their highest dose as initial drug monotherapy. Table 12.1 outlines steps in drug therapy.

Some of us in the lipid field choose a different approach. Recognizing that the "greatest bang for the buck" occurs with a statin's starting dose, we might opt to use 10 mg of rosuvastatin and then add ezetimibe 10 mg or a PCSK9 inhibitor on top of that.[39,40] Theoretically, this approach might mitigate some of the high-dose statin risks such as

Table 12.1.	Drug Therapy for Familial Hypercholesterolemia
I.	Initiate drug monotherapy with high-dose, high-intensity statin for a target >50% LDL-C reduction in 3 months time.
II.	If LDL-C does not meet target goal of >50% reduction over 3 mo, then two-drug combination is required, and ezetimibe or a PCSK9 inhibitor should be added to rosuvastatin or atorvastatin.
III.	If LDL-C does not meet target goal of >50% reduction over 3 mo, a third drug should be added. • The third drug can include a PCSK9i, ezetimibe, bile acid sequestrant or niacin.
IV.	If LDL-C does not meet target goal of >50% reduction over 3 mo, a fourth drug should be added and LDL apheresis should be considered.

myalgias and a transaminitis. If such combination therapy is subpar, we might turn to a third agent such as a bile acid sequestrant (BAS). In FH patients with very resistant LDL levels and/or ASCVD, use of lipoprotein apheresis should always be considered.[41–43]

E. **Lipoprotein apheresis** Apheresis was FDA approved in the United States in 1996, and currently, ~60 centers are dispersed within the United States (to find a center, visit www.thefhfoundation.org).

Two machines have been approved for apheresis, Kaneka's Liposorber and B. Braun's H.E.L.P. They differ in their filtration systems but both will effectively acutely drop LDL-C by 70% or more. Other substances are also acutely reduced, including inflammatory agents, fibrinogen, and Lp(a).

Over the ensuing 2 weeks after apheresis, the LDL (as well as the other aforementioned blood products) will rise toward baseline, requiring an additional treatment. Typically, HeFH patients will undergo apheresis every other week, while HoFH patients will be treated weekly.

Each procedure requires the insertion of two large bore IVs and takes ~2-3 hours to complete. As achieving venous access may at times become challenging, some patients require the creation of an AV fistula. It is imperative for doctors and patients alike to understand that apheresis differs significantly from hemodialysis. It is typically not debilitating and may in fact have the opposite result causing invigoration of patients.[44] Thus, fear of the procedure should not be a barrier to its use. Although large outcomes trials can never be performed with these patients, observational studies have demonstrated reduction in ASCVD risk by as much as 72%.[45] Apheresis is therefore a procedure/therapy that should not be ignored.

F. **New medications** In 2013, two novel agents were approved for adjunctive therapy in the treatment of HoFH, lomitapide and mipomersen (Table 12.2). In order to prescribe either of these medications, clinicians must first undergo REMS (Risk Evaluation Mitigation Strategy) certification.

1. **Indications** These medications are indicated only when in the view of the treating clinician a patient has HoFH. They are not intended to be used in the HeFH patient. Of course, this distinction can at times be quite challenging, even for the most erudite lipidologist. It is therefore important to give great consideration prior to prescribing these agents, remembering that typically HoFH patients have premature vascular disease, very high LDL-C, and a history of very high LDL-C and/or premature ASCVD on both sides of the family.

2. **Mechanisms of action** The mechanisms of action (MOA) of both medications are important to review, as they provide further insight into the pathophysiology of FH. While most of our LLTs rely upon LDLR up-regulation to achieve optimal effect, these agents act independently of the LDLR. If you recall, standard LLTs are less

Table 12.2.	Lomitapide and Mipomersen	
Drug Name	**Annual Cost (2015)**	**Side Effects**
Lomitapide	$250 000	• Diarrhea, nausea, vomiting, abdominal cramping • Flulike symptoms • Elevated liver enzymes and hepatic steatosis
Mipomersen	$176 000	• Injection site bruising • Flulike symptoms • Nausea • Headache • Elevated liver enzymes and hepatic steatosis

effective in patients with FH because FH is an LDLR disorder, and up-regulation of LDLRs that have diminished functionality results in suboptimal benefit. As lomitapide and mipomersen act independently of the LDLR, their impact is not blunted by the FH genetic defect itself.

   a. **Lomitapide**

     Lomitapide is a microsomal triglyceride transport inhibitor (MTP inhibitor). During assembly of very low density lipoproteins (VLDLs) in hepatocytes, MTP is used to stabilize the production of apoB-100 and also to add TG to the growing VLDL particle.[46] By blocking MTP, lomitapide diminishes VLDL production, along with the downstream production of LDL. The resulting drop in LDL can average 40%-50% in HoFH patients,[47] a remarkable achievement. Potential side effects include a fatty liver and GI symptoms. A very low fat diet is vital in preventing GI side effects.

   b. **Mipomersen**

     Mipomersen is an antisense oligonucleotide (ASO), which blocks the creation of apoB-100, the large structural protein on all VLDL and LDL particles. Without apoB-100, the liver cannot produce VLDL, which thereby diminishes LDL by over 25%. Mipomersen is a small nucleotide strand complementary to a portion of mRNA coding for apoB-100. When it binds this mRNA in the liver, it creates a double strand of mRNA, something the body abhors and therefore immediately destroys. Mipomersen's efficacy, like that of lomitapide, is independent of the functionality of the LDLR. Thus, these two medications are perfect candidates for the management of HoFH.

G. Proprotein convertase subtilisin/kexin type 9 (PCSK9) inhibitors

   1. **Indications** In 2015, the FDA approved two (PCSK9i), alirocumab and evolocumab. Both were approved for patients with ASCVD and/or HeFH who require greater LDL reduction on maximally tolerated statin therapy.[48] Maximally tolerated statin therapy can be as low as a dose of zero, if patients have tried and failed two or more statins. We must be cautious though. This does not mean that statin intolerance is a stand-alone indication for the PCSK9i. It means though that as long as a patient satisfies the HeFH and/or ASCVD criteria, he/she can be placed on a PCSK9i even if statin intolerance is an issue. An additional prescribing difference should be noted before describing the MOA of these wonder drugs. While both agents are indicated in HeFH, only evolocumab was approved for HoFH[49] (Table 12.3).

Table 12.3. Proprotein Convertase Subtilisin/Kexin Type 9 Inhibitors		
Drug Name	**Annual Cost (2015)**	**Side Effects**
Alirocumab (Praluent)	$14 600	• Nose and throat irritation • Injection site bruising • Flulike symptoms • Urinary tract infection • Diarrhea • Bronchitis/cough • Muscle pain • Spasms
Evolocumab	$14 100	• Runny nose • Sore throat • Flu symptoms • Back pain • Injection site bruising

2. **Mechanism of action**
   a. The mechanism of action for the PCSK9i medications is not only fascinating but also scientifically revealing. PCSK9 was discovered in 2003 and immediately recognized to be central in LDL metabolism.[50]
   b. PCSK9 is a proprotein initially comprised of 5 segments. In the endoplasmic reticulum, it undergoes autocatalysis with the top two subunits being cleaved from the proprotein. Subsequently, one of the subunits binds to and irreversibly blocks the catalytic site of PCSK9. Thus, when PCSK9 is transported into the Golgi apparatus and subsequently the blood, it serves as a binding, not a catalytic protein. And its binding target is the LDLR. It targets the receptor for degradation, preventing it from making its usual 150+ recycling journeys to and from the surface of the hepatocyte to rid the blood of LDL. Active PCSK9 therefore increases LDL levels, while PCSK9 inhibition lowers LDL levels. Of additional scientific and clinical interest, during the time of drug development, individuals were identified with gain of function PCSK9 mutations[51] (high PCSK9 and high LDL) as well as loss of function PCSK9 mutations (low PCSK9 and low LDL).[52] The former individuals were shown to have an increase in ASCVD, while the latter group, a decrease. These mendelian randomization types of data strongly suggested cause and effect between PCSK9 levels and ASCVD events.
   c. Thus, PCSK9 became a powerful potential target for therapeutic intervention. In 2007, Amgen scientists published PCSK9's crystal structure. Human monoclonal antibodies to PCSK9 were then built to block the action of this proprotein; clinical trials were performed; and the drugs were approved in 2015, just 12 years after the discovery of their target protein.

3. **Efficacy**
   a. The PCSK9i medications are extraordinarily effective as LDL-lowering agents in both ASCVD and HeFH individuals. They predictably drop LDL levels by around 60%-65% on top of statin therapy. In the setting of HoFH, however, evolocumab is less predictable, decreasing LDL by an average of only 30%.
   b. While the type of mutation causing FH is irrelevant in HeFH, it does impact efficacy in HoFH. Remember, as opposed to lomitapide and mipomersen, the PCSK9i, like other LLTs, works by impacting the LDLR. In the HeFH patient, the "normal" allele for the receptor appears to take over, resulting in predictable and intensive LDL-C lowering. Such is not the case in HoFH. In HoFH, the type of mutation matters greatly. Two general distinctions can be made between LDLR mutations—null, <2% activity, and defective, between 2% and 25% activity. Individuals with 2 defective mutations get the best response from evolocumab (~47% reduction), while those with 2 null mutations get the worst (no reduction).[53] Individuals with one null and one defective mutation fall in between (~25% reduction). As the prevalence of HoFH is probably a bit <1/160 000, this distinction doesn't have great clinical relevance. Still, it is not only scientifically interesting but also simply good to know.
   c. Also, when treating an HoFH patient with evolocumab, one should always assess drug response by measuring LDL-C within 4-8 weeks after initiating therapy.[54] This way, if the medication is ineffective, it can be stopped.

VI. Conclusion

In the final analysis, the management of patients with FH is like the management of patients with other disorders. We always treat the individual. A reasonable axiom is, the sicker the patient, the more intensive the treatment. All FH patients are to be considered high risk. Some however are unfortunately even higher risk than the rest.

References

1. Goldstein JL, Brown MS. Familial hypercholesterolemia: identification of a defect in the regulation of 3-hydroxy-3-methylglutaryl coenzyme A reductase activity associated with overproduction of cholesterol. *Proc Natl Acad Sci U S A.* 1973;70(10):2804-2808.
2. Brown MS, Goldstein JL. Familial hypercholesterolemia: defective binding of lipoproteins to cultured fibroblasts associated with impaired regulation of 3-hydroxy-3-methylglutaryl coenzyme A reductase activity. *Proc Natl Acad Sci U S A.* 1974;71(3):788-792.
3. Goldstein JL, Hobbs HH, Brown MS. Familial hypercholesterolemia. In: A. Scriver CR, Sly WS, Valle D, eds. *The Metabolic and Molecular Bases of Inherited Disease.* New York, NY: McGraw Hill; 2001:2863-2913.
4. Varret M, et al. Genetic heterogeneity of autosomal dominant hypercholesterolemia. *Clin Genet.* 2008;73(1):1-13.
5. Hopkins PN, et al. Familial hypercholesterolemias: prevalence, genetics, diagnosis and screening recommendations from the National Lipid Association Expert Panel on Familial Hypercholesterolemia. *J Clin Lipidol.* 2011;5(3 Suppl):S9-S17.
6. Borén J, et al. The molecular mechanism for the genetic disorder familial defective apolipoprotein B100. *J Biol Chem.* 2001;276(12):9214-9218.
7. Whitfield AJ, et al. Lipid disorders and mutations in the APOB gene. *Clin Chem.* 2004;50(10):1725-1732.
8. Horton JD, Cohen JC, Hobbs HH. Molecular biology of PCSK9: its role in LDL metabolism. *Trends Biochem Sci.* 2007;32(2):71-77.
9. Horton JD, Cohen JC, Hobbs HH. PCSK9: a convertase that coordinates LDL catabolism. *J Lipid Res.* 2009;(50 Suppl):S172-S177.
10. Cuchel M, et al. Homozygous familial hypercholesterolaemia: new insights and guidance for clinicians to improve detection and clinical management. A position paper from the Consensus Panel on Familial Hypercholesterolaemia of the European Atherosclerosis Society. *Eur Heart J.* 2014;35(32):2146-2157.
11. Sjouke B, et al. Homozygous autosomal dominant hypercholesterolaemia in the Netherlands: prevalence, genotype-phenotype relationship, and clinical outcome. *Eur Heart J.* 2015;36(9):560-565.
12. Vishwanath R, Hemphill LC. Familial hypercholesterolemia and estimation of US patients eligible for low-density lipoprotein apheresis after maximally tolerated lipid-lowering therapy. *J Clin Lipidol.* 2014;8(1):18-28.
13. Walzer S, et al. Homozygous familial hypercholesterolemia (HoFH) in Germany: an epidemiological survey. *Clinicoecon Outcomes Res.* 2013;5:189-192.
14. Nordestgaard BG, et al. Familial hypercholesterolaemia is underdiagnosed and undertreated in the general population: guidance for clinicians to prevent coronary heart disease: consensus statement of the European Atherosclerosis Society. *Eur Heart J.* 2013;34(45):3478-3490.
15. Seftel HC, et al. Prevalence of familial hypercholesterolemia in Johannesburg Jews. *Am J Med Genet.* 1989;34(4):545-547.
16. Humphries SE, et al. What is the clinical utility of DNA testing in patients with familial hypercholesterolaemia? *Curr Opin Lipidol.* 2008;19(4):362-368.
17. Taylor A, et al. Multiplex ARMS analysis to detect 13 common mutations in familial hypercholesterolaemia. *Clin Genet.* 2007;71(6):561-568.
18. Baum SJ, et al. The doctor's dilemma: challenges in the diagnosis and care of homozygous familial hypercholesterolemia. *J Clin Lipidol.* 2014;8(6):542-549.
19. Marais AD, et al. A dose-titration and comparative study of rosuvastatin and atorvastatin in patients with homozygous familial hypercholesterolaemia. *Atherosclerosis.* 2008;197(1):400-406.
20. Raal FJ, Santos RD. Homozygous familial hypercholesterolemia: current perspectives on diagnosis and treatment. *Atherosclerosis.* 2012;223(2):262-268.
21. Kolansky DM, et al. Longitudinal evaluation and assessment of cardiovascular disease in patients with homozygous familial hypercholesterolemia. *Am J Cardiol.* 2008;102(11):1438-1443.
22. Goldstein JL, et al. Hyperlipidemia in coronary heart disease. II. Genetic analysis of lipid levels in 176 families and delineation of a new inherited disorder, combined hyperlipidemia. *J Clin Invest.* 1973;52(7):1544-1568.
23. Neefjes LA, et al. Accelerated subclinical coronary atherosclerosis in patients with familial hypercholesterolemia. *Atherosclerosis.* 2011;219(2):721-727.
24. Choumerianou DM, Dedoussis GV. Familial hypercholesterolemia and response to statin therapy according to LDLR genetic background. *Clin Chem Lab Med.* 2005;43(8):793-801.
25. Wierzbicki AS, Lumb PJ, Chik G. Comparison of therapy with simvastatin 80 mg and 120 mg in patients with familial hypercholesterolaemia. *Int J Clin Pract.* 2001;55(10):673-675.
26. Wierzbicki AS, et al. Comparison of therapy with simvastatin 80 mg and atorvastatin 80 mg in patients with familial hypercholesterolaemia. *Int J Clin Pract.* 1999;53(8):609-611.
27. Zech LA, Hoeg JM. Correlating corneal arcus with atherosclerosis in familial hypercholesterolemia. *Lipids Health Dis.* 2008;7:7.
28. Srimannarayana I, et al. Supravalvular aortic stenosis and coronary ostial stenosis in homozygous familial hypercholesterolemia. *Indian Heart J.* 2004;56(2):152-154.

29. Khera AV, et al. Lipoprotein(a) concentrations, rosuvastatin therapy, and residual vascular risk: an analysis from the JUPITER Trial (Justification for the Use of Statins in Prevention: an Intervention Trial Evaluating Rosuvastatin). *Circulation.* 2014;129(6):635-642.
30. Erqou S, et al. Lipoprotein(a) concentration and the risk of coronary heart disease, stroke, and nonvascular mortality. *JAMA.* 2009;302(4):412-423.
31. Alonso R, et al. Lipoprotein(a) levels in familial hypercholesterolemia: an important predictor of cardiovascular disease independent of the type of LDL receptor mutation. *J Am Coll Cardiol.* 2014;63(19):1982-1989.
32. O'Brien EC, et al. Rationale and design of the familial hypercholesterolemia foundation CAscade SCreening for Awareness and DEtection of Familial Hypercholesterolemia registry. *Am Heart J.* 2014;167(3):342-349.e17.
33. Alonso R, et al. Early diagnosis and treatment of familial hypercholesterolemia: improving patient outcomes. *Expert Rev Cardiovasc Ther.* 2013;11(3):327-342.
34. van Aalst-Cohen ES, et al. Diagnosing familial hypercholesterolaemia: the relevance of genetic testing. *Eur Heart J.* 2006;27(18):2240-2246.
35. Baum S, Soffer D, Duell B. Emerging treatments for heterozygous and homozygous familial hypercholesterolemia. *Rev Cardiovasc Med.* 2016;17:17-27.
36. Watts GF, et al. Integrated guidance on the care of familial hypercholesterolemia from the International FH Foundation. *J Clin Lipidol.* 2014;8(2):148-172.
37. Gidding SS, et al. The agenda for familial hypercholesterolemia: a scientific statement from the American Heart Association. *Circulation.* 2015;132(22):2167-2192.
38. Eckel RH, et al. 2013 AHA/ACC guideline on lifestyle management to reduce cardiovascular risk: a report of the American College of Cardiology/American Heart Association Task Force on Practice Guidelines. *J Am Coll Cardiol.* 2014;63(25 Pt B):2960-2984.
39. Charles Z, Pugh E, Barnett D. Ezetimibe for the treatment of primary (heterozygous-familial and non-familial) hypercholesterolaemia: NICE technology appraisal guidance. *Heart.* 2008;94(5):642-643.
40. Hamilton-Craig I, et al. Combination therapy of statin and ezetimibe for the treatment of familial hypercholesterolemia. *Vasc Health Risk Manag.* 2010;6:1023-1037.
41. Leebmann J, et al. Lipoprotein apheresis in patients with maximally tolerated lipid-lowering therapy, lipoprotein(a)-hyperlipoproteinemia, and progressive cardiovascular disease: prospective observational multicenter study. *Circulation.* 2013;128(24):2567-2576.
42. Schettler V, et al. Current view: indications for extracorporeal lipid apheresis treatment. *Clin Res Cardiol Suppl.* 2012;7:15-19.
43. Thompson GR. The evidence-base for the efficacy of lipoprotein apheresis in combating cardiovascular disease. *Atheroscler Suppl.* 2013;14(1):67-70.
44. Lappegard K. Side effects in LDL apheresis: types, frequency and clinical relevance. *J Clin Lipidol.* 2011;6:717-722.
45. Mabuchi H, et al. Long-term efficacy of low-density lipoprotein apheresis on coronary heart disease in familial hypercholesterolemia. *Am J Cardiol.* 1998;82:1489-1495.
46. Berriot-Varoqueaux N, et al. The role of the microsomal triglyceride transfer protein in abetalipoproteinemia. *Annu Rev Nutr.* 2000;20:663-697.
47. Rader DJ, Kastelein JJ. Lomitapide and mipomersen: two first-in-class drugs for reducing low-density lipoprotein cholesterol in patients with homozygous familial hypercholesterolemia. *Circulation.* 2014;129(9):1022-1032.
48. Robinson JG, et al. Efficacy and safety of alirocumab in reducing lipids and cardiovascular events. *N Engl J Med.* 2015;372(16):1489-1499.
49. Markham A. Evolocumab: first global approval. *Drugs.* 2015;75(13):1567-1573.
50. Abifadel M, et al. Mutations in PCSK9 cause autosomal dominant hypercholesterolemia. *Nat Genet.* 2003;34(2):154-156.
51. Alves AC, et al. Characterization of the first PCSK9 gain of function homozygote. *J Am Coll Cardiol.* 2015;66(19):2152-2154.
52. Benn M, Nordestgaard B, Grande P, Schnohr P, Tybjærg-Hansen A. PCSK9 R46L, low-density lipoprotein cholesterol levels, and risk of ischemic heart disease. *J Am Coll Cardiol.* 2010;55(25):2833-2842.
53. Dias CS, et al. Effects of AMG 145 on low-density lipoprotein cholesterol levels: results from 2 randomized, double-blind, placebo-controlled, ascending-dose phase 1 studies in healthy volunteers and hypercholesterolemic subjects on statins. *J Am Coll Cardiol.* 2012;60(19):1888-1898.
54. Repatha [package insert]. Thousand Oaks, CA.

CHAPTER *13*

Complex Dyslipidemias

Vanessa Hurta and Matthew C. Weiss

Key Points

- Since Fredrickson's classification of primary hyperlipidemias, many other complex lipid disorders have been identified.
- Genetic mutations that result in complex dyslipidemias can cause both cardiovascular and noncardiac medical problems.
- Providers may consider a complex or uncommon dyslipidemia when the patient's lipid levels are extremely high or low, resistant to standard treatment, present in several family members, or accompanied by other unexplained abnormal features.
- Considering the primary lipid derangement may be the simplest way to initially approach diagnosis.
- Genetic testing may not be necessary and is not always covered by insurance companies.
- Patients with complex dyslipidemias can be referred to lipid specialists certified by the American Board of Clinical Lipidology or the Accreditation Council for Clinical Lipidology.

I.   Complex Dyslipidemias

A. Introduction Knowledge of patients' lipid levels is essential to accurately estimating their global cardiovascular risk. In addition to being a critical element in the development of cardiovascular disease, lipid abnormalities can result in noncardiac medical problems including those that affect the neurological system and precipitate life-threatening pancreatitis. While the vast majority of dyslipidemias that clinicians will see are common and relatively simple to treat, it is important to recognize the less common and more complex abnormalities.

B. Classification Many genetic mutations that affect lipid levels have been identified. In 1965, Fredrickson published a classification of hyperlipidemias, which included types I, II, III, IV, and V (Table 13.1).[1] See Chapter 10 for a description of types I, IIb, and IV that result in hypertriglyceridemia. Type IIa, familial hypercholesterolemia, is delineated in Chapter 12. Type III, dysbetalipoproteinemia, is addressed here. Unaccounted for in Fredrickson's classification are alpha lipoproteins, or HDLs. Since Fredrickson's initial classification, many other dyslipidemias have been described. It may be more relevant today to organize these genetic disorders by the major pathways of lipoprotein

Table 13.1. Fredrickson Classification of Hyperlipoproteinemias		
Type (Common Name)	**Total Cholesterol**	**Triglycerides**
Type I (familial hyperchylomicronemia)	⇑	⇑⇑
Type II (familial hypercholesterolemia)	⇑	⇔
Type III (dysbetalipoproteinemia)	⇑	⇑
Type IV (familial hypertriglyceridemia)	⇑⇔	⇑
Type V (hyperchylomicronemia with environmental influences)	⇑	⇑

Data from Fredrickson DS, Lees RS. A system for phenotyping hyperlipoproteinemia. *Circulation.* 1965;31:321-327.

metabolism, hepatic, intestinal, and reverse cholesterol transport,[2] or by the predominant lipoprotein level elevation or depression with recognition of the rare genetic disorders.[3] Using the latter approach, 13 complex dyslipidemias are addressed here including their pathophysiology, presentation, and treatment.

C. General approach

1. When managing dyslipidemia, providers typically begin by examining a patient's particular lipid derangement (Table 13.2). Providers may consider a complex or uncommon dyslipidemia when the patient's lipid levels are extremely high or low, resistant to standard treatment, abnormal from birth, or accompanied by other unexplained abnormal features or several family members are affected.

2. Use of genetic testing is discussed below and may assist in the diagnosis. Several issues can complicate genetic testing. Patients can have more than one monogenic disorder[4] or polygenic disorders or have been affected by environmental influences that alter the monogenic disorder's predicted phenotype. Additionally, in cases where a provider would expect to find a family history of a disorder, the patient actually may have a de novo mutation, resulting in an index case of the disorder. Many other deleterious mutations have yet to be identified. For this reason, it is often reasonable to treat the phenotype and see results prior to ordering genetic tests.

3. Obtaining a personal and family history, conducting a comprehensive physical exam, and performing laboratory testing are crucial to making an accurate diagnosis. (See Chapters 3–5 for review of history, exam, and lab testing). Reviewing prior medical records, including pediatric records, may help determine the lipid derangement's onset. A normal baseline (prior to presenting with a lipid abnormality) lipid profile

Table 13.2.   Lipid Profile Derangements

Primary Lipid Derangement	Gene Mutation	Inheritance Pattern	Disease
Normal to severely elevated LDL-C and total cholesterol	ABCG5 ABCG8	Autosomal recessive	Phytosterolemia
Elevated to severely elevated LDL-C and total cholesterol	LPA LDLR, APOB, and PCSK9	Autosomal dominant Autosomal dominant	Elevated Lp(a) Familial hypercholesterolemia
Triglyceride and total cholesterol ratio 1:1	APOE	Autosomal recessive	Dysbetalipoproteinemia
Low LDL-C	APOB PCSK9 MTP ANGPTL3 SAR1B	Autosomal codominant Autosomal codominant Autosomal recessive Autosomal recessive Autosomal recessive	Familial hypobetalipoproteinemia Abetalipoproteinemia Familial combined hypolipidemia Chylomicron retention disease
High HDL-C	CETP LIPG LIPC	Autosomal recessive Autosomal Autosomal recessive	CETP deficiency LIPG gene mutation Hepatic lipase deficiency
Low HDL-C	APOA1 LCAT ABCA1	Autosomal dominant Autosomal recessive Autosomal recessive	Hypobetalipoproteinemia LCAT deficiency (fish eye) Tangier disease

Autosomal recessive inheritance pattern—Two mutated copies of the gene are necessary to have disease. Therefore, both parents of an affected person will have at least one affected copy of gene, and there is a 25% probability that their offspring will have disease.
Autosomal dominant inheritance pattern—One mutated copy of gene is necessary to have disease. One parent will have disease, and there is a 50% probability that offspring will have disease.
Autosomal codominant inheritance pattern—Two different versions are expressed and both affect the trait.

generally suggests a secondary cause for the dyslipidemia. However, some diseases, such as dysbetalipoproteinemia, may manifest only with a "second hit," such as diabetes or pregnancy. Providers also should determine if patients have significant alcohol intake or strong dietary preferences that could cause values consistent with a genetic dyslipidemia.

4. If one of these disorders is diagnosed, providers are encouraged to submit case reports to promote recognition, contribute to detecting the true prevalence, and expand the existing knowledge base to further the understanding and management of complex dyslipidemias.

D. Genetic testing

1. While genetic testing is not necessary in many cases, it can be helpful when a diagnosis is ambiguous and for "cascade screening" to identify family members who may also have the genetic abnormality. It also has been hypothesized that patients who have a definitive genetic diagnosis may be more likely to adhere to treatment protocols.[5]

2. The National Institutes of Health's (NIH) genetic testing registry includes a voluntary database of laboratories conducting specific tests.[6] In addition, some university medical centers offer genetic testing conducted under research protocols. Providers should choose laboratories that have been certified according to the Clinical Laboratory Improvement Amendments (CLIA).

3. Finally, patients should be notified of possible expenses related to genetic testing, as many insurance companies do not reimburse these services. Referral to a medical geneticist or genetic counselor is also an option depending on insurance coverage and ability to pay.

4. Of note, some states, such as New York, have stricter laws than others regarding genetic testing, so the provider should be aware of requirements in their state.

II. Phytosterolemia

A. Definition
Phytosterolemia, also known as sitosterolemia, is an autosomal recessive disorder characterized by elevated serum plant sterols and stanols, known as phytosterols, and the presence of xanthomas. Approximately 100 cases have been reported in the literature, but it is thought that phytosterolemia is underreported or often misdiagnosed as familial hypercholesterolemia.[7,8] Phytosterolemia is associated with premature cardiovascular disease.

B. Pathophysiology

1. **Mutation** Phytosterolemia is caused by a mutation in either of the adenosine triphosphate–binding cassette subfamily G member 5 or 8 (ABCG5 or ABCG8) genes. Phytosterols are structurally analogous to cholesterol and act to lower intestinal absorption of cholesterol by supplanting it in micelles.[9–11] Normally, the ABCG5 and ABCG8 proteins form a heterodimer that restricts intestinal absorption and facilitates biliary excretion of phytosterols.[12] A mutation in *ABCG5* or *ABCG8* causes increased intestinal absorption and restricted biliary excretion of plant sterols, such as campesterol, sitosterol, stigmasterol, and stanols. LDL receptor activity is also decreased.[2] Phytosterols and cholesterol accumulate in the blood and tissues, causing the clinical findings of phytosterolemia. Heterozygous patients can eat a normal diet without a requisite increase in their plasma phytosterol levels and do not appear to

have any clinical sequelae.[13] An *ABCG5* defect has been identified in the Japanese, Chinese, and Indian population and an *ABCG8* defect in the Caucasian population.[11,14–16] The Amish/Mennonites also are known to be a founder population.[17]

2. **Phytosterol absorption** Phytosterol consumption, dependent on the type of diet, usually varies between 150 and 450 mg/d.[11] Of that, <5% is absorbed under normal conditions,[16] resulting in a phytosterol concentration of 1 mg/dL or less in human plasma. In contrast, patients with phytosterolemia absorb a higher percentage (>50%) of phytosterols causing their plasma levels to reach 20-30 mg/dL.[12,17]

C. Presentation and diagnosis

1. **Initial findings** Patients with phytosterolemia have normal to moderately elevated total cholesterol and normal triglyceride levels. LDL-C levels vary from normal to 500 mg/dL.[2] Most patients that are seen with severe LDL-C and total cholesterol elevations have familial hypercholesterolemia, but the phenotype of phytosterolemia can resemble familial hypercholesterolemia. Phytosterolemia is a distinct disorder that requires specific management. In contrast to familial hypercholesterolemia, a family history will usually be noncontributory, and a personal history may reveal no improvement in lipid levels despite using statins and adhering to a healthy diet.

2. **Examination** On physical exam, tuberous, planar, and tendinous xanthomas may be noted, while intertriginous xanthomas have been documented in infants.[15] Hematologic abnormalities, such as hemolytic anemia, stomatocytosis, thrombocytopenia, macrothrombocytes, and bleeding, have been reported.[18] Arthritis, arthralgia, and hypersplenism[19] also have been reported. Phytosterolemia is correlated with premature cardiovascular disease and aortic stenosis. Cardiovascular disease is usually diagnosed in early to middle adulthood but has been found in patients younger than 30 years of age.[2] Differences in phenotypic severity have been attributed to factors such as concentrations of phytosterols in the blood, environmental characteristics, influences of other genes that affect plasma phytosterol levels, and gene conversion events.[8]

3. **Diagnostic Testing** Phytosterol levels should be measured when phytosterolemia is suspected. The test, usually called "plasma sterols," is not available in all commercial laboratories. Mayo Medical Laboratories and Boston Heart Diagnostics are two American laboratories that offer the test. The patient should be fasting for 12 hours or, if an infant, tested before a feeding. The sitosterol and campesterol levels must be interpreted carefully since these levels may be slightly elevated if a person eats a diet rich in plant sterols. If levels are elevated, genetic testing can confirm the diagnosis, but probably is not necessary.

D. Treatment and monitoring

1. **Medical management**
   a. Phytosterolemia management includes prescribing a regimen of bile acid sequestrants or ezetimibe, recommending a diet low in phytosterols and cholesterol, monitoring cardiovascular disease progression, and consulting with a lipid specialist. Partial ileal bypass surgeries have been conducted in the past, but they are not commonly performed now.
   b. Bile acid sequestrants decrease sterol levels in hepatocytes, allowing sterols to be removed from the circulation at a higher rate.[19] In studies, bile acid sequestrants lowered phytosterols by an average of 40%-60% in most patients, although they were not as effective in other cases.[19]

c. Ezetimibe, a sterol absorption inhibitor, often is preferred over bile acid seques-trants due to its ease of use and documented effect on multiple laboratory param-eters. Ezetimibe decreases the absorption of both cholesterol and phytosterols by blocking the Niemann-Pick C1-like 1 (NPC1L1) protein transporter. Ezetimibe has been shown to decrease phytosterol, total cholesterol, and LDL-C levels.[19] It also improved thrombocytopenia and decreased platelet size in a study of eight Hutterites with phytosterolemia.[18] Escola et al.[7] demonstrated that ezetimibe induced xanthoma regression and improved carotid bruits and cardiac murmurs. There is no data about ezetimibe's effect on cardiovascular event reduction in phytosterolemia patients.

d. Statins are not indicated in management of phytosterolemia, as HMG-CoA reductase activity is already diminished.[2] A study by Vanhehan and Miettinen reported that pravastatin and lovastatin increased stanol and sterol absorption markers.[20]

2. **Dietary therapy** The patient should consume a low cholesterol diet and avoid all dietary phytosterols.[21] Vegetable oils, margarine, nuts, seeds, avocado, and chocolate are common sources of phytosterols. Shellfish, which contains the sterol, brassicas-terol, and seaweed should also be avoided.[22] Fruit, vegetables, and cereals without wheat germ may be consumed.[23] Adherence to such a diet may be poor.[24] Tada et al. reported that weaning from breastfeeding improved total cholesterol and LDL-C levels, but not phytosterol levels, in four Japanese infants with phytosterolemia.[15]

III. Abnormalities of Lipoprotein(a)

A. Description

1. **Definition** Lipoprotein(a) [Lp(a); pronounced "LP little a"] is an inherited athero-genic lipoprotein, which has been identified as an independent risk factor for athero-sclerotic cardiovascular disease, vascular thrombosis, and calcific aortic stenosis.[25–30] Though first recognized in 1963,[31] 53 years later it continues to remain incompletely understood. Its clinical role to date has also remained limited due to the lack of a standardized reliable quantification assay to measure it, few available therapeutic options to directly lower Lp(a), and the lack of outcomes trials for treatment targeting it. Nonetheless, research surrounding Lp(a)—from its variable structure to antisense therapies to target it directly—is actively being pursued, and as a result, the clinical role for Lp(a) testing is on the rise.

2. **Particle Structure** The lipoprotein(a) particle consists of three components: a low density lipoprotein-like cholesterol-containing particle, apolipoprotein(a) [apo(a)], and apolipoprotein B-100 (apoB). The LDL-like particle contains a central core of cholesterol ester and triglyceride, which is surrounded by phospholipid and free cholesterol. ApoB, an apolipoprotein found on all atherogenic particles, is bound to apo(a) via a disulfide linkage; and apo(a) is covalently bound to the LDL-like par-ticle, chemically and structurally distinguishing it from LDL itself.[32] The structure of apo(a) is highly polymorphic—both between and within individuals.[29] Thus geneti-cally determined, varying sized isoforms of apo(a) exist, determine Lp(a) heterogene-ity,[33] and contribute to the difficulty in the development of standardized and reliably accurate quantification assays.[34,35]

3. **Measurement** Depending on geographic practice customs and local laboratory standards, Lp(a) is measured either by apo(a) mass (the amount of apo(a) presented, expressed as mg/dL), Lp(a)-P (the concentration of Lp(a) particles, which is directly

proportional to the particle number), or Lp(a)-C (the amount of cholesterol trafficked in Lp(a) itself). At present, there is a need for future international standardization of laboratory assays by which to reliably quantify Lp(a) prior to widespread clinical adoption of measurement of this cardiovascular risk factor.

B. Pathophysiology

1. Pathophysiologically, Lp(a) has been implicated in promoting thrombogenesis.[29] Lp(a)'s thrombogenicity is thought to be related to apo(a)'s homology to the plasminogen supergene family. In vitro studies have linked apo(a), and therefore Lp(a), to various procoagulant and antifibrinolytic functions, including enhanced platelet aggregation and inhibition of tPA-mediated plasminogen activation.[36–38] The extent of these effects may be inversely proportional to apo(a) and Lp(a) isoform size.[39,40] The in vivo culpability of Lp(a) for venous and/or arterial thromboembolism remains highly debated.[29] Clinical studies have shown antifibrinolytic roles of Lp(a) as a significant predictor of carotid stenosis,[41] as a predictor of resistance to endogenous thrombolysis,[42] and in the failure to recanalize after an ischemic stroke.[43] However, there is strong mendelian evidence against Lp(a) having a causal role in venous thromboembolism.[44,45] Ultimately, Lp(a) may not promote coagulation as much as it impairs fibrinolysis.

2. The relationship between Lp(a) and atherosclerotic cardiovascular disease from observational and epidemiologic studies is more well established, and elevations in Lp(a) are now widely understood to be an independent risk factor for atherosclerotic cardiovascular disease.[46] This relationship is continuous, without threshold, and independent of LDL-C and non–HDL-C. Various meta-analyses of clinical data have determined the hazard ratios for Lp(a) elevation and coronary heart disease (CHD) to range from 1.13 to 1.60, including after adjustment for traditional risk factors such as age, sex, tobacco use, and history of hypercholesterolemia and diabetes.[26,27]

3. Because Lp(a) levels are largely genetically determined via the apo(a) gene, mendelian analyses have also examined the association between Lp(a) levels and risk for CHD. Results here demonstrate hazard ratios for Lp(a) and CHD from 1.2 to 2.6, depending on Lp(a) percentile from 22nd to 66th to >95th, respectively.[28] Genetically determined kringle subtypes within apo(a) have also been associated with increased CHD risk with a hazard ratio of 2.57 for two SNPs associated with kringle IV, for example.[47]

4. Mechanistically, Lp(a) promotes atherosclerotic disease through various pathways, some of which remain incompletely understood, but include promotion of adhesion and transendothelial migration of monocytes, increased avidity for LDL-C retention in the extracellular matrix of the intimal wall, increased retention of cholesterol at sites of mechanical injury, and increased binding of proinflammatory oxidized phospholipids.[25]

C. Presentation and diagnosis
Lp(a) levels vary by ethnicity and race may be a key variable in determining Lp(a) cutoff values for CHD risk.[48] Lp(a) may be a less significant predictor of cardiovascular events in blacks, who typically have higher levels of Lp(a) as compared to their nonblack peers.[49,50] Asians, on the other hand, tend to have lower levels of Lp(a).[34] A single set of internationally established guidelines or recommendations for when to clinically test for Lp(a) does not exist. However, both the National Lipid Association and the European Atherosclerosis Society have published recommendations.[25,51] See Table 13.3 for "reasonable" candidates for Lp(a) testing based on these recommendations. Using these criteria, in one case series of consecutive patients

Table 13.3.	Candidates for Lp(a) Testing

- Patients with premature coronary artery disease (CAD) (age of myocardial infarction or percutaneous coronary intervention <55 in men and <65 in women)
- Patients with a family history of premature CAD (<55 in men and <65 in women)
- Patients with CAD at any age if traditional risk factors are well controlled (BP < 140/90 mm Hg, LDL < 70 mg/dL, A1c < 7%, nonsmoker)
- Patients of any age with evidence of disease progression despite at least moderate intensity statin therapy (simvastatin 40 mg, atorvastatin 40-80 mg, rosuvastatin 20-40 mg daily)

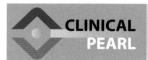

CLINICAL PEARL — Lp(a)'s associated cardiovascular risk is independent of traditional Framingham risk factors (such as LDL, etc.).

undergoing nonemergent coronary intervention, 48% of cases were found to have an elevated Lp(a) >30 mg/dL (depending on which method of analysis is used).[52] Screening moderate- and high-risk populations for Lp(a) has important clinical implications. Given Lp(a)'s known role as an independent risk factor for CHD, elevated Lp(a) is considered residual risk.

D. Treatment and monitoring

1. Several medications can lower Lp(a); however, there are no currently available therapies, which exclusively target Lp(a). Current recommendations suggest that with elevated Lp(a), there is a need for more aggressive lowering of LDL-C. Those with the combination of familial hypercholesterolemia and elevated Lp(a) are particularly at risk. Additionally, given its direct inheritance pattern, elevated Lp(a) suggests the need for appropriate cascade offspring screening.[51]

2. Multiple therapies have been shown to lower Lp(a); however, no trial data exist demonstrating that reducing Lp(a) alone results in improved clinical outcomes—in part because many therapies that affect Lp(a) also affect traditional risk factors, such as LDL-C, and thus much confounding exists. Aspirin,[53–55] niacin,[56,57] cholesterol ester transfer protein inhibitors,[58] estrogen, and PCSK9 inhibitors[59] have all been shown to reduce Lp(a) in human subjects, the latter up to 32% among patients already on standard therapy.

3. Data regarding lifestyle modification, ezetimibe use, and statin use are mixed.[60,61] Small trials of Lp(a)-specific apheresis have been successfully completed,[62] but outcome data have not been reported. Mipomersen, a second generation oligonucleotide apoB-targeting antisense technology drug, has been shown to lower Lp(a) in phase III studies.[63] Apo(a)-specific antisense therapy is in early trials.[64] For the majority of the drugs above, the exact mechanism of Lp(a) lowering remains unknown.

IV. Dysbetalipoproteinemia

A. Definition Dysbetalipoproteinemia, also known as Fredrickson type III hyperlipoproteinemia, is inherited in an autosomal recessive pattern and causes triglyceride-rich lipoproteins to accumulate in the plasma and hasten cardiovascular disease. Estimations of prevalence rates vary from 1 per 1000 to 10 000 persons.[2,65]

B. **Pathophysiology** The patient with dysbetalipoproteinemia is usually homozygous for the apolipoprotein E (apoE) e2 allele, as opposed to the wild-type e3 allele. ApoE is predominantly found in chylomicrons, VLDL and HDL.[66] It facilitates removal of chylomicron and VLDL remnants. Under normal conditions, the remnants are rapidly cleared in the liver, although some VLDL is eventually converted to LDL. A mutation in apoE hinders the proper removal of chylomicron and VLDL remnants in the liver due to defective binding of apoe2 to the LDL receptor.[66] Some clearance of these remnants continues because apoe2 is also recognized by the LDL receptor protein and heparin proteoglycans.[66] However, the surplus of chylomicron and VLDL remnants accumulate, infiltrating the vessel wall and initiating the atherosclerotic cascade.[69] Apoe2 homozygosity is not necessary to have dysbetalipoproteinemia—other variants such as apoE3 Leiden and apoE2 Christchurch have been reported.[65,67,68] Additionally, only a small percentage of patients with e2 homozygosity have phenotypic dysbetalipoproteinemia, likely because a "second hit" is usually necessary.

C. **Presentation and diagnosis**

1. **Initial findings** Total cholesterol and triglycerides are elevated, both usually >300 mg/dL.[2] HDL-C is usually low and LDL-C may be mildly elevated, but sometimes low.[69] Total cholesterol-to-triglycerides ratio of 1:1, an apoB-to-total cholesterol ratio of <0.33, or a VLDL-to-triglyceride ratio of >0.3 should raise suspicion for dysbetalipoproteinemia.[2,70]

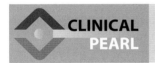 **CLINICAL PEARL** Dysbetalipoproteinemia is unique in that lipid derangements may not be apparent until later in life when the patient develops a concomitant disorder.

Dysbetalipoproteinemia may manifest only in the presence of another metabolic or endocrine disorder.

2. **Age of onset** The age at onset of abnormal lipid parameters and symptoms depends on the patient's comorbidities. It is often diagnosed as an adult when the patient develops diabetes or hypothyroidism or becomes pregnant. Obesity, menopause, systemic lupus erythematous, multiple myeloma, HIV, or antipsychotic therapy can also precipitate dysbetalipoproteinemia.[70] Hopkins, Brinton, and Nanjee estimated that patients with dysbetalipoproteinemia had a five- to eightfold increase in coronary artery disease risk.[71]

3. **Examination** Physical findings include xanthomas or yellow palmar creases (xanthoma striatum palmare), which are pathognomonic for the disease. Elevated uric acid and glucose intolerance are found in approximately half of patients with dysbetalipoproteinemia.[2]

4. **Diagnostic testing** Since dysbetalipoproteinemia diagnosis can be ambiguous, apoE genotyping should be considered and is commonly available. Cholesterol-rich VLDL or remnants seen after ultracentrifugation is also diagnostic.[69]

D. **Treatment and monitoring**

1. **Medical management** Contributing conditions such as obesity, hypothyroidism, and diabetes should be diagnosed and treated. LDL-C, non–HDL-C, and triglycerides should be targeted with fibrates, statins, and omega three fatty acids.[71] Niacin can

also be used but would not be first line. Fibrates are usually considered first-line therapy. Bile acid sequestrants should be avoided because they can increase triglycerides.[69] Patients should be monitored for progression of cardiovascular disease.

2. **Dietary therapy** A low-fat diet is recommended. Alcohol moderation or cessation should be recommended when appropriate.[69]

V. Inherited Low LDL-C

A. **Introduction** Patients with low LDL-C levels (hypobetalipoproteinemia) may benefit from their limited exposure to LDL-C, although others experience poor outcomes since cholesterol is necessary for the body to synthesize hormones, vitamin D, and bile acids and is an important component of cell membranes. Mutations in the *APOB*, *PCSK9*, *MTP*, *ANGPTL3*, and *SAR1B* genes can cause low LDL-C. Sudden onset of low LDL-C suggests a secondary cause—such as anorexia nervosa, hepatic disease, malignancies, and thyroid disease—that should be eliminated first.

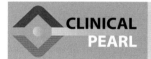

CLINICAL PEARL Secondary causes should be first ruled out when the onset of the lipid derangement is new or no baseline measurements are available.

B. **Familial hypobetalipoproteinemia**

1. **Definition** Familial hypobetalipoproteinemia (FHBL), which is inherited in an autosomal codominant pattern, results from a mutation in the *APOB* gene or a loss-of-function mutation in the *PCSK9* gene.

2. **Pathophysiology**
   a. APOB mutation
      The APOB gene encodes for the proteins apoB-48 and apoB-100. ApoB-48 is synthesized in the intestine and used in the assembly of chylomicrons. ApoB-100 is synthesized in the liver and used in the assembly of VLDL, IDL, and LDL. More than 90 APOB gene mutations have been found to cause FHBL.[72] Most mutations result in truncated versions of both apoB-100 and apoB-48. When FHBL is caused by an APOB mutation, decreased apoB secretion results in fewer triglycerides being released from the liver. The surplus triglycerides remain in the liver and accumulate in the hepatocytes, which can result in the development of hepatic steatosis.
   b. PCSK9 mutation
      Because the PCSK9 protein facilitates degradation of the LDL receptors before they reach the cell surface, the PCSK9 gene is integral to regulating the number of LDL receptors. Therefore, patients with gain-of-function PCSK9 gene mutations have phenotypic familial hypercholesterolemia with extremely elevated LDL-C levels. Patients with loss-of-function mutations have FHBL.

3. **Presentation and diagnosis**
   a. Heterozygote patients with FHBL from an *APOB* mutation are likely to have LDL-C levels 30% lower than normal for their age and sex.[73] Oral fat intolerance and malabsorption also have been reported.[74] An *APOB* mutation is associated with a poor prognosis, for example, from hepatic disease. Patients who are homozygotes or compound heterozygotes for *APOB* gene mutations have very low LDL-C levels and are referred to as having homozygous hypobetalipoproteinemia.

b. Their clinical presentation and disease course resembles injurious abetalipoproteinemia, and they should be treated as such.[73,74] See Section B for information about abetalipoproteinemia and homozygous hypobetalipoproteinemia and their management.

c. Patients with FHBL caused by PCSK9 mutations may have LDL-C levels that are 30%-70% lower than expected depending on whether they are heterozygote or homozygote.[73,74] In contrast to FHBL from an *APOB* mutation, a *PCSK9* mutation appears to be associated with decreased risk for coronary artery disease and does not seem to be associated with liver disease.[74] Kwiterovich reported that a loss-of-function *PCSK9* mutation could result in an 80% lifetime reduction in cardiovascular disease.[2]

d. Since patients with FHBL have varying prognoses based on the causative mutation, testing of *APOB* and *PCSK9* would help providers make a definitive diagnosis. If genetic testing is not available, a hepatic ultrasound should be conducted.

4. **Treatment and monitoring** If the hepatic ultrasound reveals steatosis, an *APOB* mutation should be presumed, and the patient should be monitored for progression of hepatic steatosis to steatohepatitis. However, absence of steatosis on initial ultrasound does not preclude an *APOB* mutation in these patients. If oral fat intolerance is noted, a low-fat diet and vitamin supplementation may be recommended. No treatment is recommended for FHBL from loss-of-function *PCSK9* mutations. If genetic testing cannot be performed, it may be prudent to conduct periodic hepatic ultrasounds since steatosis from an *APOB* mutation could develop at any time.

C. Abetalipoproteinemia and homozygous hypobetalipoproteinemia

1. **Definition** Abetalipoproteinemia (ABL) is inherited in an autosomal recessive pattern. Patients with homozygous hypobetalipoproteinemia (HHBL) inherit identical mutations from each parent or two nonidentical mutated alleles (compound heterozygote) resulting in a clinical phenotype identical to ABL.

2. **Pathophysiology** ABL results from a mutation in the microsomal transfer protein (MTP) gene. MTP facilitates transfer of lipids to chylomicrons in the intestine and to VLDL in the liver. When MTP is dysfunctional, triglycerides are not transferred to the developing apoB particle, and VLDL triglyceride particles cannot be assembled. Vitamin E uses chylomicrons as it travels to the liver. When this is disrupted, the patient suffers from the consequences of vitamin E deficiency. As stated previously, HHBL results from *APOB* mutations.

3. **Presentation and diagnosis** In both ABL and HHBL patients, triglycerides and total cholesterol are low, while apoB-48 and apoB-100, chylomicrons, and VLDL-C and LDL-C levels are undetectable.[2] Patients with ABL and HHBL have poor prognoses. Diarrhea and failure to thrive usually are present in infancy.[75] Oral fat intolerance, steatorrhea, fat malabsorption, retinal disorders, and vitamin deficiencies all have been reported. Anemia and acanthocytosis of red blood cells also can be observed. Fewer triglycerides are released from the liver; instead, they accumulate in the hepatocyte, potentiating hepatic steatosis. Serious consequences—such as central nervous system degeneration, ataxia, retinitis pigmentosa, and death—can result.[74] Parents of patients with ABL usually have normal lipids. Parents of patients with HHBL have reduced LDL-C levels.

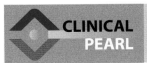
CLINICAL PEARL Pediatric providers should be alert to the signs and symptoms of ABL and HHBL. Early treatment can prevent central nervous system damage, retinitis.

4. **Treatment and monitoring** ABL and HHBL must be treated early and should be managed with a lipid specialist. A low-fat diet (5-20 g/d)[2] and supplementation of fat-soluble vitamins and fatty acids are the mainstays of treatment. Hepatic ultrasound, echocardiography, bone mineral density, and neurological and ophthalmological exams should be conducted regularly.[12,74] Yearly laboratory tests, which include measuring lipids, hepatic function, and vitamin levels, are recommended.[12,74]

D. Familial combined hypolipidemia

1. **Definition** In contrast to the normal HDL-C levels expected in a patient with FHBL, HDL-C levels are more likely to be low in familial combined hypolipidemia, an autosomal recessive disorder. All lipoprotein levels are reduced in patients who are heterozygotes, compound heterozygotes, or homozygotes for this disorder.[73,76]

2. **Pathophysiology** Familial combined hypolipidemia results from a mutation in the angiopoietin-like 3 (ANGPTL3) gene. ANGPTL3 inhibits lipoprotein and endothelial lipases, lowering triglycerides, LDL-C, and HDL-C.[74] It is unclear whether this mutation leads to significant disease.

3. **Presentation and diagnosis** Hepatic disease was reported in one study,[74] and homozygotes had a higher carotid intima-media thickness in another study, raising the question of a potential correlation with cardiovascular disease.[73] Another study found no instances of hepatic steatosis, diabetes, or cardiovascular disease in homozygotes, causing the authors to conclude that homozygosity may protect patients from these diseases.[76] Low insulin and glucose levels have also been reported in homozygote patients.[77]

4. **Treatment and monitoring** Until more data are collected about this disorder, it may be prudent to conduct intermittent hepatic ultrasounds, especially for patients with elevated hepatic function tests, and monitor for subclinical and clinical atherosclerosis.

E. Chylomicron retention disease

1. **Definition** Chylomicron retention disease, also known as Anderson disease, is inherited in an autosomal recessive pattern.

2. **Pathophysiology** Chylomicron retention disease results from a mutation in the secretion-associated, Ras-related GTPase 1B (SAR1B) gene. *SAR1B* is responsible for transporting chylomicrons. Patients with chylomicron retention disease do not properly secrete chylomicrons, leading to accumulation of lipids within the enterocytes.[73] The expression of this gene also affects the skeletal muscles, liver, heart, kidneys, and placenta accounting for the extraintestinal symptoms possible in chylomicron retention disease.[78]

3. **Presentation and diagnosis** In addition to having low LDL-C levels, apoB-48 particles are absent from the plasma in these patients. Triglyceride levels are normal and no postprandial chylomicrons are found.[2] Clinical manifestations, apparent from birth, include fat malabsorption, diarrhea, vomiting, fat-soluble vitamin deficiencies, abdominal upset, and failure to thrive. While hepatomegaly and hepatic steatosis can develop, progression to serious hepatic disease has not been reported.[73] Increased creatine kinase levels, cardiomyopathy, and poor bone mineralization and maturation have been reported.[78,79]

4. **Treatment and monitoring** The treatment for this disorder is a low-fat diet, with the fat component comprised primarily of polyunsaturated fatty acids.[78] Vitamins A and E

should be supplemented. Oral supplementation should decrease symptoms even in the setting of fat malabsorption, although vitamin E levels may remain low.[78] Hepatic ultrasound should be conducted in the setting of abnormal hepatic function testing, although Silvain et al. hypothesized that transaminitis might be related to muscle involvement, instead of hepatic dysfunction.[79] Children's growth should be tracked. Regular neurological, ophthalmological, bone mineralization, and echocardiology exams have been suggested.[78]

F. **Summary of inherited low LDL-C** Hepatic disease is a primary concern when a patient has hypobetalipoproteinemia. With the exception of a PCSK9 mutation, hepatic steatosis has been reported in all causes of hypobetalipoproteinemia. Therefore, hepatic function testing, ultrasounds, and, until more data are collected, monitoring for subclinical and clinical atherosclerosis in these patients may be prudent. Patients with ABL or HHBL have poor prognoses and may experience serious neurological and ophthalmological consequences. A low-fat diet, perhaps with vitamin and fatty acid supplementation, is recommended for patients with chylomicron retention disease, ABL, and HHBL.

VI. Inherited High HDL-C

A. **Introduction** In inherited high HDL-C or hyperalphalipoproteinemia (HALP), HDL-C levels measure in the 90th percentile. HALP can result from mutations in the *CETP*, *LIPG*, and *LIPC* genes. Secondary causes include alcohol intake, physical activity, hormonal disorders, or supplementation. Primary elevations in LDL-C can also cause high HDL-C levels that will decrease with treatment.

B. **CETP deficiency**

1. **Definition** HALP can result from mutations in cholesteryl ester transfer protein (CETP) gene.

2. **Pathophysiology** CETP facilitates transfer of cholesteryl esters from HDL to VLDL, IDL, and LDL. When a loss-of-function *CETP* mutation occurs, more cholesteryl esters remain in HDL and HDL-C levels rise. Homozygosity has been well documented in the Japanese population in which HDL levels 4 times greater than average were reported.[80] One study concluded that CETP activity was not correlated with HALP in Caucasians.[80] Heterozygotes demonstrate moderately increased HDL-C and normal LDL-C levels.[2]

3. **Presentation and diagnosis** HDL-C levels may be 120 mg/dL or higher. ApoA-1 and apoA-2 are catabolized at a slower rate, leading to elevated levels of these apolipoproteins in the plasma. Triglycerides and LDL-C may be slightly lower than average. The effect of CETP deficiency on cardiovascular risk is inconclusive, although some data have suggested a minimally reduced cardiovascular risk.[81] It has been hypothesized that the HDL formed under these conditions is dysfunctional and therefore does not effectively facilitate reverse cholesterol transport.

4. **Treatment and monitoring** LDL-C and non–HDL-C levels should be targeted for treatment in this disorder.

C. **LIPG gene mutation**

1. **Definition** HALP also can result from a mutation in the lipase, endothelial (LIPG) gene.

2. **Pathophysiology** The *LIPG* gene encodes for a protein that assembles endothelial lipase. Endothelial lipase hydrolyzes HDL; therefore, a loss-of-function mutation results in elevated HDL-C. Edmondson et al. suggested that although LIPG affects HDL-C levels, it might not have a significant effect in HDL metabolism.[82]

D. **Hepatic lipase deficiency**

1. **Definition** Another cause of HALP is hepatic lipase deficiency, which is inherited in an autosomal recessive pattern.

2. **Pathophysiology** Hepatic lipase, which is also encoded by the *LIPC* gene, is secreted by hepatocytes and degrades triglycerides and phospholipids. Hepatic lipase is necessary to convert IDLs to LDLs and postprandial triglyceride-rich HDL to triglyceride-poor HDL.[83]

3. **Presentation and diagnosis** This disorder should be suspected when the patient has elevated triglycerides and HDL-C levels and abnormally large HDL particles. VLDL remnants also are elevated, while LDL-C may be low. Eruptive xanthomas, premature atherosclerosis, and pancreatitis have been reported with this disorder. In contrast, another study revealed no premature atherosclerosis.[83] Persons with hepatic lipase deficiency may have a family history of hypertriglyceridemia or consanguinity.[84] Heparin lipase would be seen in postheparin blood in these patients.

4. **Treatment and monitoring** Results of heparin lipase testing may not affect treatment since managing LDL-C and non–HDL-C levels is the primary objective in patients with hepatic lipase deficiency.

E. **Summary of inherited high HDL-C** In general, it should not be inferred that an elevated level of HDL-C prevents atherosclerosis. The quantity of HDL-C may not correlate with functionality. Until HDL-C functionality can be elucidated, a patient's global cardiovascular risk and LDL-C and non–HDL-C levels should be the focus of treatment.[85]

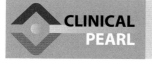
CLINICAL PEARL The functionality of HDL cannot be inferred from HDL-C levels. ApoB-containing particles, not HDL-C, should be the focus of treatment.

VII. **Inherited Low HDL-C**

A. **Introduction** HDL-C below the 10th percentile without secondary causes constitutes hypoalphalipoproteinemia. This is usually caused by mutations in *APOA1*, *LCAT*, or *ABCA1* genes.[86] Secondary causes include infections, smoking, obesity, low-fat diet, hyperthyroidism, diabetes, chronic kidney disease, cancer, and certain drugs.[87]

B. **Familial hypoalphalipoproteinemia**

1. **Definition** This disorder is inherited in an autosomal dominant pattern. Familial hypoalphalipoproteinemia is caused by decreased apoA-1 production or increased apoA-1 degradation. With this condition, there may be no clinical findings or a patient may develop atherosclerosis.

2. **Pathophysiology** Patients heterozygous for *ABCA1* or *APOA1* mutations develop familial hypoalphalipoproteinemia. See Section C for a discussion of Tangier disease

resulting from homozygosity for *ABCA1* mutation. APOA1 facilitates cholesterol efflux from cells and is necessary for LCAT to esterify cholesterol.

3. **Presentation and diagnosis** It results in low HDL-C and normal total cholesterol, triglycerides, apoB, VLDL, and LDL-C levels. Heterozygous mutations in ABCA1 cause depressions in HDL that are 50% less than normal, yet do not seem to be associated with cardiovascular disease. Homozygous *APOA1* mutations result in HDL of <5 mg/dL and heterozygous *APOA1* mutations result in an HDL reduced by ~50% compared to normal.[87] Most *APOA1* mutations are associated with increased rates of cardiovascular disease, although two variants have been associated with lower risk for cardiovascular disease.[88]

C. Lecithin-cholesterol acyltransferase deficiency (LCAT)

1. **Definition** LCAT deficiency is diagnosed when a patient's low HDL-C is accompanied by corneal opacities (see Fig. 13.1). Patients may have either complete LCAT deficiency or partial LCAT deficiency, known as fish eye disease.

2. **Pathophysiology** The *LCAT* gene encodes for a protein that facilitates removal of cholesterol from the blood and tissues through cholesterol esterification. LCAT is crucial to synthesizing mature, spherical HDL, and reverse cholesterol transport. LCAT is predominantly made in the liver, and its concentration in plasma is ~5 μg/mL under normal conditions. When a deficiency of LCAT occurs, cholesterol and phospholipids are not removed correctly, and cholesterol esters are deposited in adipose tissue.

3. **Presentation and diagnosis**
   a. Complete LCAT deficiency
      Complete LCAT deficiency is autosomal recessive. HDL-C levels can be expected to be <10 mg/dL. The HDLs are cholesterol ester poor and do not

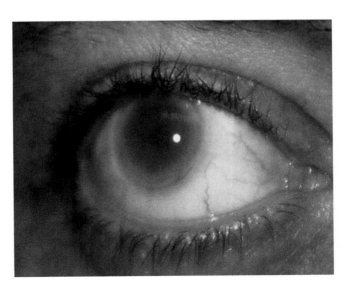

FIGURE 13.1: Corneal opacification in LCAT deficiency. (Reprinted with permission from Roshan B, Ganda OP, Desilva R, et al. Homozygous lecithin: cholesterol acyltransferase (LCAT) deficiency due to a new loss of function mutation and review of the literature. *J Clin Lipidol.* 2011;5(6):493-499.)

mature into spherical HDLs. Additionally, the LDL particles tend to be small and triglyceride enriched.[90] Lipoprotein X (LpX) occurs in complete LCAT deficiency, but not in partial LCAT deficiency. LpX is an abnormal lipoprotein particle and hypothesized to be the cause of renal disease in complete LCAT deficiency.[92] The clinical phenotype of complete LCAT deficiency includes accumulation of cholesterol in the corneas, kidneys, and other tissues. Renal disease, hepatomegaly, splenomegaly, lymphadenopathy, nephrotic syndrome, and corneal arcus have been reported.[90] Thrombocytopenia and stomatocytosis may be seen on a complete blood count. Anemia often is present.[89] The data regarding LCAT deficiency and atherosclerosis are mixed; it is still unclear as to whether these patients are at higher risk for atherosclerosis.[90] Peripheral atherosclerosis has been reported.[2]

   b. Partial LCAT deficiency

     HDL-C levels can be expected to be <27 mg/dL in partial deficiency. LDL-C levels vary but usually are low to normal, while triglycerides and VLDL are elevated.[89] The clinical phenotype of partial LCAT deficiency includes clouding of the corneas but is generally less severe than with complete LCAT deficiency. The opacities can manifest at any age but usually begin around age 20.[89] Anemia and renal disease may still be seen,[90] but premature atherosclerotic disease is not associated with partial LCAT deficiency.[2]

  4. Treatment and monitoring Treatment of both types of LCAT deficiency includes managing LDL-C and non–HDL-C levels. A low-fat diet is recommended. Keratoplasty may be necessary for corneal opacities.[91] The renal disease associated with complete LCAT deficiency may necessitate dialysis or transplant. However, even with transplant, the disease will return within years.[92] Angiotensin-converting enzyme inhibitors are recommended to treat the renal disease, but there are no definitive data that these are an effective treatment.[93] Recombinant human LCAT infusions are in development.[94]

D. Tangier disease

  1. Definition Tangier disease is an autosomal recessive disorder resulting in low HDL-C and apoA-1 levels and accumulation of cholesterol ester in the tissues. The disease, described in 1961 by Fredrickson and colleagues, is named for the Tangier Islands in Virginia, where a founder population exists.[95]

  2. Pathophysiology Tangier disease results from a mutation in the ATP-binding cassette family A member 1 (*ABCA1*) gene. The *APOA1* gene is normal.[2] When *ABCA1* is dysfunctional, apoA-1 is cleared from the circulation rapidly, so HDL is not properly formed. Reverse cholesterol transport is disrupted, causing the clinical manifestations of cholesterol accumulation in the tissues. Brunham recently reported a de novo mutation of this disorder.[96] Heterozygotes have intermediate HDL-C levels, do not experience any of the symptoms resulting from cholesterol ester accumulation, but may have an increased risk for coronary artery disease.[97] This disease is extremely rare; only about 100 cases have been reported worldwide.[98]

  3. Presentation and diagnosis HDL-C is absent or close to absent (<5 mg/dL) and apoA-1 is very low.[95] The LDL-C level may be reduced and triglycerides usually are elevated. Peripheral neuropathy and yellow-orange tonsils are hallmark signs of Tangier disease.[95] (see Fig. 13.2). Hypersplenism, hepatosplenomegaly, hepatic steatosis, lymphadenopathy, thrombocytopenia, corneal opacifications, stomatocytosis, and

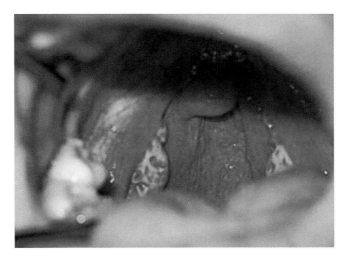

FIGURE 13.2: Yellow-orange tonsils in Tangier disease. (Reprinted with permission from Puntoni M, Sbrana F, Bigazzi F, Sampietro T. Tangier disease. Epidemiology, pathophysiology and management. *Am J Cardiovasc Drugs.* 2012;12(5):303-311.)

increased risk for cardiovascular disease also have been reported.[97,99,100] Accumulation of cholesterol in the Schwann cells, liver, thymus, spleen, tonsils, bone marrow, gastrointestinal mucosa, and cutaneous fibroblasts has been found.[99] Investigation of abdominal symptoms led to diagnoses of two children, although it is unknown whether these symptoms were caused by Tangier disease.[96] Pichit reported a large diversity in phenotypes and Tangier influence of development of cardiovascular disease remains unclear.[101] ABCA1 testing is possible.

4. **Treatment and monitoring** Currently, there is no treatment available to increase HDL-C or treat Tangier disease specifically. An apoA-1 mimetic peptide developed by Fukuoka University, known as FAMP, is under investigation and appears to enhance antiatherogenic effect of HDL without increasing HDL-C levels.[97] It is important to measure LDL-C and non–HDL-C levels in these patients and treat accordingly. A low-fat diet may help reduce hepatic steatosis and cause particles rich in cholesteryl esters to disappear.[102]

E. **ApoA-1 Milano** This is a mutation where carriers are heterozygotes and have very low HDL-C levels, normal to elevated LDL-C levels, and moderately elevated triglycerides. Persons with this mutation do not have premature ACSVD due to an enhanced capacity for cholesterol efflux (the first step in reverse cholesterol transport) despite low HDL-C.

F. **Summary of inherited low HDL-C** Numerous epidemiological studies have demonstrated a correlation between low HDL-C and cardiovascular disease, yet cardiovascular disease in hypoalphalipoproteinemia is not inevitable. There has been minimal success and even deleterious results from increasing HDL-C with medications. Currently, HDL research is focusing more on enhancing functional capacity of HDL to promote an antiatherogenic effect and increase reverse cholesterol transport, which will hopefully result in more treatments available to patients with hypoalphalipoproteinemia.

References

1. Fredrickson DS, Lees RS. A system for phenotyping hyperlipoproteinemia. *Circulation.* 1965;31:321-327.
2. Kwiterovich PO Jr. Diagnosis and management of familial dyslipoproteinemias. *Curr Cardiol Rep.* 2013;15(6):371.
3. Sullivan D, Lewis B. A classification of lipoprotein disorders: implications for clinical management. *Clin Lipidol.* 2011;6(3):327-338.
4. Li Y, Salfelder A, Schwab KO, et al. Against all odds: blended phenotypes of three single-gene defects. *Eur J Hum Genet.* 2016;24(9):1274-1279.
5. Goldberg AC, Hopkins PN, Toth PP, et al. Familial hypercholesterolemia: screening, diagnosis and management of pediatric and adult patients: clinical guidance from the National Lipid Association Expert Panel on familial hyper-cholesterolemia. *J Clin Lipidol.* 2011; 5(3):133-140.
6. National Institute of Health. *Genetic Testing Registry [Internet].* Bethesda, MD; [cited 2016 March 1]. Available from: http://www.ncbi.nlm.nih.gov/gtr/
7. Escola-Gil JC, Quesada H, Julve J, Martin-Campos JM, Cedo L, Blanco-Vaca F. Sitosterolemia: diagnosis, investigation and management. *Curr Atheroscler Rep.* 2014;16(7):424.
8. Colima Fausto AG, Gonzalez Garcia JR, Wong Ley Madero LE, Magana Torres MT. Two novel mutations in the ABCG5 gene, c.144-1G>A and c.1523delC, in a Mexican family with sitosterolemia. *J Clin Lipidol.* 2016;10(1):204-208.
9. Ostlund RE Jr. Phytosterols, cholesterol absorption and healthy diets. *Lipids.* 2007;42(1):41-45.
10. Ostlund RE Jr. Phytosterols and cholesterol metabolism. *Curr Opin Lipidol.* 2004;15(1):37-41.
11. Izar MC, Tegani DM, Kasmas SH, Fonseca FA. Phytosterols and phytosterolemia: gene-diet interactions. *Genes Nutr.* 2011;6(1):17-26.
12. Ramasamy I. Update on the molecular biology of dyslipidemias. *Clin Chim Acta.* 2016;454:143-185.
13. Myrie SB, Mymin D, Triggs-Raine B, Jones PJ. Serum lipids, plant sterols, and cholesterol kinetic responses to plant sterol supplementation in phytosterolemia heterozygotes and control individuals. *Am J Clin Nutr.* 2012;95(4):837-844.
14. Lee M, Lu K, Patel, S. Genetic basis of sitosterolemia. *Curr Opin Lipidol.* 2001;12(2):141-149.
15. Tada H, Kawashiri M, Takada M, et al. Infantile cases of sitosterolemia with novel mutations in the ABCG5 gene: extreme hypercholesterolemia is exacerbated by breastfeeding. *JIMD Rep.* 2015;21:155-122.
16. Weingartner O, Bohm M, Laufs U. Controversial role of plant sterol esters in the management of hypercholesterol-aemia. *Eur Heart J.* 2009;21:2009.
17. Solca C, Stanga Z, Pandit B, Diem P, Greeve J, Pateel SB. Sitosterolemia in Switzerland: molecular genetics links the US Amish-Mennonites to their European roots. *Clin Genet.* 2005;68(2):174-178.
18. Othman RA, Myrie SB, Mymin D, et al. Ezetimibe reduces plant sterol accumulation and favorably increases platelet count in sitosterolemia. *J Pediatr.* 2015;166(1):125-131.
19. Ajagbe BO, Othman RA, Myrie SB. Plant sterols, stanols and sitosterolemia. *J AOAC Int.* 2015;98(3):716-723.
20. Vanhahan H, Miettinen TA. Pravastatin and lovastatin similarly reduce serum cholesterol and its precursor levels in familial hypercholesterolemia. *Eur J Clin Pharmacol.* 1992;42(2):127-130.
21. Pollin TI, Quartuccio M. What we know about diet, genes, dyslipidemia: is there potential for translation. *Curr Nutr Rep.* 2013;2(4):236-242.
22. Gregg RE, Connor WE, Lin DS, Brewer HB Jr. Abnormal metabolism of shellfish sterols in a patient with sitosterol-emia and xanthomatosis. *J Clin Invest.* 1986;77(6):1864-1872.
23. Tsubakio-Yamamoto K, Nishida M, Nakagawa-Toyama Y, Masuda D, Ohama T, Yamashita S. Current therapy for patients with sitosterolemia-effect of ezetimibe on plant sterol metabolism. *J Atheroscler Thromb.* 2010;17(9):891-900.
24. Yoo EG. Sitosterolemia: a review and update on pathophysiology, clinical spectrum, diagnosis and management. *Ann Pediatr Endocrinol Metab.* 2016;21(1):7-14.
25. Nordestgaard B, Chapman J, Ray K, et al. Lipoprotein(a) as a cardiovascular risk factor: current status. *Eur Heart J.* 2010;31:2844-2853.
26. Bennet A, Di A, Erqou S, et al. Lp(a) levels and risk of future coronary heart disease: large-scale prospective data. *Arch Intern Med.* 2008;168:598-608.
27. Erqou S, Kaptoge S, Perry P, et al. Lipoprotein(a) concentration and the risk of coronary heart disease, stroke, and nonvascular mortality. *JAMA.* 2009;302:412-423.
28. Kamstrup P, Tybjaerg-Hansen A, Steffensen R, Nordestgaard B. Genetically elevated lipoprotein(a) and increased risk of myocardial infarction. *JAMA.* 2009;301:2331-2339.
29. Boffa MB, Koschinsky ML. Lipoprotein(a): truly a direct prothrombotic factor in cardiovascular disease? *J Lipid Res.* 2016;57(5):745-757.
30. Rogers MA, Aikawa E. A not-so-little role for lipoprotein(a) in the development of calcific aortic valve disease. *Circulation.* 2015;132:621-623.
31. Berg K. A new serum type system in man: the Lp system. *Acta Pathol Microbiol Scand.* 1963;59:369-382.
32. Koschinsky ML, Marcovina SM. Structure-function relationships in apolipoprotein(a): insights into lipoprotein(a) assembly and pathogenicity. *Curr Opin Lipidol.* 2004;15:167-174.

33. Rader DJ, Cain W, Ikewaki K, et al. The inverse association of plasma lipoprotein(a) concentrations with apolipoprotein(a) isoform size is not due to differences in Lp(a) catabolism but to differences in production rate. *J Clin Invest.* 1994;93:2758-2763.

34. Marcovina SM, Albers JJ. Lipoprotein (a) measurements for clinical application. *J Lipid Res.* 2016;57(4):526-537.

35. McConnell JP, Guadagno PA, Dayspring TD, et al. Lipoprotein (a) mass: a massively misunderstood metric. *J Clin Lipidol.* 2014;8:550-553.

36. Loscalzo J, Weinfeld M, Fless BM, Scanu AM. Lipoprotein(a), fibrin binding, and plasminogen activation. *Arteriosclerosis.* 1990;10:240-245.

37. Edelberg JM, Gonzalez-Gronow M, Pizzo SV. Lipoprotein(a) inhibition of plasminogen activation by tissue-type plasminogen activator. *Thromb Res.* 1990;57:155-162.

38. Sangrar W, Bajzar L, Nesheim ME, Koschinsky ML. Antifibrinolytic effect of recombinant apolipoprotein(a) in vitro is primarily due to attenuation of tPA-mediated Glu-plasminogen activation. *Biochemistry.* 1995;34:5151-5157.

39. Knapp JP, Herrmann W. In vitro inhibition of fibrinolysis by apolipoprotein(a) and lipoprotein(a) is size- and concentration-dependent. *Clin Chem Lab Med.* 2004;42:1013-1019.

40. Kronenberg F, Kronenberg MF, Kiechl S, et al. Role of lipoprotein(a) and apolipoprotein(a) phenotype in atherogenesis: prospective results from the Bruneck study. *Circulation.* 1999;100:1154-1160.

41. Klein JH, Hegele RA, Hackam DG, Koschinsky ML, Huff MW, Spence JD. Lipoprotein(a) is associated differentially with carotid stenosis, occlusion, and total plaque area. *Arterioscler Thromb Vasc Biol.* 2008;28:1851-1856.

42. Moliterno DJ, Lange RA, Meidell RS, et al. Relation of plasma lipoprotein(a) to infarct artery patency in survivors of myocardial infarction. *Circulation.* 1993;88:935-940.

43. Ribo M, Montaner J, Molina CA, Arenillas FJ, Santamaria E, Alvarez-Sabin J. Admission fibrinolytic profile predicts clot lysis resistance in stroke patients treated with tissue plasminogen activator. *Thromb Haemost.* 2004;91:1146-1151.

44. Helgadottir A, Steganssson K, et al. Apolipoprotein(a) genetic sequence variants associated with systemic atherosclerosis and coronary atherosclerotic burden but not with venous thromboembolism. *J Am Coll Cardiol.* 2012;60:722-729.

45. Kamstrup PR, Tybjaerg-Hansen A, Nordestgaard BG. Genetic evidence that lipoprotein(a) associates with atherosclerotic stenosis rather than venous thrombosis. *Arterioscler Thromb Vasc Biol.* 2012;32:1732-1741.

46. Utermann G. Lipoprotein(a). In: Scriver CR, Beaudet AL, Sly WS, Valle D, eds. *The Metabolic and Molecular Basis of Inherited Disease.* 8th ed. New York: McGraw-Hill; 2001:2753-2787.

47. Clarke R, Peden JF, Hopewell JC, et al. Genetic variants associated with Lp(a) lipoprotein level and coronary disease. *N Engl J Med.* 2009;361:2518-2528.

48. Guan W, Cao J, Steffen BT, et al. Race is a key variable in assigning lipoprotein(a) cutoff values for coronary heart disease risk assessment: the Multi-Ethnic Study of Atherosclerosis. *Arterioscler Thromb Vasc Biol.* 2015;35:996-1001.

49. Sharrett AR, Ballantyne CM, Coady SA, et al. Coronary heart disease prediction from lipoprotein cholesterol levels, triglycerides, lipoprotein(a), apolipoproteins A1 and B, and HDL density subfractions. The Atherosclerosis Risk in Communities (ARIC) Study. *Circulation.* 2001;104:1108-1113.

50. Virani SS, Brautbar A, Davis BC, et al. Associations between lipoprotein(a) levels and cardiovascular outcomes in black and white subjects: the Atherosclerosis Risk in Communities (ARIC) Study. *Circulation.* 2012;125:241-249.

51. Davidson MH, Ballantyne CM, Jacobson TA, et al. Clinical utility of inflammatory markers and advanced lipoprotein testing: advice from an Expert Panel of lipid specialists. *J Clin Lipidol.* 2011;5:338-367.

52. Weiss MC, Berger JS, Gianos E, et al. Lipoprotein(a) screening in patients with controlled traditional risk factors undergoing percutaneous coronary intervention. *J Clin Lipidol.* 2017;11:1177-1180.

53. Kagawa A, Azuma H, Akaike M, Kanagawa Y, Matsumoto T. Aspirin reduces apolipoprotein(a) (apo(a)) production in human hepatocytes by suppression of apo(a) gene transcription. *J Biol Chem.* 1999;274:43111-43115.

54. Akaike M, Azuma H, Kagawa A, et al. Effect of aspirin treatment on serum concentrations of lipoprotein(a) in patients with atherosclerotic diseases. *Clin Chem.* 2002;48:1454-1459.

55. Chasman DI, Shiffman D, Zee RY, et al. Polymorphism in the apolipoprotein(a) gene, plasma lipoprotein(a), cardiovascular disease, and low-dose aspirin therapy. *Atherosclerosis.* 2009;203:371-376.

56. Knopp RH, Alagona P, Davidson M, Goldber AC, Marcovina S. Equivalent efficacy of a time-release form of niacin (Niaspan) given once-a-night versus plain niacin in the management of hyperlipidemia. *Metabolism.* 1998;47:1097-1104.

57. Maccubbin D, Bays HE, Olsson AG, Elinoff V, Ells A, Paolini JF. Lipid-modifying efficacy and tolerability of extended-release niacin/laropiprant in patients with primary hypercholesterolaemia or mixed dyslipidaemia. *Int J Clin Pract.* 2008;62:1959-1970.

58. Cannon CP, Shah S, Dansky HM, et al. Safety of anacetrapib in patients with or at high risk for coronary heart disease. *N Engl J Med.* 2010;363:2406-2415.

59. Desai NR, Kohil P, Giugliano RP, et al. AMG145, a monoclonal antibody against proprotein convertase subtilisin/kexin type 9, significantly reduces lipoprotein(a) in hypercholesterolemic patients receiving statin therapy: an analysis from the LDL-C Assessment with Proprotein Convertase Subtilisin Kexin Type 9 Monoclonal Antibody Inhibition Combined with Statin Therapy (LAPLACE)-Thrombolysis in Myocardial Infarction (TIMI) 57 trial. *Circulation.* 2013;128:962-969.

60. Koschinsky ML. Lipoprotein(a). In: Ballantyne CM, ed. *Clinical Lipidology. A Companion to Braunwald's Heart Disease.* 2009:130-143.
61. Gonbert S, Malinsky S, Sposito AC, et al. Atorvastatin lowers lipoprotein(a) but not apolipoprotein(a) fragment levels in hypercholesterolemic subjects at high cardiovascular risk. *Atherosclerosis.* 2002;164:305-311.
62. Safarova MS, Ezhov MV, Afanasieva OI, Matchin YG, Atanesyan RV, Pokrovsky SN. Effect of specific lipoprotein(a) apheresis on coronary atherosclerosis regression by quantitative coronary angiography. *Atheroscler Suppl.* 2013;14:93-99.
63. Tsimikas S, Witztum J, Catapano A. Effect of mipomersen on lipoprotein(a) in patients with hypercholesterolemia across four phase III studies. *J Am Coll Cardiol.* 2012;59:494.
64. Tsimikas S, Viney NJ, Hughes SG, et al. Antisense therapy targeting apolipoprotein(a): a randomised, double-blind, placebo-controlled phase 1 study. *Lancet.* 2015;386:1472-1483.
65. Koopal C, Retterstol K, Sjouke B, et al. Vascular risk factors, vascular disease, lipids and lipid targets in patients with familial dysbetalipoproteinemia: a European cross-sectional study. *Atherosclerosis.* 2015;240:90-97.
66. Phillips M. Apolipoprotein E isoforms and lipoprotein metabolism. *IUBMB Life.* 2014;66(9):616-623.
67. Wardell MR, Brennan SO, Jaus ED, Fraser R, Carrell RW. Apolipoprotein E2-Christchurch (136 Arg----Ser). New variant of human apolipoprotein E in a patient with type III hyperlipoproteinemia. *J Clin Invest.* 1987;80(2):483-490.
68. Havekes L, de Wit E, Leuven JG, et al. Apolipoprotein E3-Leiden. A new variant of human apolipoprotein E associated with familial type III hyperlipoproteinemia. *Hum Genet.* 1986;73(2):157-163.
69. Marais D. Dysbetalipoproteinemia: an extreme disorder of remnant metabolism. *Curr Opin Lipidol.* 2015;26(4): 292-297.
70. Kei A, Miltiadous G, Bairaktari E, Hadjivassiliou M, Cariolou M, Elisaf M. Dysbetalipoproteinemia: two cases report and a diagnostic algorithm. *World J Clin Cases.* 2015;3(4):371-376.
71. Hopkins P, Brinton E, Nanjee MN. Hyperlipoproteinemia type 3: the forgotten phenotype. *Curr Atheroscler Rep.* 2014;16:440.
72. Genetics home reference. https://ghr.nlm.nih.gov/gene/APOB
73. Hooper A, Burnett J. Update on primary hypobetalipoproteinemia. *Curr Atheroscler Rep.* 2014;16:423.
74. Welty F. Hypobetalipoproteinemia and abetalipoproteinemia. *Curr Opin Lipidol.* 2015;25(3):161-168.
75. Singh A, Prasad R, Mishra OP. An infant with chronic diarrhoea and failure to thrive: familial hypobetalipoproteinemia. *J Clin Diagn Res.* 2015;9(12):1-2.
76. Minicocci I, Montali A, Robciuc MR, et al. Mutations in the ANGPTL3 gene and familial combined hypolipidemia: a clinical and biochemical characterization. *J Clin Endocrinol Metab.* 2012;97(7):E1266-E1275. doi:10.1210/jc.2012-1298.
77. Robciuc MR, Maranghi M, Lahikainen A, et al. Angptl3 deficiency is associated with increased insulin sensitivity, lipoprotein lipase activity, and decreased serum free fatty acids. *Arterioscler Thromb Vasc Biol.* 2013;33(7):1706-1713. doi:10.1161/ATVBAHA.113.301397.
78. Peretti N, Sassolas A, Roy CC, et al. Guidelines for the diagnosis and management of chylomicron retention disease based on a review of the literature and experience of two centers. *Orphanet J Rare Dis.* 2010;5:24.
79. Silvain M, Bligny D, Laforet L, et al. Anderson's disease (chylomicron retention disease): a new mutation in the SARA2 gene associated with muscular and cardiac abnormalities. *Clin Genet.* 2008;74:546-552.
80. Van der Steeg WA, Hovingh GK, Klerkx AH, et al. Cholesteryl ester transfer protein and hyperalphalipoproteinemia in Caucasians. *J Lipid Res.* 2007;48(3):674-682.
81. Thompson A, Di Angelantonio E, Sarwar N, et al. Association of cholesteryl ester transfer protein genotypes with CETP mass and activity, lipid levels, and coronary risk. *JAMA.* 2008;299(23):2777-2788.
82. Edmondson A, Brown R, Kathiresan S, et al. Loss of function variants in endothelial lipase are a case of elevated HDL cholesterol in humans. *J Clin Invest.* 2009;119(4):1042-1050.
83. Kobayashi J, Miyashita K, Nakajima K, Mabuchi H. Hepatic lipase: a comprehensive view of its role on plasma lipid and lipoprotein metabolism. *J Atheroscler Thromb.* 2015;22(10):1001-1011.
84. Al Riyami N, Al-Ali AM, Al-Sarraf AJ, et al. Hepatic lipase deficiency in a Middle Eastern Arabic male. *BMJ Case Rep.* 2010;12:2010.
85. Vigna GB, Satta E, Bernini F, et al. Flow-mediated dilation, carotid wall thickness and HDL function in subjects with hyperalphalipoproteinemia. *Nutr Metab Cardiovasc Dis.* 2014;24:777-783.
86. Tietjen I, Hovingh GK, Singaraja R, et al. Increased risk of coronary artery disease in Caucasians with extremely low HDL due to mutations in ABCA1, APOA1 and LCAT. *Biochim Biophys Acta.* 2012;1821:416-424.
87. Moutzouri E, Elisaf M, Liberopoulos EN. Hypocholesterolemia. *Curr Vasc Pharmacol.* 2011;9(2)200-212.
88. Xuming D, Szymon W, Evans J, Runge M. Genetics of coronary artery disease and myocardial infarction. *World J Cardiol.* 2016;8(1):1-23.
89. Ossoli A, Simonelli S, Vitali C, Franceschini C, Calabresi L. Role of LCAT in atherosclerosis. *J Atheroscler Thromb.* 2016;23(2):119-127.
90. Sahay M, Vali PS, Ismal K, Gowrishankar S, Padua MD, Swain M. An unusual case of nephrotic syndrome. *Indian J Nephrol.* 2016;26(1):55-56.

91. Kapoor S. Fish-eye disease: another under-recognized cause of familial corneal opacification. *Ophthalmic Genet.* 2016;37(3):349.
92. Ossoli A, Neufeld EB, Thacker SG, et al. Lipoprotein X causes renal disease in LCAT deficiency. *PLoS One.* 2016;11(2):e0150083.
93. Aranda P, Valdivielso P, Pisciotta L, et al. Therapeutic management of a new case of LCAT deficiency with a multifactorial long-term approach based on high doses of angiotensin II receptor blockers (ARBs). *Clin Nephrol.* 2008;69(3):213-218.
94. Shamburek R, Bakker-Arkema R, Shamburek A, et al. Safety and tolerability of ACP-501, a recombinant human Lecithin:cholesterol Acyltransferase, a phase 1 single dose escalation study. *Circ Res.* 2016;118(1):73-82.
95. Fredrickson DS, Altrocchi P, Avioli L, Goodman DW, Goodman H. Tangier disease. Combined clinical staff conference at the National Institutes of Health. *Ann Intern Med.* 1961;55(6):1016-1031.
96. Brunham LR, Kang MH, Van Karnebeek C, et al. Clinical, biochemical and molecular characterization of novel mutations in ABCA1 in families with Tangier disease. *JIMD Rep.* 2015;18:51-62.
97. Uehara Y, Ando S, Yahiro E, et al. FAMP, a novel ApoA-1 mimentic peptide suppresses aortic plaque formation through promotion of biological HDL function in ApoE-deficient Mice. *J Am Heart Assoc* 2013;2(3):e000048.
98. National Institute of Health. *Genetic Testing Registry [Internet].* Bethesda, MD; [cited 2016 March 1]. Available from: ghr.nlm.nih.gov/condition/tangier-disease#statistics
99. Nagappa M, Taly AB, Mahadevan A, et al. Tangier's disease: an uncommon cause of facial weakness and non-length dependent demyelinating neuropathy. *Ann Indian Acad Neurol.* 2016;19(1):137-139.
100. Ravesloot MJ, Bril H, Braamskamp MJ, Wiegman A, Wong Chung RP. The curious case of the orange coloured tonsils. *Int J Pediatr Otorhinolaryngol.* 2014;78(12):2305-2307.
101. Pichit P, Quillard M, Couvert P, et al. Tangier disease phenotype diversity in dizygous twin sisters. *Rev Neurol.* 2010;166:534-537.
102. Puntoni M, Sbrana F, Bigazzi F, Sampietro T. Tangier disease. Epidemiology, pathophysiology and management. *Am J Cardiovasc Drugs.* 2012;12(5):303-311.

CHAPTER 14

Children and Adolescents Step-by-Step Evaluation and Management Plan

Don P. Wilson, Catherine McNeal, and Piers R. Blackett

◆ Key Points

- Lipid disorders are common in children, often caused by genetic mutations in cholesterol metabolism, acquired cardiovascular risk factors such as obesity and insulin resistance, or both.

- Of those with genetic mutations, heterozygous familial hypercholesterolemia (HeFH) is common, occurring in 1:200-1:500 individuals. Children with HeFH are asymptomatic, usually of normal weight, and have no physical signs of hypercholesterolemia. Most are detected by routine cholesterol screening.

- Although events rarely occur in children and adolescents, elevated levels of cholesterol play a dominant role in the initiation and progression of atherosclerosis, starting in childhood, especially in those with FH.

- In individuals with FH, elevated blood cholesterol levels are present from birth, and surrogate markers of adverse atherosclerotic vascular changes can be demonstrated in youth, necessitating the need for early efforts aimed at primary prevention of atherosclerotic cardiovascular diseases (ASCVD).

- In addition to adopting a lifelong, heart-healthy lifestyle for all youth, those with inherited disorders of lipid metabolism and, in selected cases, those with acquired risk factors and conditions, pharmaceutical intervention is often necessary to reduce or postpone morbidity and premature mortality attributable to ASCVD in adulthood.

- Youth with milder elevation of LDL-C and non–HDL-C, as well as those with elevated TG, should also be recognized and appropriately addressed, including an emphasis on lifestyle changes, monitoring, and, when indicated, pharmacologic treatment.

I. Introduction

A. Lipid disorders are common in children, often caused by genetic mutations in cholesterol metabolism, acquired ASCVD risk factors and conditions, or both. Acquired risk factors are often associated with adverse lifestyle habits, such as poor nutrition and low levels of physical activity, leading to obesity, insulin resistance, and type 2 diabetes (T2D). In addition to the use of tobacco, a variety of medications, and conditions, such as renal disease and lupus erythematosus, contribute to increased ASCVD risk.

B. Perhaps the most common dyslipidemia encountered in children and adolescences is atherogenic dyslipidemia, characterized by elevated levels of TG, low HDL, and increased number of small dense LDL particles. This pattern is often found in children with excessive weight gain and insulin resistance. Long-term moderate-to-high levels of TG (150-499 mg/dL) may increase risk of premature ASCVD during adulthood.

C. As a consequence of lifelong exposure to elevated levels of atherogenic lipoproteins (ie, non–HDL-C and LDL-C) and low HDL-C, affected children are at increased risk of developing premature ASCVD, that is, coronary artery disease and cerebrovascular disease, in adulthood. The goal of identification and treatment of dyslipidemia in youth is sustained reduction of atherogenic lipoproteins, starting as early as possible. The foundation of all interventions, including those with genetic dyslipidemias, is TLC in parallel with counseling aimed at preventing the acquisition of additional risk factors such as tobacco use, hypertension, and diabetes. While sufficient reduction in atherogenic lipoproteins can be attained in some with lifestyle changes alone, judicious use of cholesterol-lowering agents is effective in those with higher cholesterol levels, especially in those with FH and/or multiple risk factors or risk conditions. Since most children with FH are of normal weight and are asymptomatic, it is important to perform lipid screening of all children, regardless of general health or the presence or absence of ASCVD risk factors.

D. Inherited disorders of lipid and lipoprotein metabolism are caused by mono- or polygenic mutations (Table 14.1). Those that result in hypercholesterolemia most often affect the LDL-C receptor. HeFH is a common (1 in 200-500) genetic cause of hypercholesterolemia. It is most frequently inherited as an autosomal codominant trait resulting in lack of or reduced removal of LDL particles from the plasma, causing elevated LDL-C and

Table 14.1.	**Classification of Disorders in Lipid and Lipoprotein Metabolism**			
Diagnosis	**Fredrickson Classification**	**Primary Lipid Change**	**Primary Lipoprotein Change**	**Genetics**
Familial Hyperchylomicronemia	Type 1	↑ TG	↑ chylomicrons	Monogenic; autosomal recessive due to two mutant alleles of LPL, APOC2, APOA5, LMF1, GPIHBP1, or GPD1; presentation mainly in children and young adults
Familial Hypercholesterolemia	Type 2A	↑ TC	↑ LDL	Monogenic; autosomal codominant; heterozygous form results from one mutant allele of LDLR, APOB, or PCSK9. Homozygous form results from two mutant alleles of these genes or of LDLRAP1 (recessive).
Familial Combined Hyperlipoproteinemia	Type 2B	↑ TC, ↑ TG	↑ VLDL, ↑ LDL	Polygenic; high GRS[a] for hypertriglyceridemia; excess of rare variants in hypertriglyceridemia-associated genes; high GRS for LDL cholesterol
Dysbetalipoproteinemia	Type 3	↑ TC, ↑ TG	↑ IDL	Polygenic; high GRS for hypertriglyceridemia; excess of rare variants in hypertriglyceridemia-associated genes; APOE E2/E2 homozygosity; or heterozygous rare mutations in APOE
Primary Hypertriglyceridemia	Type 4	↑ TG	↑ VLDL	Polygenic; high GRS for hypertriglyceridemia; excess of rare variants in hypertriglyceridemia-associated genes
Mixed Hypertriglyceridemia	Type 5	↑ TC, ↑ TG	↑ VLDL, ↑ chylomicrons	Polygenic; high GRS for hypertriglyceridemia; excess of rare variants in hypertriglyceridemia-associated genes, with higher burden of risk alleles than for hyperlipoproteinemia type 4

[a]GRS, polygenic genetic risk score.
(Adapted with permission from Hegele RA. Plasma lipoproteins: genetic influences and clinical implications. *Nat Rev Genet*. 2009;10(2):109-121.)

premature ASCVD during adulthood. Homozygous (HoFH) and recessive types of FH occur but are rare (~1:1,000,000). Recent publications, however, suggest that the prevalence of HoFH may be more frequent than previously reported.

E. The most common mutations in autosomal codominant FH are in the low-density lipoprotein receptor (LDLR), apolipoprotein B (APOB), and proprotein convertase subtilisin/kexin type 9 (PCSK9) genes. While genetic testing is available, it only identifies a small fraction of the defects. Therefore, while informative if known, it should be noted that identifying a monogenic cause of FH is not always possible. FH is less likely to be attributed to known single gene mutations in certain ethnic groups, especially in African Americans.

F. Defects in the LDLR gene are estimated to cause up to 90% of autosomal codominant FH. HeFH can cause a functional loss of 50% or more of LDL receptors, due to a quantitative or qualitative defect. In HoFH, affected individuals have little or no LDLR functionality, and ASCVD-related events can occur very early in life, even in childhood, without treatment. Early diagnosis and treatment of FH is imperative for timely treatment and prevention of premature ASCVD and related events.

G. Because genetic testing only identifies a small number of FH mutations, a presumptive diagnosis is typically made based on the LDL-C value. In adults with untreated HeFH, the LDL-C is generally >190 mg/dL, with levels >160 mg/dL in children and adolescents (Table 14.2). In a US population <18 years of age, there is a wide distribution of LDL-C levels in affected individuals, with overlap between those with and without FH. When screening for only a few of the possible genetic causes of FH, the probability of having genetically confirmed FH with a LDL-C above 164 mg/dL has been estimated to be 1.8%. The probability of having FH with a level above 190 mg/dL was 57.6%, but in first-degree relatives of a known proband with FH, the chances of having FH at the same levels are 90% and 99.9%.

H. Studies on European populations also show overlap between LDL-C levels in FH compared to unaffected relatives, which increases with age and results in missed diagnoses or false negatives. Diagnosis of FH is improved when age-specific cut points for LDL-D are combined with genetic testing. If genetic testing is not available, a good family history and serial evaluation of LDL-C levels, after implementation of TLC, is helpful in suspected cases and to help inform clinical decision-making. Published criteria for diagnosis of FH are listed in Figure 14.1. Although genetic causes of hypercholesterolemia

Table 14.2.	LDL-C Diagnostic Categories				
				Minimum LDL-C, mg/dL	
Category	Description	Age < 20 y	Age 20-29 y	Age 30+ y
1	General population 95th percentile	130	160	190
2	80% have FH in first-degree relatives[a]	150	170	200
3	80% have FH in general population[b]	190	220	260
4	99% have FH in general population	220	240	280
5	99.9% have FH in general population	240	260	300

[a]Used for cascade screening.
[b]NHLBI Pediatric Guidelines.
(Data from Hopkins PN, Toth PP, Ballantyne CM, Rader DJ; National Lipid Association Expert Panel on Familial Hypercholesterolemia. Familial hypercholesterolemias: prevalence, genetics, diagnosis and screening recommendations from the National Lipid Association Expert Panel on Familial Hypercholesterolemia. *J Clin Lipidol.* 2011;5(3 suppl):S9-S17.)

Table 2. Diagnostic tools for FH.

a. US MedPed Program diagnostic criteria.

Age (years)	Total cholesterol (mmol/L)			
	First-degree relative	Second-degree relative	Third-degree relative	General population
<20	5.7	5.9	6.2	7.0
20-29	6.2	6.5	6.7	7.5
30-39	7.0	7.2	7.5	8.8
>40	7.5	7.8	8.0	9.3

Diagnosis of FH if total cholesterol level exceeds the cutpoint in table above.

b. The Simon Broome register criteria

Criteria	
A	Plasma cholesterol measurement of either:
	Total cholesterol >7.5 mmol/L (adult) or >6.7 mmol/L (child <16 years)
	LDL cholesterol >4.9 mmol/L (adult) or >4.0 mmol/L (child <16 years)
B	Presence of tendon xanthomata in patient or in a first- or second-degree relative
C	DNA-based evidence of a mutation in the *LDLR* or other FH-related gene
D	Family history of myocardial infarction in a second-degree relative <50 years of age or in a first-degree relative <60 years of age
E	Family history of plasma total cholesterol of >7.5 mmol/L in a first- or second-degree relative

Diagnosis	Criteria required
Definite FH	A + B OR C
Probable FH	A + D OR A + E

c. The Dutch Lipid Clinic Network criteria

Criteria	Points
1 Family history	
First-degree relative with known premature coronary and vascular disease	1
First-degree relative with known plasma LDL cholesterol concentration greater than 95th percentile for age and sex in an adult relative	1
First-degree relative with known plasma LDL cholesterol concentration greater than 95th percentile for age and sex in a relative <18 years of age	2
First-degree relative with known tendon xanthomata or corneal arcus	2
2 Clinical history	
Presence of coronary artery disease	2
Presence of cerebral or peripheral vascular disease	1
3 Physical examination	
Presence of tendon xanthomata	6
Presence of cerebral arcus in a patient <45 years of age	4
4 LDL cholesterol level (mmol/L)	
≥8.5	8
6.5-8.4	5
5.0-6.4	3
4.0-4.9	1
5 DNA analysis	
Functional mutation in the LDLR gene or other FH-related gene	8

Diagnosis	Total points
Definite FH	>8
Probable FH	6-8
Possible FH	3-5

FIGURE 14.1: Criteria for the clinical diagnosis of familial hypercholesterolemia. (Reprinted with permission from Fahed AC, Nemer GM. Familial hypercholesterolemia: the lipids or the genes? *Nutr Metab.* 2011;8(1):1.)

are common and are of major concern, it should be noted that elevated blood levels of LDL-C also commonly occur in children with poor health habits, unrecognized conditions such as hypothyroidism, and with use of a variety of medications.

I. Because affected children are asymptomatic, often of normal weight, and the family history unavailable, incomplete, or unreliable, systematic screening (universal, targeted, and cascade; see below) is recommended in the United States to facilitate early identification of youth with dyslipidemia. In 2011, US practice guidelines recommended universal cholesterol screening once at 10 years of age (range 9-11 years) and, if normal, repeated once between 17 and 20 years of age. To simplify screening and be consistent with screening recommendations for adults, after the initial screening at 10 year of age, it seems reasonable to repeat screening once every 5 years thereafter. Lipid screening during adolescence may also detect those with dyslipidemia caused by poor dietary habits, lack of physical activity, and use of medications, such as oral contraceptives.

II. **STEP I. CVD Risk Assessment**

A. Lipid screening: Who to screen

1. Targeted screening in all children ≥2 years of age in whom:
    - One or both biologic parents are known to have hypercholesterolemia or are receiving lipid-lowering medications
    - Who have a family history of premature cardiovascular disease (defined below), that is, men <55 years of age and women <65 years of age
    - Whose family history is unknown (eg, children who were adopted)

2. Universal screening of all children 10 years of age (range 9-11), regardless of general health or the presence/absence of CVD risk factors and, if normal, repeat every 5 years thereafter.

3. Cascade screening involves systematic testing of all first-degree relatives (parents, siblings, and children) of an FH index case, followed by testing of second- and third-degree relatives if any of the first-degree relatives are affected. The most practical approach to cascade screening is biochemical testing of cholesterol, which is inexpensive and readily available. However, up to 25% of family members may be misdiagnosed as being either affected or unaffected when screening is based on cholesterol levels alone. Testing for a known genetic mutation in the family combined with LDL-C levels will yield a definitive diagnosis. The family history may also be unknown, incomplete, or inaccurate.

B. Lipid screening: When to screen

1. Lipid testing is recommended during scheduled clinic visits, such as with childhood immunizations and well-child visits.

C. Lipid screening: What to order

1. Either a fasting or nonfasting lipid profile is acceptable although a fasting lipid panel is usually suggested for targeted screening and a nonfasting non–HDL-C level for general (universal) screening.

2. Blood samples can be drawn by venipuncture or fingerstick. If available, point of care lipid testing (eg, tabletop analyzer) has proven reliable and correlates well with standard laboratory results.

3. The non-HDL-C (i.e., TC - HDL-C) should be calculated. In addition to LDL-C, non–HDL-C is recommended as a target of therapy since it is an estimate of all atherogenic lipoprotein particles. Non–HDL-C has been shown to be a better predictor of CVD risk than LDL-C.

4. If the initial non–HDL-C level from a nonfasting sample is ≥145 mg/dL (95th percentile), two fasting lipid profiles should be obtained and the results averaged for evaluation of the most appropriate action. It should be noted that the desirable level

for non-HDL is <120 mg/dL (<75th percentile). Therefore, levels of 120-145 should be followed closely, especially if other risk factors are present.

5. Routine measurement of lipoprotein (a) [Lp(a)], apoB, apoA1, and lipoprotein subclasses and their sizes by advanced lipoprotein analysis is not recommended at this time but may be helpful in selected cases.

   a. If the nonfasting TG is ≥150 mg/dL, a fasting lipid profile should be performed since triglycerides are largely distributed in non-HDL particles that also contain cholesterol. LDL-C cannot be calculated if TG > 400 mg/dL. If TG remain elevated (>400 mg/dL), LDL-C level can be measured directly.

D. Lipid screening: Which family members to screen?

1. **First-degree relatives:** Biological parents and siblings

2. **Second-degree relatives:** Biological grandparents, aunts, and uncles

E. Lipid screening: Which conditions?

1. Treated angina

2. Myocardial infarction (MI)

3. Percutaneous coronary catheter intervention procedure

4. Coronary artery bypass grafting (CABG)

5. Stroke or sudden cardiac death (before 55 years of age in men or 65 years of age in women

F. Lipid screening: Physical examination

1. Children, including those with HeFH, rarely have physical stigmata of hyperlipidemia, such as xanthoma, xanthelasma, or corneal arcus. Exceptions include children with HoFH, sitosterolemia, and cerebrotendinous xanthomatosis, all of whom may have manifestations at a very young age.

2. In children with severe hypertriglyceridemia, eruptive xanthomas may occur on the trunk, buttocks, palms, and extensor surfaces of the extremities. Lipemia retinalis may also be visible on retinal exam.

3. The physical examination should look for signs of other risk conditions, such as T2D (acanthosis nigricans), hypothyroidism (goiter), nephrotic syndrome (edema), polycystic ovarian syndrome in females (hirsutism and excessive acne), and chronic inflammatory conditions, such as lupus erythematosus (malar rash).

G. Medical History

1. Identify the presence of risk factors or risk conditions that confer moderate-to-high risk of premature ASCVD (Table 14.3).

H. Family History

1. A family history of premature ASCVD represents the net effect of genetic, biochemical, behavioral, and environmental components. However, reliance on family history alone as a basis for lipid screening fails to identify as many as 30%-60% of children and adolescents with elevated lipid levels. Despite its limitations, the presence of a positive family history and/or risk factors should lead to evaluation of all family members, especially the biological parents, for ASCVD risk factors. The family history should be updated regularly as a part of routine pediatric care.

Table 14.3.   Factors and Conditions That Increase Risk of Premature Cardiovascular Disease

Criteria	Moderate Risk	High Risk
Body mass index	≥95th percentile to 96th percentile	≥97th percentile
Hypertension	High blood pressure without medication	High blood pressure with medication
Cigarette smoking	—	Current smoker
HDL-C	<40 mg/dL	—
Predisposing medical conditions	Kawasaki disease with regressed coronary aneurysms Chronic inflammatory disease[a] HIV infection Nephrotic syndrome	Kawasaki disease with current coronary aneurysms Type 1 and type 2 diabetes mellitus Post orthotopic heart transplant Chronic kidney disease/end-stage renal disease/postrenal transplant

[a]Systemic lupus erythematosus, rheumatoid arthritis.
(Data from Expert Panel on Integrated Guidelines for Cardiovascular Health and Risk Reduction in Children and Adolescents, National Heart, Lung, and Blood Institute. Expert panel on integrated guidelines for cardiovascular health and risk reduction in children and adolescents: summary report. *Pediatrics*. 2011;128(suppl 5):S213-S256.)

III.   STEP 2. Determine Risk Category

A. Although use of LDL-C cut points vs pooled ASCVD risk estimates in adults has recently been questioned, determining non–HDL-C and LDL-C goals in youth is useful in helping select appropriate interventions. In the absence of outcome studies that help define goals, percentile-based cut points are recommended and should be considered as the upper limits for valid therapeutic goal ranges for managing children and adolescents.

B. Determine the need for TLC.

C. Assess non–HDL-C, LDL-C, and TG levels for consideration of a lipid-lowering drug (Table 14.4).

IV.   STEP 3. Clinical Interventions: Lifestyle, Medications

A. Initiate TLC if non–HDL-C and LDL-C are above goal

1. Weight management, if overweight (body mass index [BMI] 85-94th percentile) or obese (BMI ≥ 95th percentile).

Table 14.4.   Lipid Goals and Cut Points for Therapeutic Lifestyle Changes (TLC) and Drug Therapy[a]

Lab Test	Acceptable	Borderline	Mild	Abnormal Moderate	High to Severe
LDL-C	≤110	110-129	130-159	160-189	≥190
Non–HDL-C	≤140	140-159	160-189	190-219	≥220
TG	≤110	110-149	150-249	250-499	≥500
Intervention	• TLC • CHILD 1 diet	• TLC • CHILD 1 diet • Other risk factor interventions as appropriate	• TLC • CHILD 2 diet (see below) • Other risk factor interventions as appropriate		• TLC • CHILD 2 diet (see below) • Other risk factor interventions as appropriate • Lipid-lowering drug
Reevaluate and referral	In 5 y	In 1 y	In 6 mo if levels remain abnormal, consider appropriate treatment or referral to a lipid specialist.		Consider referral to a lipid specialist.

[a]Youth <18 years of age.
TLC, therapeutic lifestyle changes; CHILD, cardiovascular health integrated lifestyle diet.

Diet	Age[a]	Total[b]	SFA	MUFA	PUFA	Trans	Chol[c]	Supportive Measures
Table 14.5.	**Dietary Recommendations for Children and Adolescents with Dyslipidemia**							
				Daily Dietary Fat				
CHILD 2-LDL Lowering	2-21	25%-30%	≤7%	~10%	~10%	Avoid	<200	• Plant sterol esters and/or plant stanol esters[d] up to 2 g/d as replacement for usual fat sources can be used after age 2 y in children with familial hypercholesterolemia. • Water-soluble fiber psyllium can be added to a low-fat, low–saturated fat diet as cereal enriched with psyllium at a dose of 6 g/d for children 2-12 y and 12 g/d for those ≥12 y of age. • Recommend 1 h/d of moderate to vigorous physical activity and <2 h/d of sedentary screen time.

CHILD 2-TG Lowering	2-21	25%-30%	≤7%	~10%	~10%	Avoid	<200	• Decrease sugar intake:
								  ◦ Replace simple with complex carbohydrates.
								  ◦ No sugar-sweetened beverages
								• Increase dietary fish to increase omega-3 fatty acids.[e]
								• Recommend 1 h/d of moderate to vigorous physical activity and <2 h/d of sedentary screen time.

CHILD, cardiovascular health integrated lifestyle diet; SFA, saturated fatty acid; MUFA, monounsaturated fatty acid; PUFA, polyunsaturated fatty acid; Trans, trans fats; Total, total fat.

[a]Years.

[b]% daily kcal/estimated energy requirements from fat.

[c]mg/dL.

[d]If child is obese, nutrition therapy should include calorie restriction, and increased activity (beyond that recommended for all children) should be prescribed.

[e]The Food and Drug Administration (FDA) and the Environmental Protection Agency (EPA) are advising women of child-bearing age who may become pregnant, pregnant women, nursing mothers, and young children to avoid some types of fish and shellfish and eat fish and shellfish that are low in mercury. For more information, call the FDA's food information line toll free at 1–888–SAFEFOOD or visit http://www.cfsan.fda.gov/~dms/admehg3.html.

(Data from Expert Panel on Integrated Guidelines for Cardiovascular Health and Risk Reduction in Children and Adolescents, National Heart, Lung, and Blood Institute. Expert panel on integrated guidelines for cardiovascular health and risk reduction in children and adolescents: summary report. *Pediatrics.* 2011;128 (suppl 5):S213-S256.)

2. 60 minutes of moderate to vigorous physical activity per day.

3. Cardiovascular Health Integrated Lifestyle Diet (CHILD 1) is the recommended initial diet for all children and adolescents at elevated risk of ASCVD. Age- and gender-appropriate recommendations from birth to 21 years of age can be found at the National Heart, Lung, and Blood Institute's *Integrated Guidelines for Cardiovascular Health and Risk Reduction in Children and Adolescents* Web site at http://www.nhlbi.nih.gov/health-pro/guidelines/current/cardiovascular-health-pediatric-guidelines/summary.

4. Cardiovascular Health Integrated Lifestyle Diet (CHILD 2) LDL-C and TG-lowering diets (Table 14.5): The CHILD 2 diet recommendations are for ages 2-21 years with elevated LDL-C, non–HDL-C, and/or TG levels.

B. Consider adding drug therapy if non-HDL-C and LDL-C exceed cut points

1. Consider adding drug to TLC after 3-6 months.

2. Consider drug therapy simultaneously with TLC for HoFH, sitosterolemia, and cerebrotendinous xanthomatosis. For HoFH, more aggressive therapy is often needed, such as use of emerging lipid-lowering drugs (see Table 14.6), plasma apheresis, and liver transplantation. It is recommended that individuals with these disorders

Table 14.6.   Newer Drug Therapies that Affect Lipids and Lipoprotein Metabolism for use in those with Severely Elevated LDL-C and/or Those at Very High Risk

Medication	Pediatric Dosing	Adult Dosing	Side Effects	Comments
Microsomal Transport Protein (MTP) Inhibitors				
Lomitapide (Juxtapid)	Dose: Not currently available	Dose: Initially 5 mg/d; titrate to 10–40 mg/d; max dose 60 mg/d. Titrate in 4-wk intervals.	Diarrhea, nausea, vomiting, dyspepsia, abdominal pain. Increased hepatic fat with or without concomitant increases in transaminases	Initiate low-fat diet (<20% of energy from fat); titrate dose based on acceptable safety/tolerability. Maintenance dose should be individualized. Before treatment, measure ALT, AST, alkaline phosphatase, and total bilirubin. Obtain a negative pregnancy test in females. Dose adjustment required for persistent LFTs >3X ULN.
Antisense Inhibitor of apoB Synthesis				
Mipomersen (Kynamro)	Dose: Not currently available	Dose: 200 mg SC once weekly; max dose, same	Injection site reactions; flu-like symptoms; nausea; diarrhea; headaches; elevations in serum transaminases, specifically ALT; and increases in hepatic fat with or without concomitant increases in transaminases	SC injection given on the same day every week; if a dose is missed, injection should be given at least 3 d from the next weekly dose. Avoid in moderate to severe hepatic impairment or active liver disease, including unexplained persistent elevations of LFTs.
Monoclonal Antibodies to PCSK9				
Alirocumab (Praluent)	Dose: Not currently available	Dose: 75 mg SC every 2 wk. May increase to 150 mg SC every 2 wk after 4–8 wk as needed. May also give 300 mg every 4 wk.	Nasopharyngitis, injection site reactions, and influenza	SC injection given on the same day every 2 wk; if a dose is missed, injection should be given within 7 d from the missed dose and then resume the original schedule. If the missed dose is not administered within 7 d, wait until the next dose on the original schedule.
Evolocumab (Repatha)	Dose: For 13 y of age and older, 140 mg SC every 2 wk or 420 mg SC once monthly	Dose: 140 mg SC every 2 wk or 420 mg SC once monthly	Nasopharyngitis, upper respiratory tract infections, and influenza	SC injection given on the same day every 2 wk or once a month; if a dose is missed, administer as soon as possible if there are >7 d until the next schedule dose or omit the missed dose and administer the next dose according to the original schedule. To administer the 420 mg dose, give three injections consecutively within 30 min.
Enzyme Replacement Therapy				
Sebelipase alfa (Kanuma)	Dose: Rapidly progressing lysosomal acid lipase (LAL) deficiency presenting within the first 6 mo of life 1 mg/kg as an intravenous infusion once weekly. For patients that do not achieve an optimal clinical response, increased to 3 mg/kg once weekly	Dose: LAL deficiency, give 1 mg/kg as an IV infusion once every other week	Rapidly progressive disease within the first 6 mo of life: diarrhea, vomiting, fever, rhinitis, anemia, cough, nasopharyngitis, and urticaria Pediatric and adults: Headache, fever, oropharyngitis, nasopharyngitis, asthenia, constipation, and nausea	Infuse over at least 2 h; consider prolonged infusion for the 3 mg/kg dose or if a hypersensitivity reaction occurs. Consider 1-h infusion for 1 mg/kg dose, as tolerated. Patients should be observed for hypersensitivity reactions, including anaphylaxis. Consider the risk and benefits of treatment in patients with known systemic hypersensitivity reactions to eggs and egg products. Pretreatment with antipyretics and/or antihistamines may prevent subsequent reactions.

Omega-3-Carboxylic Acids

Epanova	Dose: Not FDA approved for use in children; safety and efficacy not established	Dose: 2 g (2 capsules) or 4 g (4 capsules) once daily	In patients with hepatic impairment, ALT and AST levels should be monitored periodically during therapy. Use with caution in patients with known hypersensitivity to fish and/ or shellfish. Omega-3 fatty acids have been demonstrated to prolong bleeding time in some patients.	FDA approved spring 2014. Anticipated availability is currently unknown.

Gene Replacement Therapy

Alipogene tiparvovec (Glybera)	Dose: Not FDA approved for use in children; safety and efficacy not established	Dose: Given as a single treatment involving multiple injections into the muscles of the upper and lower legs. The dose and number of injections is dependent upon the patient's weight.	The most common side effect reported in clinical trials was pain in the legs following the injections in a third of patients. Other common side effects reported include headache, tiredness, hyperthermia, and contusion.	Approved by the European Commission in October 2012 for treatment of adults diagnosed with familial lipoprotein lipase deficiency (LPLD) confirmed by genetic testing and suffering from severe or multiple pancreatitis attacks despite dietary fat restrictions.

(Adapted with permission from Wilson DP, de la Torre A, Brautbar A, Hamilton L. Screening for genetic mutations in children and adolescents with dyslipidemia: importance of early identification and implications of missed diagnoses. *Expert Opin Orphan Drugs.* 2016;4(7):699-710.)

be referred to a lipid specialist with access to multidisciplinary care for treatment and follow-up. A list of lipid specialists can be found at http://www.lipidfoundation.org/professionals.

C. Establish goals of therapy

1. Although long-term outcome data are lacking, the case for managing children and adolescents based on their percentiles is strengthened by mendelian randomization studies showing that lower levels of LDL-C and non–HDL-C may be more advantageous for cardiovascular health when maintained over a lifetime.

D. For children with high-risk lipid abnormalities, the presence of additional risk factors or high-risk conditions (see Table 14.3) may lower the recommended LDL-C and non–HDL-C level for initiation of drug therapy, and lower the desired goal LDL-C and non–HDL-C levels and, in selected cases, may prompt consideration for initiation below the age of 10 years. Select appropriate drug therapy (see Tables 14.7-14.9).

1. Review available drugs that affect lipids and lipoprotein metabolism with the parent or caregiver.

2. Age- and developmentally appropriate information should be provided to the child and the literacy level and learning style considered in providing information to the parent or caregiver.

3. Explore the child's/parent's/caregiver's knowledge and experience with lipid-lowering medications.

4. Address fears, concerns, and preferences. Often, parental preferences are based upon personal experiences, drug-related side effects, and cost.

5. Advise about potential medication interactions. In females, provide information about concerns with pregnancy, contraindication of using most lipid-lowering agents, especially statins, during pregnancy, and breastfeeding, and address the need for appropriate contraception.

6. Provide handouts and links to informative Web sites, such as *Learn Your Lipids* (http://www.learnyourlipids.com/) and *Familial Hypercholesterolemia* (https://thefh-foundation.org/).

E. Long-term safety The preferred pharmacotherapy algorithm for adults with HeFH is listed in Figure 14.2. Although studies in children demonstrating long-term safety and efficacy are lacking, given the significant risk of premature ASCVD in individuals with FH, aggressive therapy should be considered, but used with caution. The decision to use a third-line agent must take into account multiple factors, including disease severity, patient/family preference, cost, and outcome data, if available.

F. When to refer Children and adolescents who respond poorly to therapeutic lifestyle changes only or who have severe elevations of LDL-C (≥190 mg/dL) and/or non–HDL-C (≥220 mg/dL) should be referred to a pediatric lipid specialist (http://www.lipidfoundation.org/professionals). These youth often have complex disorders of lipid metabolism, for example, HeFH and HoFH or genetic mutations in TG metabolism. Successful treatment may require aggressive management and/or use of investigational drugs. Table 14.6 illustrates some new and emerging drugs for treatment of hypercholesterolemia and hypertriglyceridemia.

Table 14.7.	Cholesterol-Lowering Medications			
Medication	**Pediatric Dosing**	**Adult Dosing**	**Side Effects**	**Indication/Comments**
HMG-CoA–Reductase Inhibitors				
Atorvastatin	Age 10-17 Dose: 10-20 mg/d	Dose: 10-80 mg/d	Headache; nausea; sleep disturbance; elevations in hepatocellular enzymes and alkaline phosphatase. Myositis and rhabdomyolysis, primarily when given with gemfibrozil or cyclosporine; myositis is also seen with severe renal insufficiency (CrCl < 30 mL/min).	Heterozygous familial hypercholesterolemia May be titrated at ≥4 wk intervals
Fluvastatin	Age 10-16 Dose: 20-80 mg/d	Dose: 20-80 mg/d		Heterozygous familial hypercholesterolemia May be titrated at ≥6 wk intervals. Adjust dose amount for insufficiency (CrCl < 30 mL/min); not to exceed 40 mg/d
Lovastatin	Age 10-17 Dose: 10-40 mg/d	Dose: 20-80 mg/d		Heterozygous familial hypercholesterolemia Initiated at 20 mg/d for ≥20% LDL reduction; may be titrated at ≥4 wk intervals. Doses >20 mg/d should be carefully considered with severe renal impairment (CrCl < 30 mL/min).
Pitavastatin	Dose: Not currently available. Pediatric safety and efficacy not established. Not FDA approved for use in children	Dose: 1-4 mg/d		Heterozygous familial hypercholesterolemia Initiate at 1 mg/d and maximum of 2 mg/d in moderate renal impairment (CrCl 30<60 mL/min) or end-stage renal disease on hemodialysis.
Pravastatin	Age 8-13: 20 mg/d Age 14-18: 40 mg/d Dose: 20-40 mg/d	Dose: 10-40 mg/d		Heterozygous familial hypercholesterolemia Use with caution in patients with renal and hepatic impairment; contraindicated in active liver disease
Rosuvastatin	Age 10-17 Dose: 5-20 mg/d	Dose: 10-40 mg/d		Heterozygous familial hypercholesterolemia May be titrated at ≥4 wk intervals. Used with caution in renal insufficiency; contraindicated in active liver disease
Simvastatin	Age 10-17 Dose: 10-40 mg/d	Dose: 10-40 mg/d		Heterozygous familial hypercholesterolemia May be titrated at ≥4 wk intervals. Used with caution in patients with renal insufficiency. The FDA is recommending limiting the use of simvastatin (80 mg) because of increased risk of muscle damage. Simvastatin 80 mg should be used only in patients who have been taking this dose for 12 mo or more without evidence of muscle injury (myopathy).
Cholesterol Absorption Inhibitors				
Ezetimibe	Age ≥10 Dose: 10 mg/d	Dose: 10 mg/d	Increased transaminases in combination with statins	Homozygous familial hypercholesterolemia Sitosterolemia No dosage adjustment for renal impairment or mild hepatic impairment. Avoid use with moderate to severe hepatic impairment. Although not approved, it has been shown to be effective and safe for cholesterol lowering in children in a small study.

Adapted from Miller ML, Wright CC, Browne B. Lipid-lowering medications for children and adolescents. *J Clin Lipidol*. 2015;9(5 suppl):S67-S76; Expert Panel on Integrated Guidelines for Cardiovascular Health and Risk Reduction in Children and Adolescents, National Heart, Lung, and Blood Institute. Expert panel on integrated guidelines for cardiovascular health and risk reduction in children and adolescents: summary report. *Pediatrics*. 2011;128(suppl 5):S213-S256; Gidding SS, Ann Champagne M, de Ferranti SD, et al. The agenda for familial hypercholesterolemia: a scientific statement from the American Heart Association. *Circulation*. 2015;132(22):2167-2192.

Table 14.8. Medications for Primarily Lowering Cholesterol

Medication	Pediatric Dosing	Adult Dosing	Side Effects	Indication/Comments
Bile Acid Sequestrants				
Colesevelam	Age 10-17 Dose: 1.875 g twice daily or 3.75 g daily. Can be administered as an oral suspension or tabs	Dose: 1.875 g twice daily or 3.75 g daily	Nausea, bloating, cramping, and constipation; elevations in hepatic transaminases and alkaline phosphatase. Impaired absorption of fat-soluble vitamins and coadministered medications. Interaction can be minimized by taking other medications at least 1 h before or 4 h after bile acid sequestrant.	Heterozygous familial hypercholesterolemia May be used as monotherapy or in combination with a statin. No dosage adjustment for renal or hepatic impairment
Colestipol	Age 7-12 Dose: Pediatric safety and efficacy not established. Not FDA approved for use in children. If used, suggested dose 5 g twice daily, 10 g daily, or 125-500 mg/kg/d Age ≥12 Ped dose: Pediatric safety and efficacy not established. Not FDA approved for use in children. If used, suggested dose 10-15 g/d	Dose: Tabs: 2-16 g/d Granules: 5-30 g/d Dose: Tabs: 2-16 g/d Granules: 5-30 g/d		Primary hypercholesterolemia Tabs: 2 g daily or every 12 h; increase of 2 g at 1-2 mo intervals Granules: 5 g daily; increase of 5 g at 1-2 mo intervals (max 30 g/d)
Cholestyramine	Age 6-12 Dose: Pediatric safety and efficacy not established. Not FDA approved for use in children. If used, suggested dose 240 mg/kg/d divided three times daily before meals Age ≥12 Dose: Pediatric safety and efficacy not established. Not FDA approved for use in children. If used, suggested dose 8 g/d divided twice daily before meals	Dose: 4-24 g daily Dose: 4-24 g daily		Hypercholesterolemia Initiate at 2-4 g twice daily

Adapted from Miller ML, Wright CC, Browne B. Lipid-lowering medications for children and adolescents. *J Clin Lipidol.* 2015;9(5 suppl):S67-S76; Gidding SS, Ann Champagne M, de Ferranti SD, et al. The agenda for familial hypercholesterolemia: a scientific statement from the American Heart Association. *Circulation.* 2015;132(22):2167-2192.

Table 14.9. Medications for Primarily Lowering Triglycerides

Medication	Pediatric Dosing	Adult Dosing	Side Effects	Indication/Comments
Fibric Acid Derivatives				
Fenofibrate (many generic preparations available)	Dose: Pediatric safety and efficacy not established. Not FDA approved for use in children	Dose: Product specific Generally employ full dose in the setting of normal renal function	Skin rash, gastrointestinal (nausea, bloating, cramping) myalgia; lowers blood cyclosporine levels; potentially nephrotoxic in cyclosporine-treated patients. Avoid in patients with CrCl < 30 mL/min.	Hypertriglyceridemia Monitor renal function; avoid in the presence of severe renal function. Regular monitoring of liver function test is required. Discontinue if persistent elevation of LFTs >3X ULN.
Gemfibrozil (Lopid)	Dose: Pediatric safety and efficacy not established. Not FDA approved for use in children	Dose: 1200 mg po daily, divided bid, 30 min before breakfast and dinner	Potentiates warfarin action. Absorption of gemfibrozil diminished by bile acid sequestrants	Hypertriglyceridemia Use with caution in patients with renal impairment; contraindicated with severe renal impairment; use contraindicated with hepatic impairment. Avoid with concurrent statin therapy.

Table 14.9.	Medications for Primarily Lowering Triglycerides (*Continued*)				
Medication	**Pediatric Dosing**	**Adult Dosing**	**Side Effects**	**Indication/Comments**	
Nicotinic Acid					
Niacin (multiple preparations available)	Age ≥10 Dose: Pediatric safety and efficacy not established. Not FDA approved for use in children. If used, suggested dose. Initial: 100-250 mg/d (max: 10 mg/kg/d) divided 3 times daily with meals	Dose: Slowly titrate to max dose of intermediate-release niacin (3 g/d) or slow-release niacin (2 g/d)	Prostaglandin-mediated cutaneous flushing, headache, warm sensation, and pruritus; dry skin; nausea; vomiting; diarrhea; and myositis	Adjunct therapy to reduce high TG For pediatric dosing may titrate weekly by 100 mg/d or every 2-3 wk by 250 mg/d. No dosing adjustment has been provided by the manufacturer for renal or hepatic impairment. Contraindicated in the presence of significant unexplained hepatic dysfunction, active liver disease, or unexplained persistent LFT elevation.	
Omega-3 Fatty Acids					
Ethyl esters (Lovaza)	Dose: Pediatric safety and efficacy not established. Not FDA approved for use in children	Dose: 2-4 g EPA + DHA daily, divided bid	Eructation, dyspepsia. Diarrhea (7%-15%) most commonly reported. May enhance anticoagulant and antiplatelet effects of other medications	Adjunct therapy to reduce high TG No dosage adjustments required for impaired renal or hepatic function. Periodic monitoring of ALT and AST is recommended for patients with hepatic impairment.	
Icosapent (Vascepa)	Dose: Pediatric safety and efficacy not established. Not FDA approved for use in children.	Dose: 2-4 g EPA daily, divided bid	Arthralgia, oropharyngeal pain		

Renal insufficiency is indicated by a creatinine clearance of <30 mL/min; agents known to decrease HMG-CoA−reductase inhibitor clearance include grapefruit juice, gemfibrozil, ritonavir, cyclosporine, danazol, amiodarone, azole antifungals, macrolide antibiotics, and verapamil.
(Adapted from Miller ML, Wright CC, Browne B. Lipid-lowering medications for children and adolescents. *J Clin Lipidol.* 2015;9(5 suppl):S67-S76; Expert Panel on Integrated Guidelines for Cardiovascular Health and Risk Reduction in Children and Adolescents, National Heart, Lung, and Blood Institute. Expert panel on integrated guidelines for cardiovascular health and risk reduction in children and adolescents: summary report. *Pediatrics.* 2011;128(suppl 5):S213-S256; Gidding SS, Ann Champagne M, de Ferranti SD, et al. The agenda for familial hypercholesterolemia: a scientific statement from the American Heart Association. *Circulation.* 2015;132(22):2167-2192.)

V. STEP 4: Identify MetS and, if Persistent, Treat After 3-6 months of TLC

A. Clinical identification of the MetS

1. In adults, the presence of the MetS is associated with a fivefold increased risk of developing T2D and a threefold increased risk of developing ASCVD. The importance of diagnosing MetS in the pediatric population is less certain since considerable flux in the individual MetS components may occur over time. Nonetheless, children with components of the MetS are considered to be at increased risk.

2. Overweight and obesity are associated with insulin resistance and the MetS. However, the presence of abdominal obesity is more highly correlated with the syndrome criteria than is an elevated BMI. Therefore, the simple measure of waist circumference is recommended to identify the body weight component of the MetS. Some male patients can develop multiple metabolic risk factors when the waist circumference is only marginally increased, for example, 94-102 cm (37-39 in.). Such patients may have a strong genetic contribution to insulin resistance. They should benefit from changes in lifestyle habits, similarly to males with categorical increases in waist circumference. Asians have a lower waist circumference threshold for association with cardiometabolic risk.

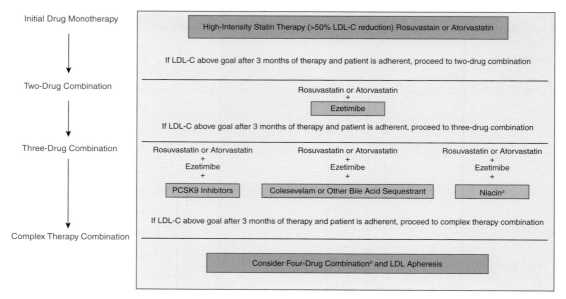

Initial Drug Monotherapy

High-Intensity Statin Therapy (>50% LDL-C reduction) Rosuvastain or Atorvastatin

If LDL-C above goal after 3 months of therapy and patient is adherent, proceed to two-drug combination

Two-Drug Combination

Rosuvastatin or Atorvastatin
+
Ezetimibe

If LDL-C above goal after 3 months of therapy and patient is adherent, proceed to three-drug combination

Three-Drug Combination

| Rosuvastatin or Atorvastatin
+
Ezetimibe
+
PCSK9 Inhibitors | Rosuvastatin or Atorvastatin
+
Ezetimibe
+
Colesevelam or Other Bile Acid Sequestrant | Rosuvastatin or Atorvastatin
+
Ezetimibe
+
Niacin[a] |

If LDL-C above goal after 3 months of therapy and patient is adherent, proceed to complex therapy combination

Complex Therapy Combination

Consider Four-Drug Combination[b] and LDL Apheresis

FIGURE 14.2: Preferred pharmacotherapy algorithm for adults with heterozygous familial hypercholesterolemia. The decision to use a third-line agent must take into account multiple factors, including disease severity, patient preference, cost, and outcomes data if available. Future research on PCSK9 inhibitors and other new agents will also inform the choice of a third agent, particularly in the context of statin intolerance. HoFH indicates homozygous familial hypercholesterolemia; LDL, low-density lipoprotein; LDL-C, low-density lipoprotein cholesterol; and PCSK9, proprotein convertase subtulisin/kexin type 9. [a]Prescription niacin preferred. [b]Consider lomitapide or mipomersen in HoFH subjects. (Reprinted with permission from Gidding SS, Ann Champagne M, de Ferranti SD, et al. The agenda for familial hypercholesterolemia: a scientific statement from the American Heart Association. *Circulation.* 2015;132(22):2167-2192.)

B. Treatment of the MetS

1. **Obesity:** Decrease total calories as part of weight management using multicomponent interventions.

2. **Lipids:** Manage atherogenic dyslipidemia according to TG, HDL-C, and non–HDL-C levels and cut points.

3. **Glucose intolerance:** Manage elevations in fasting glucose according to cut points for prediabetes and diabetes.

4. **Blood pressure elevations:** Manage hypertension according to percentile-based guidelines.

5. **Lifestyle behaviors:** Diet, exercise, and smoking status should be assessed before recommending changes and/or referral for medical nutrition treatment (MNT) by qualified professionals.

6. **Treat lipid and nonlipid risk factors if they persist despite lifestyle therapies.**
   a. Treat hypertension, if present.
   b. Smoking avoidance/cessation, including use of e-cigarettes.
   c. Consider treating elevated TG and/or low HDL-C (see below).

VI. STEP 5. Treat Elevated TG

Elevated levels of TG are commonly encountered in clinical practice. Very high levels of TG (>1000 mg/dL) are usually genetic and may increase the risk of gallstones and pancreatitis, while moderate-to-high levels (<1000 mg/dL) are often associated with

Table 14.10.	Classification of Triglyceride Levels
Classification	**Range (mg/dL)**
Acceptable	<110
Borderline	110-149
Mild	150-249
Moderate	250-499
High	500-999
Severe	1000-1999
Very severe	≥2000

(Adapted with permission from Shah AS, Wilson DP. Primary hypertriglyceridemia in children and adolescents. *J Clin Lipidol*. 2015;9(5 suppl):S20-S28.)

lower levels of HDL-C and higher non–HDL-C levels, increasing the risk of premature ASCVD. While this atherogenic dyslipidemia pattern occurs most frequently in youth who are obese and insulin resistant, concomitant polygenic mutations that alter lipid metabolism are common. As noted, those with severe elevation of TG (>1000 mg/dL) are likely to have a monogenic cause. Because the severe hypertriglyceridemia in monogenic hypertriglyceridemia, such as lipoprotein lipase deficiency, is the result of failure to clear dietary-derived chylomicrons, standard lipid-lowering therapies, such as omega-3 fatty acids, niacin, and fibrates, are generally ineffective. Successful management requires life-long restriction of dietary fat while assuring adequate intake of essential fatty acids and fat-soluble vitamins. Hyperchylomicronemia, an additional genetic cause of very high TG levels, is discussed below.

A. **Classification of serum TGs (mg/dL)**

    1. Table 14.10 provides a clinically useful classification of hypertriglyceridemia, based upon the TG level.

B. **Treatment of hypertriglyceridemia**

    1. An algorithm for treatment of hypertriglyceridemia can be found in Table 14.11.

Table 14.11.	Algorithm for Treatment of Hypertriglyceridemia			
TG (mg/dL) Level	**Acceptable-Borderline** <150	**Mild-Moderate** 150-499	**High** 500-999	**Severe-Very Severe** ≥1000
Objective	Health Maintenance	CVD Risk Prevention	Avoid Pancreatitis	
Target/Goal	TG < 150	Non–HDL-C < 130	TGs < 500, ideally <150	
Diet				
Fat[a]	25%-30%	25%-30%	15%-30%	<10%-15%
CHO[a]	55%-60%	Avoid excessive consumption		
Physical Activity	60 min of moderate to vigorous physical activity a day			
TG-Lowering Therapy	None	Consider statin as 1st-line therapy	[b]Consider Fibrate; O3FA[c]; niacin	Usually ineffective

[a]% of daily kcal/estimated energy requirements per day for age/gender.
[b]Not FDA approved for use in children.
[c]O3FA, omega-3 fatty acid.

C. **Treatment of low HDL-C (<40 mg/dL)** HDL-C has been inversely associated with risk of CVD but is currently not a target of treatment in either adults or children since evidence from clinical trials has not been supportive. Other than lifestyle changes, there are no drugs recommended to raise HDL-C that have been shown to have beneficial in clinical outcomes studies. While niacin has been shown to raise HDL-C, it is not FDA approved for use in children and there are no long-term studies in children demonstrating its efficacy and safety. Forevermore, the frequent side effects that are associated with niacin, such as flushing and pruritis, limit compliance. Functional assays of HDL-C activity are not clinically available. It appears clear, however, that the function of the HDL particle is more important than the level of cholesterol content of the HDL particle, and it is unclear if existing medications improve functionality. Lifestyle changes, especially when associated with TLC, TG lowering, and smoking avoidance/ cessation, often raise HDL-C and may restore HDL composition and function to normal.

1. First reach non–HDL-C and LDL-C goals.

2. Intensify TLC, that is, weight management and increase physical activity.

3. If TG are 150-499 mg/dL, the therapeutic goal is prevention of premature ASCVD by achieving the non–HDL-C goal.

4. Currently, there are drugs to increase HDL-C that have been shown to reduce future ASCVD in the adult population.

5. The primary treatment for isolated low HDL-C is with lifestyle changes intended to decrease insulin resistance and lower TG.

D. **Treatment of familial chylomicronemia syndrome (FCS)**

1. Familial chylomicronemia syndrome (FCS) is an inherited disorder characterized by severe hypertriglyceridemia, with levels generally >1000 mg/dL. Differentiating FCS from hypertriglyceridemia due to causes discussed above is often based on the absence or suboptimal response to TG-lowering medications.

2. Standard lipid-lowering therapies, such as omega-3 fatty acids, niacin, and fibrates, are generally ineffective.

3. TG may be substantially lowered by restricting dietary fat to <15% of the total daily caloric intake (Table 14.12).

4. If TG are not lowered to goal, further dietary fat restriction may be necessary while ensuring daily essential fat intake.

5. Goal: 10%-15% calories from fat, 60% calories from complex carbohydrates, and 25%-30% calories from protein while avoiding concentrated carbohydrates.

6. If dietary fat is limited to essential fatty acids, supplemental medium-chain TG (MCT), oil-containing fatty acids of 8-12 carbon atoms in length, should be considered to improve macronutrient balance while providing additional fat and calories (Table 14.13). MCTs are directly metabolized by the liver and do not contribute to triglyceride levels.

7. Adequate intake of linoleic acid, alpha linolenic acid and fat-soluble vitamins (A, D, E, and K) should be monitored. Supplement as needed.

Table 14.12.	Formula Comparison Chart					
Formula Manufacturer (kcal/mL)	**Grams/100 mL (% kcals)**			**% Fat as MCT**	**Source**	**Comments**
	CHO	**Fat**	**Protein**			
Recommended						
Monogen Nutricia (22 kcal/30 mL)	11.9 (64)	1.9 (24)	2.2 (12)	80%	CHO—corn syrup solids FAT—fractionated coconut oil, walnut oil PRO—whey protein concentrate (milk, soy lecithin), free amino acids	• Approved for children over 1 y of age • Ratio of essential fatty acids: N6:n3 ratio of 6.2:1 • Provides recommended intake of vitamins and minerals, including trace elements • Available in powder only • Beneficial for FCS due to high MCT concentration with adequate LCT to meet essential fat needs
Enfaport Mead Johnson (30 kcal/30 mL)	10.2 (40)	5.6 (460)	3.6 (14)	84%	CHO—corn syrup solids FAT—MCT and soy oils, DHA, ARA PRO—calcium and sodium caseinates (from milk)	• Approved for infants • Ratio of essential fatty acids: N6:n3 ratio of 2:1 • Nutritionally complete at 30 kcal/30 mL. Can be diluted to desired concentration • Available in ready-to-feed only • Must ensure that formula provides adequate LCTs to meet essential fat needs
Recommended with Modification						
Human milk, term (20 kcal/30 mL)	8 (47)	3.5 (47)	0.9 (5)	Varies	CHO—lactose FAT—human milk PRO—human milk–whey predominate	• Nutrient content varies among women. • Not recommended for FCS unless skimmed and fortified to meet essential fat and MCT needs
Not Recommended						
Portagen Mead Johnson (30 kcal/30 mL)	11.5 (46)	4.8 (40)	3.5 (14)	87%	CHO—corn syrup solids, sugar FAT—MCT and corn oils PRO—sodium caseinate	• Not recommended for infants • Not nutritionally complete. Essential fatty acid and micronutrient supplementation recommended with long-term use • Not recommended as sole nutrition for FCS as it is not nutritionally complete
Similac Advance Abbott nutrition (19 kcal/30 mL)	6.9 (42)	3.6 (50)	1.3 (8)	Unk	CHO—lactose, galactooligosaccharides (GOS) FAT—high oleic safflower, soy and coconut oils, DHA, ARA PRO—nonfat milk and whey protein concentrate	• Standard infant formula • Portion of fat from coconut oil, providing unknown MCT • Available in powder and ready-to-feed • Not recommended for FCS due to high fat and low MCT content

Reprinted with permission from Williams L, Wilson DP. Editorial commentary: dietary management of familial chylomicronemia syndrome. *J Clin Lipidol*. 2016;10(3):462-465.

VII. Step 6: Assessing Response to Therapy and Monitoring

The goal of lipid lowering in individuals with moderate-to-high elevation of LDL-C and non–HDL-C is prevention of premature ASCVD and prevention of pancreatitis in those with high to severe elevations of TG. In general, pancreatitis can be avoided in those with chylomicronemia if the TG level is maintained below 2000 mg/dL. Levels of TG < 500 mg/dL may be necessary in those with acquired CVD risk factors, such as obesity and insulin resistance, and elevated non–HDL-C, to lower risk of both CVD and pancreatitis. Recommendations for monitoring and follow-up can be found in Table 14.14.

Table 14.13. Modular Additives: Fat

Liquid Products

Additives	Grams/100 mL (% kcals) CHO	Fat	Protein	Source	Comments
MCT oil	0	95 (100)	0	Modified palm kernel oil and/or coconut oil (MCTs)	• Nonemulsified. Must be bolus doses • Cannot be placed in plastic bottles or tubing
Liquigen Nutricia	0	50 (100)	0	Refined palm kernel and/or coconut oil	• Emulsified for improved mixing • Unflavored. Mixes well with many foods and beverages • Opened bottles may be stored in the refrigerator for 14 d.

Powder

Additive	Grams/100 g (% kcals) CHO	Fat	Protein	Source	Comments
MCT Procal	21 (12)	63 (80)	13 (8)	CHO—glucose syrup FAT—fractionated coconut oil PRO—sodium caseinates, whey protein concentrate	• 99% fat from MCT • Suitable from 1 y of age • Can be added to hot or cold food or beverages. Not suitable to mix with fruit juice • Not suitable for milk protein allergies or lactose intolerance • Open packets must be used within 24 h

Reprinted with permission from Williams L, Wilson DP. Editorial commentary: dietary management of familial chylomicronemia syndrome. *J Clin Lipidol*. 2016;10(3):462-465.

Table 14.14. Monitoring and Follow-Up

Drug Therapy	Baseline	First Year 1-1/2 mo	q3-4 mo	Second Year q6-12 mo	Targets
Laboratory Monitoring					
Lipid profile	X	X	X	X	Ideal LDL-C <110 mg/dL; minimal LDL-C <130 mg/dL
ALT[a]	X	X[b]	X[b]	X[b]	<3X ULN
AST[a]	X	X[b]	X[b]	X[b]	<3X ULN
CK	X	X[b]	X[b]	X[b]	<10 ULN
Physical Examination					
Height	X	—	X	X	Assess other risk factors regularly:
Weight	X	—	X	X	• Weight gain
BMI	X	—	X	X	• Smoking
BP	X	—	X	X	• Physical inactivity
Sexual maturation	X	—	X	X	
Medication Monitoring					
Compliance	X	X	X	X	Advise females about:
Tolerance	X	X	X	X	• Contraindication in pregnancy and breastfeeding • Need for appropriate contraception
Side effects	X	X	X	X	Advise females and males about: • Proper drug administration • Potential medication interactions

Comments:
[a]Elevated ALT/AST at baseline suggests the need to consider comorbid or concomitant liver disease (eg, NASH, LAL-D, etc.)
[b]Retest if symptomatic. If laboratory abnormalities are noted or symptoms are reported, temporarily withhold medication and repeat the blood work in 2 weeks. When the abnormalities resolve, the medication may be restarted with close monitoring.
ULN, upper limit of normal.

Acknowledgments

The authors would like to acknowledge Luke Hamilton, Dena Hanson, Lorrainea Williams and Lauren Williams for their assistance in preparing and editing this article.

Suggested Readings

American Academy of Pediatrics. *Bright Futures*. Updated 2016. Accessed March 17, 2016. Available at: https://brightfutures.aap.org

American Academy of Pediatrics. *Recommendations for Preventive Health Care*. Updated October 2015. Accessed March 17, 2016. Available at: https://www.aap.org/en-us/Documents/periodicity_schedule.pdf

American Diabetes Association. Standards of medical care in diabetes—2016. *Diabetes Care*. 2016;39(suppl 1):S1-S112.

Cohen JC, Boerwinkle E, Mosley TH Jr, Hobbs HH. Sequence variations in PCSK9, low LDL, and protection against coronary heart disease. *N Engl J Med*. 2006;354(12):1264-1272.

Dennison BA, Kikuchi DA, Srinivasan SR, Webber LS, Berenson GS. Parental history of cardiovascular disease as an indication for screening for lipoprotein abnormalities in children. *J Pediatr*. 1989;115(2):186-194.

Eckel RH, Jakicic JM, Ard JD, et al. 2013 AHA/ACC guideline on lifestyle management to reduce cardiovascular risk: a report of the American College of Cardiology/American Heart Association Task Force on Practice Guidelines. *J Am Coll Cardiol*. 2014;63(25 Pt B):2960-2984.

Expert Panel on Integrated Guidelines for Cardiovascular Health and Risk Reduction in Children and Adolescents, National Heart, Lung, and Blood Institute. Expert panel on integrated guidelines for cardiovascular health and risk reduction in children and adolescents: summary report. *Pediatrics*. 2011;128(suppl 5):S213-S256.

Familial Hypercholesterolemia Foundation. *Familial Hypercholesterolemia*. Accessed March 23, 2016. Available at: https://thefhfoundation.org/familial-hypercholesterolemia-2015/

Ference BA, Yoo W, Alesh I, et al. Effect of long-term exposure to lower low-density lipoprotein cholesterol beginning early in life on the risk of coronary heart disease: a Mendelian randomization analysis. *J Am Coll Cardiol*. 2012;60(25):2631-2639.

Foundation of the National Lipid Association. *Learn Your Lipids: Patient Information from the Foundation of the National Lipid Association*. Accessed March 23, 2016. Available at: http://www.learnyourlipids.com/

Freedman DS, Byers T, Sell K, Kuester S, Newell E, Lee S. Tracking of serum cholesterol levels in a multiracial sample of preschool children. *Pediatrics*. 1992;90(1 Pt 1):80-86.

Gidding SS, Champagne MA, de Ferranti SD, et al. The agenda for familial hypercholesterolemia: a scientific statement from the American Heart Association. *Circulation*. 2015;132(22):2167-2192.

Griffin TC, Christoffel KK, Binns HJ, McGuire PA. Family history evaluation as a predictive screen for childhood hypercholesterolemia. Pediatric Practice Research Group. *Pediatrics*. 1989;84(2):365-373.

Hegele RA. Plasma lipoproteins: genetic influences and clinical implications. *Nat Rev Genet*. 2009;10(2):109-121.

Hoelscher DM, Kirk S, Ritchie L, Cunningham-Sabo L; Academy Positions Committee. Position of the Academy of Nutrition and Dietetics: Interventions for the prevention and treatment of pediatric overweight and obesity. *J Acad Nutr Diet*. 2013;113(10):1375-1394.

Hopkins PN, Toth PP, Ballantyne CM, Rader DJ; National Lipid Association Expert Panel on Familial Hypercholesterolemia. Familial hypercholesterolemias: prevalence, genetics, diagnosis and screening recommendations from the National Lipid Association Expert Panel on Familial Hypercholesterolemia. *J Clin Lipidol*. 2011;5(3 suppl):S9-S17.

Jacobson TA, Maki KC, Orringer CE, et al. National Lipid Association recommendations for patient-centered management of dyslipidemia: part 2. *J Clin Lipidol*. 2015;9(6 suppl):S1-S122.e1.

Leren TP, Finborud TH, Manshaus TE, Ose L, Berge KE. Diagnosis of familial hypercholesterolemia in general practice using clinical diagnostic criteria or genetic testing as part of cascade genetic screening. *Community Genet*. 2008;11(1):26-35.

Marks D, Wonderling D, Thorogood M, Lambert H, Humphries SE, Neil HA. Cost effectiveness analysis of different approaches of screening for familial hypercholesterolaemia. *BMJ*. 2002;324(7349):1303.

McCrindle BW, Urbina EM, Dennison BA, et al. Drug therapy of high-risk lipid abnormalities in children and adolescents: a scientific statement from the American Heart Association Atherosclerosis, Hypertension, and Obesity in Youth Committee, Council of Cardiovascular Disease in the Young, with the Council on Cardiovascular Nursing. *Circulation*. 2007;115(14):1948-1967.

Miller ML, Wright CC, Browne B. Lipid-lowering medications for children and adolescents. *J Clin Lipidol*. 2015;9(5 suppl):S67-S76.

National Heart, Lung, and Blood Institute. *Integrated Guidelines for Cardiovascular Health and Risk Reduction in Children and Adolescents*. Updated January 2013. Accessed March 22, 2016. Available at: http://www.nhlbi.nih.gov/health-pro/guidelines/current/cardiovascular-health-pediatric-guidelines

National Institutes of Health. *Fact Sheet: Point-of-Care Diagnostic Testing*. Updated October 2010. Accessed March 23, 2016. Available at: https://report.nih.gov/nihfactsheets/Pdfs/PointofCareDiagnosticTesting(NIBIB).pdf

Naughton MJ, Luepker RV, Strickland D. The accuracy of portable cholesterol analyzers in public screening programs. *JAMA*. 1990;263(9):1213-1217.

Shah AS, Wilson DP. Primary hypertriglyceridemia in children and adolescents. *J Clin Lipidol*. 2015;9(5 suppl):S20-S28.

Starr B, Hadfield SG, Hutten BA, et al. Development of sensitive and specific age- and gender-specific low-density lipoprotein cholesterol cutoffs for diagnosis of first-degree relatives with familial hypercholesterolaemia in cascade testing. *Clin Chem Lab Med*. 2008;46(6):791-803.

Stone NJ, Robinson JG, Lichtenstein AH, et al. 2013 ACC/AHA guideline on the treatment of blood cholesterol to reduce atherosclerotic cardiovascular risk in adults: a report of the American College of Cardiology/American Heart Association Task Force on Practice Guidelines. *J Am Coll Cardiol*. 2014;63(25 Pt B):2889-2934.

Whitehead SJ, Ford C, Gama R. A combined laboratory and field evaluation of the Cholestech LDX and CardioChek PA point-of-care testing lipid and glucose analysers. *Ann Clin Biochem*. 2014;51(Pt 1):54-67.

Williams RR, Hunt SC, Schumacher MC, et al. Diagnosing heterozygous familial hypercholesterolemia using new practical criteria validated by molecular genetics. *Am J Cardiol*. 1993;72(2):171-176.

Williams L, Wilson DP. Editorial commentary: dietary management of familial chylomicronemia syndrome. *J Clin Lipidol*. 2016;10(3):462-465.

Zimmet P, Alberti G, Kaufman F, et al. The metabolic syndrome in children and adolescents. *Lancet*. 2007;369(9579):2059-2061.

Lipid Management in Special Populations

Diagnosis and Management of Dyslipidemia in Human Immunodeficiency Virus

Merle Myerson

> ### Key Points
>
> - Antiretroviral therapy has changed HIV from a fatal disease to a chronic disease where extended and productive life spans are possible.
> - People living with HIV are at increased risk for cardiovascular disease due in part to the HIV itself, use of ART, and people living to an age where cardiovascular disease is more prevalent.
> - HIV produces metabolic abnormalities including dyslipidemia that are exacerbated by ART; however, newer medications have fewer of these effects.
> - Diagnosis and management of dyslipidemia for patients living with HIV are needed to help prevent manifest cardiovascular disease.
> - There are no comprehensive guidelines for treatment of dyslipidemia in this population. Existing guidelines for the general population are currently used with modification for use with patients living with HIV.
> - The National Lipid Association Recommendations for Patient-Centered Management of Dyslipidemia Part 2 state that risk stratification be assessed as for the general population with HIV infection considered as an additional risk factor.
> - The LDL-C and non–HDL-C goals described in NLA Part 1. Recommendations should be followed for HIV-infected patients.

I. Introduction

A. There is no cure for HIV and most of those who became infected did not live. In 1987, the FDA approved the first antiretroviral drug (ART), zidovudine. This began a new era for those infected with HIV. Opportunistic infections and death were no longer inevitable, and longer and productive life spans were possible. HIV has become a chronic disease.

B. With the advent of ART also came a new spectrum of diseases for patients living with HIV. These included diseases related to the metabolic changes brought about by the virus itself, side effects of ART, and people infected with HIV living to ages where other diseases, such as cardiovascular disease (CVD), were more prevalent.

C. Epidemiologic studies have shown that people infected with HIV have an increased risk of CVD at all ages compared to the general population, which remains even after control of traditional risk factors.[1] This population also has higher rates of smoking, behavioral, and social factors that increase risk.[2] It is anticipated that CVD will be the leading cause of morbidity and mortality in this patient population making diagnosis and management of CVD risk factors, in particular dyslipidemia, essential to patient care. It is important to note that this need is not yet universal as access to the more basic needs of diagnosis and treatment with ART remain limited in areas such as Sub-Saharan Africa and many parts of Asia.

D. Currently, there are no specific and comprehensive cardiovascular disease guidelines or risk stratification schemes for management of dyslipidemia in patients infected with HIV, but existing recommendations as well as those for the general population are discussed here with suggestions as to how they may be applied to this patient population.

II. HIV and Risk for Cardiovascular Disease

A. Infection with HIV produces a cardiometabolic syndrome consisting of insulin resistance, lipodystrophy (fat maldistribution including increase in abdominal visceral fat), and abnormal lipids (elevated triglycerides and low HDL-C). Therapy with ART exacerbates these abnormalities. The mechanisms of these metabolic abnormalities are complex and interdependent with the impaired glucose metabolism and dyslipidemia due in part to abnormal fat distribution (especially abdominal fat) and inflammation.[3–5]

B. The role of inflammation in the pathogenesis of atherosclerosis is well known in the general population and is felt to play a significant and unique role in the development cardiovascular disease and increased risk in patients infected with HIV. In the Strategies for Management of Antiretroviral Therapy (SMART) study, patients with CD4 cell counts >350 cells/mm[3] were randomized to either continuous or intermittent antiretroviral therapy. The trial was stopped early as those in the intermittent group had greater opportunistic disease, death from any cause, and major cardiovascular disease.[6] Follow-up analysis of stored samples from the SMART study showed that inflammatory and coagulation biomarkers, IL-6, and D-dimer levels were significantly increased in the intermittent compared to the continuous therapy group and that these levels were strongly related to all-cause mortality.[7] It was hypothesized that therapies that reduce the inflammation response to HIV may be relevant to care for patients infected with HIV.[7]

C. More research is needed to better define the role of inflammation in HIV and how this influences risk for CVD. The NIH has initiated the REPRIEVE study, a multicenter, prospective, randomized clinical trial of HIV-infected individuals who are at low risk according to the 2013 ACC/AHA Guideline on the Treatment of Blood Cholesterol to Reduce Atherosclerotic Cardiovascular Risk in Adults.[8] Participants will be randomized to either statin therapy (pitavastatin) or placebo and followed to investigate how statins may reduce the risk for CVD through non–LDL-lowering benefits including anti-inflammatory properties. The study is sponsored by the National Heart, Lung, and Blood Institute and collaboration with the National Institute of Allergy and Infectious Diseases.

III. Antiretroviral Therapy

A. At the present time, there is no cure for HIV. The ART provide viral suppression, but not elimination of the virus, and allow the body to maintain higher CD4 counts and better immune function. The virus can still be transmitted while on ART. The various classes of ART prevent viral replication in different ways and are used in combination. Newer drugs with higher potency, lower toxicity, better dosing, and fewer side effects now exist facilitating early and long-term treatment.

B. Treatment progress is monitored by measuring CD4 count and viral load. CD4 counts of ≥300 cells/µL were found to be associated with good immune function.[9] Healthy persons who are not infected with HIV generally have CD4 counts in the 800-1200 cells/µL. Viral suppression is achieved when plasma RNA levels are below detectable limits.[10]

C. There are various classes of ART, each interfering with a different step in the replication of the virus. These include entry inhibitors, fusion inhibitors, nucleoside/nucleotide reverse transcriptase inhibitors (NRTI), nonnucleoside reverse transcriptase inhibitors (NNRTI), integrase inhibitors, and protease inhibitors (PI). Combination regimens are standard.

D. As noted previously, infection with HIV confers metabolic changes that may be exacerbated by ART. Protease inhibitors are the agents that produce the most adverse effects, but nucleoside reverse transcriptase inhibitors and nonnucleoside/nucleotide reverse transcriptase inhibitors also influence lipids.

E. Lipid changes with HIV infection and ART Acute infection lowers LDL-C, but levels may return to baseline after virologic suppression with ART. Chronically, there is often a pattern of low HDL and elevated TG that results from the metabolic perturbances (insulin resistance, central adiposity, low HDL, and high TG) clustered in these patients and often worsened by specific antiretrovirals, many of which are now less commonly prescribed. The magnitude of these changes is also reflective of ethnicity, race, gender, lifestyle factors, and genomic traits. As noted above, the PI and the NNRTI are the ART that most significantly influence lipid levels. Tables 15a.1 and 15a.2 provide detail on the changes that are seen with use of medications in each of these classes of ART.[11–13]

Table 15a.1. Lipid Changes Associated with Protease Inhibitor Use

Protease Inhibitor	Total Cholesterol	HDL-C	Lipids LDL-C	Triglycerides
Atazanavir	↔	↔	↔ by 16%	↓ by 12%
Atazanavir + ritonavir and atazanavir/cobicistat	↔	↔	↑	↑
Darunavir+ritonavir	↔	↔	↑	↑
Fosamprenavir + ritonavir	↑↑	↔	↑	↑↑
Lopinavir/ritonavir (coformulated)	↑↑ (additional increase over ritonavir alone)	↔ no change	↑ no additional increase over ritonavir alone	↑↑ no additional increase over ritonavir alone
Nelfinavir	↑	↔	↑↑	↑
Ritonavir (low dose for boosting)	↑ by 10%	↓ by 5%	↑ by 16%	↑↑ by 26%
Saquinavir + ritonavir	↑↑	↔	↑	↑
Tipranavir + ritonavir	↑↑	Not known	Not known	↑↑↑

Key:
↑, some increase; ↑↑, moderate increase; ↑↑↑, large increase; ↓, some decrease; ↔, no significant change; HDL-C, high-density lipoprotein cholesterol; LDL-C, low-density lipoprotein cholesterol.
(Adapted from Malvestutto CD, Aberg JA. Coronary heart disease in people infected with HIV. *Cleve Clin J Med*. 2010;77:547-556.)

Table 15a.2.	Lipid Changes Associated with Nonnucleoside Reverse Transcriptase Inhibitor Use			
	Lipids			
NNRTI	**Total Cholesterol**	**HDL-C**	**LDL-C**	**Triglycerides**
Efavirenz	↑	↑	↑	↑
Etravirine	↔	↔	↔	↔
Nevirapine	↑	↑↑ (larger increase with efavirenz)	↑	↑ (lower increase than with efavirenz)
Rilpivirine	↑	Not known	↑ (lower increase than with efavirenz)	↑ (lower increase than with efavirenz)

Key:
↑, some increase; ↑↑, moderate increase; ↑↑↑, large increase; ↓, some decrease; ↔, no significant change; HDL-C, high-density lipoprotein cholesterol; LDL-C, low-density lipoprotein cholesterol.
(Adapted from Malvestutto CD, Aberg JA. Coronary heart disease in people infected with HIV. *Cleve Clin J Med.* 2010;77:547-556.)

IV. Guidelines for the Management of Dyslipidemia in Patients Infected With HIV

A. Guidelines There are currently no comprehensive and specific guidelines for risk stratification and the diagnosis and management of dyslipidemia in patients infected with HIV. In 2003, The HIV Medical Association (HIVMA) of the Infectious Disease Society of American (IDSA) and AIDS Clinical Trials Group (ACTG)[14] recommended using NCEP ATP III, as did the 2013 HIVMA IDSA Primary Care Guidelines.[15] The National Lipid Association Recommendations for Patient-Centered Management of Dyslipidemia, Part 2 includes a section for patients infected with HIV.[16]

B. Risk stratification and scores

1. No validated risk score or stratification scheme currently exists for patients infected with HIV although two groups have proposed scoring systems. The Data Collection on Adverse Effects of Anti-HIV Drugs (D:A:D) study group has developed a risk calculator that includes both traditional risk factors and exposure to individual antiretroviral drugs.[17] The Veterans Aging Cohort Study (VACS) was used to develop the "VACS Index" to predict overall mortality. The index includes age, CD4 count, viral load, hemoglobin, aspartate and alanine transaminase, platelets, creatinine, and hepatitis C status. The VACS Index has been used in studies predicting CHD risk but has not been validated for this use.[18]

2. Use of Framingham Risk Score, although not validated in patients with HIV is endorsed by HIVMA of the IDSA[14] and the European AIDS Clinical Society (EACS)[19]; however, it is unclear if Framingham, the ACC/AHA Pooled Cohort Equations, and other risk scores are appropriate for this patient population.

3. Measures of subclinical atherosclerosis including coronary artery calcium, high-sensitive C-reactive protein (CRP), and ultrasound measure of carotid intima-media thickness (CIMT) have been studied in small numbers of patients with HIV.[20,21] In the Multicenter AIDS Cohort Study (MACS), participants who were infected with HIV and underwent coronary CT angiography had a greater prevalence of coronary artery calcium, of any plaque, and noncalcified plaque compared to participants who were not infected.[22] At this time, there is not enough information to consider these measures for use in this patient population (Box 15a.1).

BOX 15a.1 | The NLA Recommendations for Patient-Centered Management of Dyslipidemia

- A fasting lipid panel should be obtained in all newly-identified HIV-infected patients before and after starting ART.
- Risk stratification should be based on number of major ASCVD risk factors, the use of risk prediction tools such as the ATP III Framingham Risk Score or the ACC/AHA Pooled Cohort Equations if two risk factors are present.

- The presence of HIV infection may be counted as an additional risk factor.

From Jacobson TA, Maki KC, Orringer CE, et al. National lipid association recommendations for patient-centered management of dyslipidemia: part 2. *J Clin Lipidol.* 2015;9 (6 suppl):S1.e121-S122.e121.

C. Lipid targets and goals for patients living with HIV

1. Patients infected with HIV currently have lipid targets and goals as those for the general population. Note that the 2013 ACC/AHA Guidelines do not address management for this patient population.

2. Residual risk:
   a. As discussed in Chapter 5, recent guidelines for management of dyslipidemia in the general population have introduced the concept of "residual risk." Low-density lipoprotein cholesterol is highly associated with CVD, but does not reflect the total amount of atherosclerotic particles, meaning all particles that have an apolipoprotein B (apoB) (very low density lipoprotein, intermediate density lipoprotein, LDL, and lipoprotein (a)). Measures of residual risk including non–HDL-C (total cholesterol minus HDL-C), apoB, or LDL particle number (LDL-P) better predict risk for CVD than LDL-C with apoB and LDL-P performing better than non–HDL-C.[23,24]
   b. Certain populations of patients such as those with diabetes are felt to have discordance between LDL-C and these other measures, which may result in under- or overtreatment.[25] Patients infected with HIV may also have a discordance between measures with LDL-C lower than LDL-P and apoB therefore underestimating risk and treatment targets.[26,27]
   c. Although measures of residual risk are being increasingly incorporated into diagnosis and management plans, LDL-C continues to be used in the general population and for patients infected with HIV.

V. Management of Dyslipidemia in Patients Infected With HIV

Chapter 5 outlines a step-by-step plan for diagnosis and management of dyslipidemia. This should be followed for patients infected with HIV but with certain modifications that are discussed below.

A. History and physical examination

1. History of lipid abnormalities prior to diagnosis of HIV, at time of diagnosis or after treatment with antiretrovirals

2. Diet history including who buys and prepares food, whether patient is institutionalized or living without a kitchen area

3. Cigarette smoking (personal history, living with people who smoke, exposure to second hand smoke)

4. Hormone history: menopausal status, use of oral contraceptives, hormone replacement therapy, testosterone therapy, and hormone therapy for gender reassignment

5. Medication history, including ART, psychiatric medications, hepatitis B or C medications, methadone, anabolic steroids, immunosuppression medications (cyclosporine), and selective estrogen receptor modulators (SERMs).

6. Substance use: illicit drugs and alcohol

B. Physical examination

1. Presence of lipohypertrophy and/or lipoatrophy

2. Measurement of waist circumference (to assist in making diagnosis of metabolic syndrome)

C. Laboratory evaluation

1. When to use measures of residual risk
   a. Practical considerations limit the use of apoB and LDL-P measurements as not all labs are equipped to measure these and insurance coverage for these measurements is not universal.
   b. Non–HDL-C is calculated from the basic lipid panel and is recommended as a measure of residual risk for patients infected with HIV with consideration for measurement of apolipoprotein B in selected patients.
   c. At present, there is no clear indication for measurement of hs-CRP or inflammatory factors.

D. Therapeutic lifestyle modification

Therapeutic lifestyle changes are advised for all patients regardless of their level of risk. Caring for patients living with HIV has many unique and challenging aspects. Access to healthy food choices and options for exercise and physical activity can be limited by availability, knowledge, or finances. Prevalence of smoking is higher than the general population as is alcohol and illicit drug use and addiction. To address this, more medical centers now have comprehensive HIV clinics with nutrition counselors and smoking cessation programs. Educational materials can be provided to patients that reflect language and cultural aspects of the local patient population.

VI. Medications

A. Statins

1. Many issues regarding statin use in patients infected with HIV are still unclear including metabolism and efficacy, not only for LDL-C lowering but also regarding their effect on CVD events and mortality in this population. The REPRIEVE study mentioned above is expected to provide information on statin use in this population. Table 15a.3 outlines statin and ART use.

2. Pravastatin was the main statin option for HIV-infected patients in early studies due to the favorable safety profile and limited interactions with ART. Rosuvastatin and atorvastatin are more potent statins and have been used in clinical trials.[28,29]

3. Pitavastatin is the newest FDA-approved statin although it had been used in Japan for many years. Pitavastatin has been studied in patients with HIV. The INTREPID study was a phase 4, multicenter randomized, double-blind, double-dummy superiority study comparing pitavastatin 4 mg to pravastatin 40 mg in adults 18-70 years of age on stable ART with viral load <200 copies/mL and CD4 count >200 cells/mm^3.

Table 15a.3. Interactions Between Antiretroviral Therapy and Statins

Statin	Antiretroviral Therapy Drug Class	
	Protease Inhibitor	**Nonnucleoside Reverse Transcriptase Inhibitor**
Atorvastatin	• AUC ↑↑ • Use lowest starting dose and titrate carefully. • Do not exceed 20 mg daily with DRV/r, FPV/r, SQV/r. • AUC ↑↑ 488% with LPV/r • ↑↑↑ 836% with TPV/r and should not be coadministered	• AUC ↓ 43% with efavirenz • ↔ but C_{max} ↓ 37% with etravirine • No data for nevirapine • May need higher starting dose with efavirenz and etravirine • No dose adjustments for rilpivirine
Fluvastatin	• Use not recommended with nelfinavir	• AUC ↑with etravirine • May require higher starting dose with etravirine
Lovastatin	• Contraindicated with all PIs (AUC ↑↑↑)	• AUC ↓↓with efavirenz. May require higher starting dose • No adjustment needed for rilpivirine
Pitavastatin	• Modest AUC ↑ with ATV/r (31%) • Modest ↓ AUC with DRV/r (20%-26%) and LPV/r (20%). No dose adjustment required	• ↔ with efavirenz and no dose adjustment needed • No dose adjustment needed for rilpivirine
Pravastatin	• ↓ AUC of except with DRV/r and LPV/r, which ↑ AUC by 81% and 33%, respectively. Use lowest possible starting dose.	• AUC ↓ 40% with efavirenz • ↔ with etravirine. May need higher starting dose
Rosuvastatin	• AUC ↑↑213% and C_{max} ↑↑↑ 600% with LPV/r • AUC ↑↑ 108% and C_{max} ↑↑↑ 366% with ATV/r • AUC ↑ 48% and C_{max} ↑ 139% with DRV/r. Do not exceed 10 mg daily. With DRV/r, use lowest necessary dose. • AUC ↔ and C_{max} ↑ 123% with TPV/r • ↔ with FPV/r. Titrate dose carefully with LPV/r or ATV/r	• Allowed. ↔. No reported interactions
Simvastatin	• Contraindicated with PIs (AUC ↑↑↑)	• AUC ↓ 58% with efavirenz and ↓with etravirine • No data for nevirapine. May require higher starting dose

Key:
↑, some increase; ↑↑, moderate increase; ↑↑↑, large increase; ↓, some decrease; ↔, no significant change; ATV/r, atazanavir/ritonavir; AUC, area under the concentration-time curve; C_{max}, maximum drug concentration; DRV/r, darunavir/ritonavir; FPV/r, fosamprenavir/ritonavir; LPV/r, lopinavir/ritonavir; SQV/r, saquinavir/ritonavir.
(Adapted from Malvestutto CD, Aberg JA. Coronary heart disease in people infected with HIV. *Cleve Clin J Med*. 2010;77:547-556.)

This study demonstrated that pitavastatin 4 mg was superior to pravastatin 40 mg in LDL-C and non–HDL-C reduction at 52 weeks in HIV-infected patients with dyslipidemia.[30] In a post-hoc analysis of the INTREPID trial, at 12 weeks, pitavastatin significantly reduced LDL-C (31.6%), apoB (23.8%), and non–HDL-C (26.8%) more than pravastatin in men ≥ 45 years old. In women ≥ 55 years old, pitavastatin also showed significant reductions in these measures (LDL-C 29.5%, apoB 20.4%, and non–HDL-C 29.1%), but this did not reach significance when compared to pravastatin due to small numbers.[31] In an additional analysis of the INTREPID study, there were no significant effects on glucose homeostasis.[31]

4. **Statin use with ART pharmacokinetic enhancers** Some of the ART may be administered with pharmacokinetic "enhancer" often referred to as "boosters." These drugs enhance the effectiveness of a medication. Ritonavir is a potent inhibitor of CYP3A and is primarily used as a pharmacokinetic enhancer for other protease inhibitors. Ritonavir should be used with caution in patients taking PI. Cobicistat is another potent CYP3A4 inhibitor and used as an enhancer for the integrase inhibitor elvitegravir. Since several statins also depend on CYP3A for metabolic clearance, the coadministration of cobicistat with simvastatin and lovastatin can result in markedly

elevated plasma levels of statins and is contraindicated. Atorvastatin can be used with cobicistat but must be started at the lowest dose (10 mg daily) and titrated up carefully while monitoring for safety.

5. **Treatment for patients coinfected with hepatitis C** As coinfection with hepatitis C (HCV) is common in HIV-infected patients, care should also be taken when HCV antiviral medication is used with statins.

6. **Other classes of ART** Prescribing statins with ART in other (non-PI) classes is generally safe as there are few if any significant drug interactions. The integrase inhibitor, elvitegravir, must be prescribed with cobicistat, which has interactions as noted above.

7. **Side effects of statin drugs** There are no specific guidelines for patients infected with HIV, but because patients are generally on other medications with potential side effects and interactions in addition to other comorbidities, caution is advised.
   a. Liver side effects. The ART influence liver function, and there is increased prevalence of hepatitis and alcohol abuse all of which can increase the risk for liver abnormalities.
   b. Muscle
      i. Muscle soreness, or "statin myopathy," is a frequent complaint by patients taking statin medications. Serum creatine kinase (CK) may or may not be elevated in those with symptoms. Rhabdomyolysis is an uncommon, but serious condition with marked elevations in CK and acute renal failure.
      ii. Baseline measurement and routine monitoring of CK are not advised for the general population unless a patient has renal dysfunction, complaints of muscle soreness, or other clinical indications. Patients infected with HIV often have other indications including medications, medical conditions, and substance abuse that can increase the risk of myopathy (alcohol, cocaine, opioids, ART, fibrates, infectious and immune disorders, hypothyroidism) and would merit monitoring in a patient, especially those with symptoms.[32] (See Box 15a.2.)

BOX 15a.2 Monitoring Muscle and CK Side Effects of Statins

Mild elevations in CK (≤3 times the upper limit of normal) in the absence of symptoms → continue statin therapy with monitoring.

- Higher CK (>3 times the upper limit of normal), symptoms, renal insufficiency, and dark-colored urine → stop statin and proceed with further evaluation.
- Muscle soreness and normal CK options:
  ○ Hold statin and see if symptoms resolve, and then rechallenge to see if symptoms return.
  ○ Hold statin and if symptoms resolve, and rechallenge with lower dose of same statin or another statin.

○ No strong evidence that one statin over another produces fewer symptoms but small studies have suggested that pitavastatin may be better tolerated.

Consider alternate-day dosing: statins with longer half-lives (atorvastatin, rosuvastatin, and pitavastatin) can be effective in less than daily dosing.

Rosenson RS, Baker SK, Jacobson TA, Kopecky SL, Parker BA. An assessment by the Statin Muscle Safety Task Force: 2014 update. *J Clin Lipidol.* 2014;8(3 suppl):S58-S71.

Duggan ST. Pitavastatin: a review of its use in the management of hypercholesterolaemia or mixed dyslipidaemia. *Drugs.* 2012;72(4):565-584.

BOX 15a.3	**Monitoring Blood Glucose with Statin Use**

- Assess patients for risk of developing diabetes prior to starting a statin.
- Monitor blood glucose and HbA1c.

- Continue to emphasize lifestyle modifications to prevent diabetes.
- In general, continue statin treatment.

   c. Neurologic

Statin use has been associated with neurological side effects and a 2012 FDA communication described postmarketing statin adverse event reports in patients over 50 years of age who experienced memory loss or impairment that was reversible with cessation of statin therapy. This finding has not been fully supported by clinical or observational studies,[34] and larger and better-designed studies are needed to clarify the effect of statins on cognition. Patients infected with HIV often have neurocognitive changes, and although the introduction of ART has reduced the prevalence of more severe forms,[35] statin use remains an area of concern with regard to neurologic side effects.

   d. Diabetes and insulin resistance

The 2012 FDA statement also noted increased incidence of diabetes associated with statin use[34]; however, it is unclear if these patients would have progressed to manifest diabetes regardless of statin use.[36] It is felt that the cardiovascular benefits of statins outweigh these small increased risks.[34]

It is not known if patients with HIV, where insulin resistance is more prevalent, have greater risk for developing manifest diabetes due to statin use. Data from the INTREPID trial showed no significant effects on glucose homeostasis with use of Pitavastatin in patients with HIV[37] (See Box 15a.3).

8. **Nonstatin drugs for the treatment of dyslipidemia**

Chapter 9 discussed use of the nonstatin medications. Issues particular to patients infected with HIV are outlined in Table 15a.4. The newer and very potent drugs for treating familial hypercholesterolemia (PCSK9 inhibitors, lomitapide, and mipomersen) are discussed in Chapter 15 but have not been tested in patients with HIV.

Table 15a.4.	**Nonstatin Lipid Medications**			
Drug Class	**Drug Name**	**Tested in HIV**	**Interaction with ART**	**Comments**
Intestine absorption inhibitor	Ezetimibe	Yes	No	
Niacin		Yes	No significant	1. Use limited by side effects 2. Not a potent LDL-C–lowering agent 3. High doses required to lower TG
Bile acid sequestrants	Colesevelam	No	Reduces absorption of other drugs	1. Not a potent LDL-lowering medication 2. May raise TG
Fibrates	Gemfibrozil Fenofibrate	Yes	Gemfibrozil interacts with PI	1. No dose adjustment with gemfibrozil for CKD 2. Use for treatment of hypertriglyceridemia
Fish oil	Omega-3 fatty acids	Yes	No	Use for treatment of hypertriglyceridemia

9. **Other issues related to drug therapy**
    a. Cost of drugs and coverage
        This patient population often has straight Medicaid or a managed Medicaid plan with a limited formulary, or only AIDS Drug Assistance Program (ADAP), which may not offer coverage for lipid medications. Authorizations and appeals can be time-consuming but may result in coverage for a medication so providers are encouraged to submit requests if prescriptions are initially declined.
    b. Combination with other nonstatin drugs
        Patients who are not at goal on one medication or who have combined dyslipidemia (elevated LDL-C and elevated TG) may require addition of a second or third medication. For patients with very high TG (>500 mg/dL), the TG should be lowered first followed by treating LDL-C. When adding another medication, start with the lowest dose and with titration of one medication at a time. With combinations of statins, fibrates, and niacin, there is increased risk for elevation of liver enzymes, and this should be monitored, especially for patients on nonlipid medications that may influence liver function.
    c. Familial hypercholesterolemia
        Familial hypercholesterolemia (FH) is a term representing a group of genetic defects that result in markedly elevated levels of LDL-C.[38] More detail on FH can be found in Chapter 12. At present, there is no information specific to FH in patients infected with HIV and the prevalence is unknown.
    d. Switching ART
        Many ART influence lipid levels; however, changing an ART regimen to less offensive drugs may also present problems. At the time of evaluation for dyslipidemia, many patients have already undergone genotype and phenotype evaluation for ART and have been stable on a virologic effective regimen that is tolerated. Because virologic suppression is a priority, it is reasonable to treat the lipid abnormalities on an established ART regimen. Switching regimens may not significantly improve lipids and may also result in virologic failure. Switching can be considered for patients with marked lipid abnormalities, who are at very high risk or who are unable to attain reasonable response with therapy. This change should be done in consultation with the provider who is managing the patient's ART.[39,40]

10. **Monitoring and follow-up**
    a. According to the European Guidelines, recommendations for follow-up after beginning therapy "stem from consensus rather than evidence-based guidelines" and that "Response to therapy can be assessed at 6-8 weeks from initiation or dose increases for statins, but response to fibrates and lifestyle may take longer."[41]
    b. For most patients, maximum LDL and triglyceride lowering are evident by 6 weeks after starting therapy. If patients are not at goal, titrate to higher doses or add a second drug and recheck lipid levels in another 6 weeks. If a patient is already on combination therapy, only one drug should be titrated at a time. Monitoring of liver function tests, creatine kinase, glucose, and symptoms (such as muscle soreness) is as discussed above and should be performed when indicated.
    c. It is important to understand that attainment of targets for LDL-C and TG may not be reached. Care for patients living with HIV is complex with side effects of medications, problems with adherence to a multidrug regimen, and comorbidities

that impact on lipids. Review of all medical conditions and medications with the patient's other providers can help to identify priorities for the patient. Viral suppression is generally considered foremost although treatment of other conditions may also merit priority.

d. Patients with known CVD or at very high risk should aim to have LDL-C reach goal. If goal attainment is not possible, there remains an incremental benefit to lowering LDL-C even if goal cannot be reached. A triglyceride goal of <150 mg/dL may not be attainable, but attempts to lower this (with both lifestyle and medication) should be made. When levels are extremely high (>500 mg/dL), lowering to prevent pancreatitis is a priority.

VII. Conclusion

This review has provided background on HIV and how both the virus and the therapy impact cardiovascular disease and risk factors, in particular dyslipidemia. As patients infected with HIV are living longer, prevention efforts focusing on diagnosis and treatment of CVD risk factors will be an increasing need. Training for primary providers in the management of CVD and risk factors together with referral to cardiovascular and lipid specialists is becoming part of an overall management plan for these patients.

Epidemiologic studies and clinical trials are needed to establish specific and comprehensive guidelines for this patient population. Until we have the results of studies conducted in persons with HIV infection, we must rely on guidelines for non-HIV patients with extrapolation to HIV-infected patients to guide us in helping patients who are living with HIV.

References

1. Triant VA, Lee H, Hadigan C, Grinspoon SK. Increased acute myocardial infarction rates and cardiovascular risk factors among patients with human immunodeficiency virus disease. *J Clin Endocrinol Metab.* 2007;92(7):2506-2512.
2. Petoumenos K, Worm S, Reiss P, et al. Rates of cardiovascular disease following smoking cessation in patients with HIV infection: results from the D:A:D study(*). *HIV Med.* 2011;12(7):412-421.
3. Galescu O, Bhangoo A, Ten S. Insulin resistance, lipodystrophy and cardiometabolic syndrome in HIV/AIDS. *Rev Endocr Metab Disord.* 2013;14(2):133-140.
4. Reyskens KM, Fisher TL, Schisler JC, et al. Cardio-metabolic effects of HIV protease inhibitors (lopinavir/ritonavir). *PLoS One.* 2013;8(9):e73347.
5. Magkos F, Mantzoros CS. Body fat redistribution and metabolic abnormalities in HIV-infected patients on highly active antiretroviral therapy: novel insights into pathophysiology and emerging opportunities for treatment. *Metabolism.* 2011;60(6):749-753.
6. El-Sadr WM, Lundgren J, Neaton JD, et al. CD4+ count-guided interruption of antiretroviral treatment. *N Engl J Med.* 2006;355(22):2283-2296.
7. Kuller LH, Tracy R, Belloso W, et al. Inflammatory and coagulation biomarkers and mortality in patients with HIV infection. *PLoS Med.* 2008;5(10):e203.
8. Stone NJ, Robinson J, Lichtenstein AH, et al. 2013 ACC/AHA guideline on the treatment of blood cholesterol to reduce atherosclerotic cardiovascular risk in adults: a report of the American College of Cardiology/American Heart Association Task Force on Practice Guidelines. *J Am Coll Cardiol.* 2014 Jul 1;63(25 Pt B):2889-2934.
9. Gale HB, Gitterman SR, Hoffman HJ, et al. Is frequent CD4+ T-lymphocyte count monitoring necessary for persons with counts >=300 cells/μL and HIV-1 suppression? *Clin Infect Dis.* 2013;56(9):1340-1343.
10. Gunthard HF, Aberg JA, Eron JJ, et al. Antiretroviral treatment of adult HIV infection: 2014 recommendations of the International Antiviral Society-USA Panel. *JAMA.* 2014;312(4):410-425.
11. Stein JH, Komarow L, Cotter BR, et al. Lipoprotein changes in HIV-Infected antiretroviral-naive individuals after starting antiretroviral therapy: ACTG Study A5152s Stein: lipoprotein changes on antiretroviral therapy. *J Clin Lipidol.* 2008;2(6):464-471.
12. Riddler SA, Li X, Chu H, et al. Longitudinal changes in serum lipids among HIV-infected men on highly active antiretroviral therapy. *HIV Med.* 2007;8(5):280-287.

13. Riddler SA, Smit E, Cole SR, et al. Impact of HIV infection and HAART on serum lipids in men. *JAMA.* 2003;289(22):2978-2982.
14. Dube MP, Stein JH, Aberg JA, et al. Guidelines for the evaluation and management of dyslipidemia in human immunodeficiency virus (HIV)-infected adults receiving antiretroviral therapy: recommendations of the HIV Medical Association of the Infectious Disease Society of America and the Adult AIDS Clinical Trials Group. *Clin Infect Dis.* 2003;37(5):613-627.
15. Aberg JA, Gallant JE, Ghanem KG, Emmanuel P, Zingman BS, Horberg MA. Primary care guidelines for the management of persons infected with HIV: 2013 update by the HIV medicine association of the Infectious Diseases Society of America. *Clin Infect Dis.* 2014;58(1):e1-e34.
16. Jacobson TA, Maki KC, Orringer CE, et al. National lipid association recommendations for patient-centered management of dyslipidemia: part 2. *J Clin Lipidol.* 2015;9(6 suppl):S1.e121-S122.e121.
17. Friis-Moller N, Thiebaut R, Reiss P, et al. Predicting the risk of cardiovascular disease in HIV-infected patients: the data collection on adverse effects of anti-HIV drugs study. *Eur J Cardiovasc Prev Rehabil.* 2010;17(5):491-501.
18. Justice AC, Freiberg MS, Tracy R, et al. Does an index composed of clinical data reflect effects of inflammation, coagulation, and monocyte activation on mortality among those aging with HIV? *Clin Infect Dis.* 2012;54(7):984-994.
19. Lundgren JD, Battegay M, Behrens G, et al. European AIDS Clinical Society (EACS) guidelines on the prevention and management of metabolic diseases in HIV. *HIV Med.* 2008;9(2):72-81.
20. Hulten E, Mitchell J, Scally J, Gibbs B, Villines TC. HIV positivity, protease inhibitor exposure and subclinical atherosclerosis: a systematic review and meta-analysis of observational studies. *Heart.* 2009;95(22):1826-1835.
21. Hsu R, Patton K, Liang J, Okabe R, Aberg J, Fineberg N. Independent predictors of carotid intimal thickness differ between HIV+ and HIV- patients with respect to traditional cardiac risk factors, risk calculators, lipid subfractions, and inflammatory markers. *Paper presented at: 7th International AIDS Conference on HIV Pathogenesis, Treatment, and Prevention; July 3, 2013; Kuala Lumpur, Malaysia.*
22. Post WS, Budoff M, Kingsley L, et al. Associations between HIV infection and subclinical coronary atherosclerosis. *Ann Intern Med.* 2014;160(7):458-467.
23. Otvos JD, Mora S, Shalaurova I, Greenland P, Mackey RH, Goff DC Jr. Clinical implications of discordance between low-density lipoprotein cholesterol and particle number. *J Clin Lipidol.* 2011;5(2):105-113.
24. Cromwell WC, Otvos JD, Keyes MJ, et al. LDL particle number and risk of future cardiovascular disease in the Framingham Offspring Study—implications for LDL management. *J Clin Lipidol.* 2007;1(6):583-592.
25. Malave H, Castro M, Burkle J, et al. Evaluation of low-density lipoprotein particle number distribution in patients with type 2 diabetes mellitus with low-density lipoprotein cholesterol <50 mg/dL and non-high-density lipoprotein cholesterol <80 mg/dL. *Am J Cardiol.* 2012;110(5):662-665.
26. Myerson M, Lee R, Varela D, et al. Lipoprotein measurements in patients infected with HIV: is cholesterol content of HDL and LDL discordant with particle number? *J Clin Lipidol.* 2014;8(3):332-333.
27. Swanson B, Sha BE, Keithley JK, et al. Lipoprotein particle profiles by nuclear magnetic resonance spectroscopy in medically-underserved HIV-infected persons. *J Clin Lipidol.* 2009;3(6):379-384.
28. Calza L, Manfredi R, Colangeli V, et al. Two-year treatment with rosuvastatin reduces carotid intima-media thickness in HIV type 1-infected patients receiving highly active antiretroviral therapy with asymptomatic atherosclerosis and moderate cardiovascular risk. *AIDS Res Hum Retroviruses.* 2013;29(3):547-556.
29. Aslangul E, Assoumou L, Bittar R, et al. Rosuvastatin vs pravastatin in dyslipidemic HIV-1-infected patients receiving protease inhibitors: a randomized trial. *AIDS.* 2010;24(1):77-83.
30. Sponseller CA, Campbell SE, Thompson M, Aberg JA. Pitavastatin is superior to pravastatin for LDL-C lowering in patients with HIV. *Conference on Retroviruses and Opportunistic Infections; March 2014; Boston, MA.*
31. Sponseller CA, Tanahashi M, Suganami H, Aberg JA. Pitavastatin 4 mg vs. Pravastatin 40 mg in HIV: dyslipidemia: post-hoc analysis of the INTREPID trial based on the independent CHD risk factor of age. *National Lipid Association Annual Scientific Sessions; May 1-4, 2014; Orlando, FL.*
32. Rosenson RS, Baker SK, Jacobson TA, Kopecky SL, Parker BA. An assessment by the Statin Muscle Safety Task Force: 2014 update. *J Clin Lipidol.* 2014;8(3 suppl):S58-S71.
33. Duggan ST. Pitavastatin: a review of its use in the management of hypercholesterolaemia or mixed dyslipidaemia. *Drugs.* 2012;72(4):565-584.
34. Administration UFaD. FDA Drug Safety Communication: Important Safety Label Changes to Cholesterol-lowering Statin Drugs. https://www.fda.gov/drugs/drugsafety/ucm293101.htm. Accessed September 18, 2017.
35. Chan P, Brew BJ. HIV associated neurocognitive disorders in the modern antiviral treatment era: prevalence, characteristics, biomarkers, and effects of treatment. *Curr HIV/AIDS Rep.* 2014;11(3):317-324.
36. Sattar N, Ginsberg HN, Ray KK. The use of statins in people at risk of developing diabetes mellitus: evidence and guidance for clinical practice. *Atheroscler Suppl.* 2014;15(1):1-15.
37. Aberg JA, Sponseller CA. Neutral effects of pitavastatin 4 grams and pravastatin 40 mg on blood glucose levels over 12 weeks. *Prescpecified Safety Analysis from INTREPID; June 16, 2013; San Francisco, CA.*

38. Goldberg AC, Hopkins PN, Toth PP, et al. Familial hypercholesterolemia: screening, diagnosis and management of pediatric and adult patients: clinical guidance from the National Lipid Association Expert Panel on Familial Hypercholesterolemia. *J Clin Lipidol*. 2011;5(3 suppl):S1-S8.
39. Nguyen ST, Eaton SA, Bain AM, et al. Lipid-lowering efficacy and safety after switching to atazanavir-ritonavir-based highly active antiretroviral therapy in patients with human immunodeficiency virus. *Pharmacotherapy*. 2008;28(3):323-330.
40. Bain AM, White EA, Rutherford WS, Rahman AP, Busti AJ. A multimodal, evidence-based approach to achieve lipid targets in the treatment of antiretroviral-associated dyslipidemia: case report and review of the literature. *Pharmacotherapy*. 2008;28(7):932-938.
41. Catapano AL, Chapman J, Wiklund O, Taskinen MR. The new joint EAS/ESC guidelines for the management of dyslipidaemias. *Atherosclerosis*. 2011;217(1):1.

Special Topics for Lipid Management: Lipid Management in Special Populations (Women, Pregnancy, Menopause)

Sara Talken and Robert A. Wild

Key Points

- Cardiovascular disease (CVD) is a major cause of death in women, so health providers should be adept to preventing and treating this disease.
- Risk factors for dyslipidemia can be present in women during their reproductive years, and recognition and prevention should be a focus of primary care physicians.
- Cholesterol and triglyceride changes are normal during pregnancy and near delivery. They will peak to maximal levels due to placental changes. The effects are shown with increasing insulin resistance as the pregnancy continues.
- The best time to screen for and prevent lipid disorders is before conception. However, should dyslipidemia be diagnosed during pregnancy, there are options for treatment during pregnancy.
- Dyslipidemia should be considered when counseling on and prescribing contraception for patients.
- Menopause is characterized by specific changes in lipid profiles.
- Hormone replacement therapy should be initiated for symptoms, not for management of chronic disease. There are contraindications to using hormone therapy, and physicians should be aware of the risks and benefits to these treatment options.

I. Introduction

Because the major cause of death for women is CVD, health care providers should be adept in ways to reduce atherosclerotic cardiovascular disease (ASCVD). There are required practices and preventive universal principles that are commonly followed for both male and female patients; however, the diagnosis and treatment of lipid disorders in women has many unique aspects that the clinician should become familiar with. Dyslipidemia and the risk for development of ASCVD pose risk to women as well as their offspring.[1]

This section discusses some of the unique issues in women's health important for lipid management. Clinicians caring for women of reproductive age are ideally placed to begin the management of risk factors and preventing CVD. Most of women's health is practiced by primary care practitioners or gynecologists, and it is important for those as well as other providers to have a strong working knowledge about managing dyslipidemia for women. For these providers, the recognition of high-risk patients and how lipids affect, and are affected, by major reproductive issues should be of high priority.

In general, CVD in women is diagnosed ~10 years after it is recognized in men patients. In addition, prevention is inadvertently less of a priority during the female reproductive years.

II. Lipid Considerations in Women During Reproductive Years

A. Prevalence of risk factors in women According to the National Health and Nutrition Examination Survey 1999-2008 data, among women aged 18-44 years old in the United States, 2.4% had diabetes, 7.7% were estimated to have hypertension, about 25% used tobacco, 2.9% had chronic kidney disease, and 57.6% were either overweight or obese. While prevalence of some of these risk factors has remained constant over the years, the prevalence of diabetes, hypertension, chronic kidney disease, and obesity continues to significantly increase. The odds of developing a hypertensive disease complication during pregnancy are 3.5 times greater in those that have hypertension and obesity before they become pregnant.[2] Women who have a genetic cause of high LDL or high triglycerides can also be diagnosed during the reproductive years.

B. With approximately half of pregnancies being unplanned, the ability to diagnose and treat many risk factors for CVD before becoming pregnant is limited. A Kaiser Family Foundation national survey discovered that the rate of CVD screening in women ages 18-44 years old was 58% compared with 78% for women ages 45-64 years.[3] It was also found that blood pressure screening in the younger population is even lower.

C. **Provider specialty** In another national survey, it was found that in women aged 18-64 years, 15% were seen by a general medicine physician, 62% were seen by a gynecologist, and 23% were seen by both. It was found that those patients seen by a gynecologist received more counseling and preventive services.[4] An assessment of two health care policies was also very revealing. Out of the 3.6 million members covered by the policies, one-third of women were diagnosed with hypertension during their course of care. Also, irrespective of the specialty that provided care, <70% of women received lipid screening, nutritional counseling, and weight counseling. The survey also uncovered that there was limited knowledge about hypertensive diseases of pregnancy, such as preeclampsia, and their future CVD risk because of preeclampsia in reproductive-age women for all the specialties that provide care for these patients.

D. The most recent National Vital Statistics report showed that overall pregnancy rates for women aged 25-29 have not shown much change in the past several years. However, the rates of pregnancy in women in the 30s and 40s have increased. Additionally, women aged 35-44 years in the United States have had the greatest increase in obesity in the past 45 years.

E. Due to the known relationship between obesity and dyslipidemia, these results have strong implications. Currently, almost 50% of women begin pregnancy overweight or obese. Metabolic syndrome is prevalent in obese women. This statistic has almost doubled in the past 30 years. Another concerning finding is that almost half of women gain more than the recommended 20-30 lb during pregnancy. It is well known in obstetrics that maternal obesity contributes to pregnancy complications such as gestational diabetes, macrosomia, hypertensive disorders, and other perinatal complications.[5]

F. For most women, their reproductive years span three decades. This provides a prolonged period of time to diagnose and treat CVD risk factors for the health of the mother and future children.

III. Lipid Considerations in Pregnancy

A. Overview

1. Reproductive age refers to a time period in a woman's life when she is able to bear children, from the onset of menstruation until the age of menopause. With the average age of menses around age 12, most women enter menopause by age 52. The reproductive years are during the young and ideally healthy time during a women's life.

2. A large cohort study that followed women through normal pregnancy and delivery found that the average circulating values of total cholesterol, low density lipoprotein cholesterol (LDL-C), high density lipoprotein cholesterol (HDL-C), and triglycerides (TG) decreased slightly in the first trimester, and by the end of the third

month (or end of first trimester), there is a noticeable increase. There continues to be an increase in the major lipoprotein lipids through the pregnancy with the levels peaking near term.[6] Proper energy for the fetus is achieved by lipid metabolism.

3. Assessment of normal lipid values during pregnancy should include values relevant to trimester in pregnancy. When values for fasting triglycerides exceed 250 mg/dL, this should be considered abnormal, and the clinician should be aware that a potential pregnancy complication may form. Mean lipid levels have been found to be elevated (>300 mg/dL) in complicated pregnancies.[7,8] Triglyceride levels >250 mg/dL during pregnancy are associated with complications including pregnancy-induced hypertension, preeclampsia, gestational diabetes, and macrosomic infants.[5]

4. Many women have undiagnosed dyslipidemia before pregnancy and this disease is often linked to conditions that make them at risk for obstetric and fetal complications should they become pregnant. Polycystic ovarian syndrome, uncontrolled diabetes mellitus, and genetic lipid disorders can be related to problems for the mother, the fetus, and future offspring should the mother conceive again. Recent surveys have revealed about one-third of women presenting to obstetrics and gynecology practices had CVD risk factors that should be diagnosed and potentially reversed. Familial hypercholesterolemia (FH) is more common than the other genetic conditions screened for during pregnancy[9]; however, there are currently no screening recommendations for FH. Pregnancy is a cardiometabolic stress test. Maternal and fetal complications can be prevented by proper taking of an in-depth metabolic/pregnancy history to identify existing medical problems and proper screening and management before and during pregnancy.

5. **When to screen** The best time to screen for lipid disorders is before pregnancy or very early in gestation, preferably shortly after the pregnancy is diagnosed. Screening should routinely be performed postpartum, preferably at the 6-week postpartum visit. Women who experienced complicated pregnancies, obesity before or during pregnancy or had excessive weight gain during pregnancy (>25-35 lb for women whose BMI is 18.5-24.9 and less for women with higher BMI), are more likely to have abnormal cardiometabolic profiles.[10] Many women who experience complications of pregnancy are followed by a high-risk obstetrician, as opposed to their usual provider, and the lack of continuity can pose a potential risk for missing a diagnosis of hyperlipidemia. It becomes prudent to follow up and provide proper screening for detection and management of dyslipidemia after pregnancy.

B. Fetal considerations

1. **Developmental programming** There is a large amount of literature that suggests an unhealthy uterine environment can lead to difficulty adjusting to postuterine life and which some have attributed as a cause for the origin of chronic diseases such as ASCVD.[11] There are several prepregnancy components that contribute to fetal programming while in utero including genetics, metabolic disturbances of the mother and father, and genetics. Environmental factors include maternal malnutrition, maternal smoking, preeclampsia, obesity, placental function, hyperlipidemia, etc., that have important influences on the fetus. Recent animal studies have revealed that changes in DNA methylation and chromatin remodeling may be responsible for the epigenetic programming and increased atherosclerotic susceptibility.[12] However, exact mechanisms of the underlying effects of maternal hypercholesterolemia in offspring are still unclear.

2. **Epigenetic programming** Epigenetic programming of metabolism during embryonic and fetal development may be involved[13] with animal studies revealing changes

in either DNA methylation or chromatin modification, or both, may be the cause for epigenetic programming responsible for atherosclerotic susceptibility.[14] For example, maternal hypercholesterolemia in apoE-deficient mice leads to the activation of genes involved in cholesterol synthesis and LDLR activity in adult offspring.[14,15] More research is needed to reveal the exact mechanisms of how maternal dyslipidemia influences the cellular development in the fetus.

C. Treatment of dyslipidemia in pregnancy

1. **Choice of medications**
   a. For women on lipid-lowering medications to treat previously diagnosed dyslipidemia, any medication besides bile acid–sequestering agents and omega-3 fatty acids should be stopped in pregnancy.
   b. Statins should be discontinued 1-3 months before conception. However, this recommendation is based on expert opinion without definitive evidence. Although early uncontrolled case series reported congenital anomalies associated with statin use, more recent observational studies did not report an increased risk of congenital anomalies with statin exposure in pregnancy when compared to control groups or the prevalence of congenital anomalies in the general population.[16] This study concludes that statins may not be teratogenic. However, until there is more information available, statins should not be taken during pregnancy.[16] Box 15b.1 shows the FDA classification for medications during pregnancy, and Table 15b.1 provides the pregnancy classifications for widely used lipid-lowering drugs.

BOX 15b.1 | **FDA Pregnancy Drug Classifications**

Category A
Adequate and well-controlled studies have failed to show a risk to the fetus in the first trimester of pregnancy, and there is no evidence of risk in later trimesters.
  Examples of drugs or substances: levothyroxine, folk acid, magnesium sulfate, liothyronine.

Category B
Animal reproduction studies have failed to show a risk to the fetus, and there are no adequate and well-controlled studies in pregnant women.
  Examples of drugs: metformin, hydrochlorothiazide, cyclobenzaprine, amoxicillin, pantoprazole

Category C
Animal reproduction studies have shown an adverse effect on the fetus and there are no adequate and well-controlled studies in humans, but potential benefits may warrant use of the drug in pregnant women despite potential risks.
  Examples of drugs: tramadol, gabapentin, amlodipine, trazodone, prednisone

Category D
There is positive evidence of human fetal risk based on adverse reaction data from investigational or marketing experience or studies in humans, but potential benefits may warrant use of the drug in pregnant women despite potential risks.
  Examples of drugs: lisinopril, alprazolam, losartan, clonazepam, lorazepam

Category X
Studies in animals or humans have shown fetal abnormalities and/or there is positive evidence of human fetal risk based on adverse reaction data from investigational or marketing experience, and the risks involved in use of the drug in pregnant women dearly outweigh potential benefits.
  Examples of drugs: atorvastatin, simvastatin, warfarin, methotrexate, finasteride

Category N
FDA has not classified the drug.
  Examples of drugs: aspirin, oxycodone, hydroxyzine, acetaminophen, diazepam

Source: Wild R, Weedin E, Gill E. Women's health considerations for lipid management. *Cardiol Clin.* 2015;33:217-231.

Table 15b.1. Lipid Level–Lowering Agents and Pregnancy Classification	
Lipid Level–lowering Agent	**Pregnancy Class**
Statins	X
Fibrates	C
Ezetimibe	C
Niacin	C
Cholestyramine	C
Colesevelam	B
Mipomersen	B

Reprinted with permission from Wild R, Weedin E, Gill E. Women's health considerations for lipid management. *Cardiol Clin.* 2015;33:217-231.

   c. In 2015, the FDA approved a new class of medication, PCSK9 inhibitors. This medication is a monoclonal antibody that works in adjunct with diet and maximally tolerated statin therapy. At this time, PCSK9 inhibitors fall into the "not classified" category of drugs for use in pregnancy.[17]

      The FDA suggests that the risks and benefits for any medication should be understood and discussed when deciding on a treatment plan.

2. Treatment plan
   a. Lifestyle modification
     All patients with dyslipidemia in pregnancy should be treated with diet, weight management, and physical activity.
   b. Diabetes
     Careful glycemic control, if indicated. Controlling diabetes is essential to managing triglyceride levels.
   c. Treatment of elevated LDL-C
     Hypercholesterolemia can be treated with bile acid sequestrates, preferably colesevelam, previously category B in pregnancy.
   d. Treatment of hypertriglyceridemia
     Severe hypertriglyceridemia can be treated with omega-3 fatty acids, parenteral nutrition, plasmapheresis, and low-fat diets. Fenofibrate or gemfibrozil can be used early in the second trimester based on clinical judgment.[18]

3. Monitoring Lipids should be monitored every trimester or within 6 weeks of a new intervention to evaluate for effectiveness and compliance. Mothers with FH or dysmetabolic problems during pregnancy need close follow-up.[19-21]

4. Breast-feeding For mothers with lipid disorders, breast-feeding is still recommended. Medications that can be taken while breast-feeding include bile acid sequestrants, fish oil, fenofibrates, and gemfibrozil.[19-21]

IV. Contraceptive Considerations in Patients With Dyslipidemia

A. Lipid changes with contraceptives

   1. The different forms of contraception can have varied effects. Different formulations of oral contraceptives have varying amounts of estrogen and, if it is a combined formulation, of progesterone.

BOX 15b.2	CDC Compendium for Medical Conditions Best Resource for Recommendations With Comorbidities

Categories for Classifying Contraceptive Methods

1 = A condition for which there is no restriction for the use of the contraceptive method.
2 = A condition for which the advantages of using the method generally outweigh the theoretical or proven risks.

3 = A condition for which the theoretical or proven risks usually outweigh the advantages of using the method.
4 = A condition that represents an unacceptable health risk if the contraceptive method is used.

Source: http://www.cdc.gov/reproductivehealth/unintendedpregnancy/usmec.htm

2. The estrogen in these products may increase total cholesterol, HDL-C, and triglycerides and lower LDL-C. The androgenic progesterones (norgestrel and levonorgestrel) can raise LDL-C and lower HDL-C, but the other progesterones are generally lipid neutral.

3. The more estrogen that a produce contains, the greater the triglyceride-raising effect. Caution is advised for those with elevated baseline triglycerides. Transdermal formulations are less likely to produce clinically significant increases in triglycerides.

B. When choosing a contraceptive method for a patient with dyslipidemia, there are several considerations. The CDC recommendations are outlined in Box 15b.2 and Table 15b.2.

V. Menopause

A. Lipid changes

1. Lipid changes occur during the onset of menopause (ovarian insufficiency) with both LDL-C and apolipoprotein B increasing and HDL-C decreasing.[22] The changes that result are thought to be due to the decrease in estrogen production from the failing ovaries. As the ovarian follicles diminish, they secrete less estradiol. Changes in adipose tissue distribution are also noted during this time.[23] Also, a link to an increase in prevalence of metabolic syndrome has been observed during this time.[24]

2. The absolute risk for CVD significantly increases during the midlife of women due to their increasing age but also their lack of estradiol, which is well known to have cardioprotective effects. Because of this, women who were at increased risk for CVD before menopause are at an even higher risk once they enter into the menopausal transition so it is extremely important for clinicians to identify these patients early and initiate the proper treatment.

Table 15b.2.	US Medical Eligibility for Contraceptive Use					
Condition	COC Patch Ring	Progester One Only Pill	Depo-Provera	Nexplanon	LevoNG IUD (ex. Mirena)	Copper IUD
Hyperlipidemia	2/3	2*	2*	2*	2*	1*

*Please see the complete guidance for a clarification to this classification.
COC, combined oral contraception pill; LevoNG, levonorgestrel.
(Data from http://www.cdc.gov/reproductivehealth/unintendedpregnancy/usmec.htm.)

B. Recommendations for hormone replacement therapy

1. **Indications** Hormone replacement therapy (HRT) for menopausal women is used primarily to treat symptoms associated with the menopause including hot flashes, night sweats, fatigue, vaginal atrophy, and mood swings. Replacement therapy should not be prescribed to prevent or treat CVD. There is a black box warning placed by the FDA for women with known coronary artery disease and thromboembolic disorders or those who have had a stroke because hormone replacement therapy carries a risk of thrombosis and other critical events in women with a history or disorders with thrombotic pathophysiology.

2. **Confusion over benefits and risks** There has been confusion regarding safety and efficacy of HRT, in particular after the results of the Women's Health Initiative (WHI). This study was conducted in the 1990s and was a placebo-controlled randomized trial of estrogen plus progestin and estrogen alone in women aged 50-79 years without known CVD. The study found no evidence of protection from CVD and increases in breast cancer and thromboembolic events. As a result, HRT was no longer considered standard of care for postmenopausal women and those already on treatment were taken off therapy. There were many criticisms of the study design including time of treatment (average enrollee was about 12 years postmenopausal) and formulations of the HRT.[25]

3. **Identification of appropriate patients for HRT**
   a. It is important to identify the appropriate patients for HRT because of the complex profile of risks and benefits associated with HRT. The Women's Health Initiative and other randomized trials have shown that it is important to consider a woman's age, proximity to menopause, and underlying cardiovascular risk factor status when considering this therapy.
   b. It is now possible to individualize HRT and thus better predict which patients may have better outcomes vs adverse effects with HT. Once a woman is identified as a potential candidate for HRT to improve her quality of life due to menopausal symptoms, risk stratification may be an important tool for minimizing the patient's risk.[25]
   c. An individualized approach should be taken with each patient when deciding to initiate HRT.

4. **Summary of recommendations for HRT** Approved HRT for menopausal symptoms in the United States and Canada can been found in Tables 15b.3–15b.7.[26]

Table 15b.3. Oral Estrogen Agents		
Active Ingredient(s)	**Product Name(s)**	**Dosages (mg/d)**
17β-estradiol[a]	Estrace[b] Generic(s) available	0.5, 1.0, 2.0
Conjugated estrogens	Premarin	0.3, 0.45[c], 0.625, 0.9[c], 1.25
Synthetic conjugated estrogens, B	Enjuvia[c]	0.3, 0.45, 0.625, 0.9, 1.25
Conjugated estrogens, CSD[c] (synthetic)	C.E.S. pms-Conjugated estrogens, CSD	0.3, 0.625, 0.9, 1.25
Esterified estrogens	Merest[c] Estragyn[b]	0.3, 0.625, 1.25, 2.5 (administer cyclically) 0.3, 0.625
Estropipate	Generic(s) available[c]	0.625 (0.75 estropipate), 1.25 (1.5), 2.5 (3.0)

[a]Bioidentical: defined as compounds that have the same chemical and molecular structure as hormones that are produced in the body.
[b]Available in Canada but not the United States.
[c]Available in the United States but not Canada.
(Data from http://www.menopause.org/for-women.)

Table 15b.4.   Transdermal Estrogen Products

Active Ingredient(s)	Product Name	Dosage (mg E$_2$/d)
Patch, Film		
17β-estradiol[a]	Alora[b]	0.025, 0.05, 0.075, 0.1 twice/wk
	Climara	0.025, 0.0375,[b] 0.05, 0.06,[b] 0.075, 0.1 once/wk
	Estraderm[b]	0.05, 0.1 twice/wk
	Estradot[c]	0.025, 0.0375, 0.05, 0.075, 0.1 twice/wk
	Minivelle[b]	0.025, 0.0375, 0.05, 0.075, 0.1 twice/wk
	Oesclim[c]	0.025,6 0.0375, 0.05, 0.075, 0.1 twice/wk
	Vivelle-Dot[b]	0.025, 0.0375, 0.05, 0.075, 0.1 twice/wk
	Generic(s) available	
Transdermal gel		
17β-estradiol[a]	Divigel	0.25, 0.5, 1.0
	EstroGel	0.75 (*US:* single approved dose, *Canada:* adjust to control symptoms)
	Elestrin[b]	0.52 (adjust based on clinical response)
Transdermal spray		
17β-estradiol[a]	Evamist[b]	1.53 (1 spray/d initially, adjust dosage by clinical response)

[a]Bioidentical: defined as compounds that have the same chemical and molecular structure as hormones that are produced in the body.
[b]Available in the United States but not Canada.
[c]Available in Canada but not the United States.
(Data from http://www.menopause.org/for-women.)

Table 15b.5.   Vaginal Estrogen Products

Active Ingredient(s)	Product Name *Indication*	Dosage
Creams		
17β-estradiol[a]	Estrace Vaginal Cream[b] *Vulvar and vaginal atrophy*	Initial: 2-4 g/d for 1-2 wk Maintenance: 1 g 1-3 times/wk (0.1 mg estradiol/g)
Conjugated estrogens	Premarin Vaginal Cream *Atrophic vaginitis Kraurosis vulvae Dyspareunia (US: Moderate to severe)*	*US: For atrophic vaginitis and kraurosis vulvae:* 0.5-2 g/d (0.625 mg conjugated estrogens/g) for 21 d then off 7 d *For moderate to severe dyspareunia:* 0.5 g twice weekly continuous or for 21 d then off 7 d *Canada:* Low dose: 0 5 g intravaginal or topical twice/wk Maximum recommended dose: 0.5 g/d intravaginally or topically for 21 d then off 7 d. Start with 0 5 g/d. Dosage adjustments (0.5-2 g) may be made based on individual response
Estrone[a]	Estragyn Vaginal Cream[c] *Vulvovaginal atrophy*	2-4 g/d (1 mg active ingredient/g) adjusted to lowest amount that controls symptoms. Usually cyclic (for 21 d then off 7 d)
Rings		
17β-estradiol[a]	Estring *US: Moderate to severe symptoms of vulvar and vaginal atrophy due to menopause Canada: Postmenopausal urogenital complaints due to estrogen deficiency*	2 mg (releases 7.5 µg/d) for 90 d *Canada:* Maximum recommended duration of continuous therapy is 2 y
Estradiol acetate[a]	Femring[b] *Moderate to severe vasomotor symptoms due to menopause Moderate to severe vulvar and vaginal atrophy due to menopause*	0.05 mg/d, 0.10 mg/d for 90 d (both strengths release systemic levels and require consideration of a progestogen if the uterus is intact)

(Continued)

Table 15b.5.   Vaginal Estrogen Products (*Continued*)

Active Ingredient(s)	Product Name *Indication*	Dosage
Tablet		
Estradiol hemihydrate[a]	Vagifem[b] *Atrophic vaginitis due to menopause*	10 µg, 25 µg Initial: 1 tablet/d for 2 wk Maintenance: 1 tablet twice/wk
	Vagifem 10[c] *Symptoms of vaginal atrophy due to estrogen deficiency*	10 µg Initial: 1 tablet/d for 2 wk Maintenance: 1 tablet twice/wk

[a]Bioidentical: defined as compounds that have the same chemical and molecular structure as hormones that are produced in the body.
[b]Available in the United States but not Canada.
[c]Available in Canada but not the United States.
Products not marked are available in the United States and Canada.
(Data from http://www.menopause.org/for-women.)

Table 15b.6.   Combined Estrogen-Progesterone

Active Ingredient(s)	Product Name	Dosage
Oral continuous-cyclic		
Conjugated estrogens (E) + medroxyprogesterone acetate (P)	Premphase[a]	0.625 mg E + 5.0 mg P (2 tablets: E days 1-14, E + P days 15-28)
Oral continuous-combined		
Conjugated estrogens (E) + medroxyprogesterone acetate (P)	Prempro[a]	0.3 or 0.45 mg E + 1.5 mg P, 0.625 mg E + 2.5 or 5.0 mg P
Ethinyl estradiol (E) + norethindrone acetate (P)	femhrt[a], femHRT Lo[b] Generic(s) available[a] femhrt[a], femHRT[b] Generic(s) available[a]	2.5 µg E + 0.5 mg P 5 µg E + 1 mg P
17β-estradiol (E) + norethindrone acetate (P)	Activella[a] Generic(s) available[a] Activelle LD[b] Activelle[b]	0.5 mg E + 0.1 mg P, 1 mg E + 0.5 mg P 0.5 mg E + 0.1 mg P 1 mg E + 0.5 mg P
17β-estradiol (E) + drospirenone (P)	Angeliq	1 mg E + 0.5 mg P[a], 0.5 mg E + 0.25 mg P[a], 1 mg E + 1 mg P[b]
Oral intermittent-combined		
17β-estradiol (E) + norgestimate (P)	Prefest[a]	1 mg E and 1 mg E + 0.09 mg P (E alone for 3 d, followed by E+P for 3 d, repeated continuously)
Transdermal continuous-combined		
17β-estradiol (E) + norethindrone acetate (P)	CombiPatch[a] Estalis[b]	0.05 mg E + 0.14 mg P twice/wk 0.05 mg E + 0.25 mg P twice/wk
17β-estradiol (E) + levonorgestrel (P)	Climara Pro	0.045 mg E + 0.015 mg P once/wk

[a]Available in the United States but not Canada.
[b]Available in Canada but not the United States.
Products not marked are available in both the United States and Canada.
(Data from http://www.menopause.org/for-women.)

Table 15b.7.	Progestins	
Active Ingredient(s)	**Product Name**	**Dosage (mg/d)**
Medroxyprogesterone acetate	Provera Generic(s) available	5, 10 (administer cyclically 12-14 d/mo)
Micronized progesterone[a]	Prometrium	200 (administer cyclically) *US:* 12d/28-d cycle *Canada:* last 14 d/cycle

[a]Bioidentical: defined as compounds that have the same chemical and molecular structure as hormones that are produced in the body.
Products not marked are available in both the United States and Canada.
(Data from http://www.menopause.org/for-women.)

These tables have been adapted from the North American Menopause Society (NAMS) recommendations on their website. General recommendations are as follows:

- Use the lowest effective dose of HRT for symptom relief.
- Oral conjugated estrogen <0.3 mg daily does not control hot flashes in most women; however, this dose has been shown to be protective against bone loss from estrogen deficiency osteopenia.
- Transdermal and vaginal preparations of estrogens are associated with fewer effects on clotting factors, lipid metabolism, inflammatory biomarkers, and sex hormone–binding globulin synthesis.
- Effects of different HRT combinations depend on dose, route, and formulation.[16]

VI. Conclusion

In conclusion, lipid management in women, no matter which phase of life, is extremely important in the management of her overall health. Clinicians should make it a priority to counsel about, screen for, and treat dyslipidemias to prevent potential adverse health conditions for female patients now and in the future.

References

1. Palinski W, D'Armiento FP, Witztum JL, et al. Maternal hypercholesterolemia and treatment during pregnancy influence the long-term progression of atherosclerosis in offspring of rabbits. *Circ Res.* 2001;89(11):991-996.
2. Charlton F, Tooher J, Rye KA, et al. Cardiovascular risk, lipids and pregnancy: preeclampsia and the risk of later life cardiovascular disease. *Heart Lung Circ.* 2014;23(3):203-212.
3. Kjerulff LE, Sanchez-Ramos L, Duffy D. Pregnancy outcomes in women with polycystic ovary syndrome: a metaanalysis. *Am J Obstet Gynecol.* 2011;204(6):558.e1-558.e6.
4. Gunderson EP. Childbearing and obesity in women: weight before, during and after pregnancy. *Obstet Gynecol Clin North Am.* 2009;36(2):317-332, ix.
5. Wild RA, Carmina E, Diamanti-Kandarakis E, et al. Assessment of cardiovascular risk and prevention of cardiovascular disease in women with polycystic ovary syndrome: a consensus statement by the Androgen Excess and Polycystic Ovary Syndrome (AE-PCOS) Society. *J Clin Endocrinol Metab.* 2010;95(5):2038-2049.
6. Woollett LA. Where does fetal and embryonic cholesterol originate and what does it do? *Annu Rev Nutr.* 2008;28:97-114.
7. Woollett LA. Fetal lipid metabolism. *Front Biosci.* 2001;6:D36-D45.
8. Woollett LA. Maternal cholesterol in fetal development: transport of cholesterol from the maternal to the fetal circulation. *Am J Clin Nutr.* 2005;82(6):1155-1161.
9. Vuorio AF, Miettinen TA, Turtola H, et al. Cholesterol metabolism in normal and heterozygous familial hypercholesterolemic newborns. *J Lab Clin Med.* 2002;140(1):35-42.
10. Spellacy WN, Ashbacher LV, Harris GK, et al. Total cholesterol content in maternal and umbilical vessels in term pregnancies. *Obstet Gynecol.* 1974;44(5):661-665.

11. Hanson M, Godfrey KM, Lillycrop KA, et al. Developmental plasticity and developmental origins of non-communicable disease: theoretical considerations and epigenetic mechanisms. *Prog Biophys Mol Biol.* 2011;106(1):272-280.

12. Deruiter M, Alkemade F, Groot A, et al. Maternal transmission of risk for atherosclerosis. *Curr Opin Lipidol.* 2008;4:333-337.

13. Herrera E. Metabolic adaptations in pregnancy and their implications for the availability of substrates to the fetus. *Eur J Clin Nutr.* 2000;54(suppl 1):S47-S51.

14. DeRuiter MC, Alkemade FE, Gittenberger-de Groot AC, et al. Maternal transmission of risk for atherosclerosis. *Curr Opin Lipidol.* 2008;19(4):333-337.

15. Reymer PW, Groenemeyer BE, van de Burg R, et al. Apolipoprotein E genotyping on agarose gels. *Clin Chem.* 1995;41(7):1046-1047.

16. http://www.cdc.gov/reproductivehealth/unintendedpregnancy/usmec.htm. Accessed September 19, 2016.

17. Product Information. *Repatha (evolocumab).* Thousand Oaks, CA: Amgen USA.

18. Goldberg AS, Hegele RA. Severe hypertriglyceridemia in pregnancy. *J Clin Endocrinol Metab.* 2012;97(8):2589-2596.

19. Wild R, Weedin E, Gill E. Women's health considerations for lipid management. *Cardiol Clin.* 2015;33:217-231.

20. Wild R, Weedin E, Wilson D. Dyslipidemia in Pregnancy. *Cardiol Clin.* 2015;33:209-215.

21. Karalis D, Hill AN, Clifton A. The risks of statin use in pregnancy: a systematic review. *J Clin Lipidol.* 2016;10(5):1081-1090.

22. Derby CA, Crawford SL, Pasternak RC, et al. Lipid changes during the menopause transition in relation to age and weight: the Study of Women's Health Across the Nation. *Am J Epidemiol.* 2009;169(11):1352-1361.

23. Park JK, Lim YH, Kim KS, et al. Changes in body fat distribution through menopause increase blood pressure independently of total body fat in middle-aged women: the Korean National Health and Nutrition Examination Survey 2007-2010. *Hypertens Res.* 2013;36(5):444-449.

24. Mendes KG, Theodoro H, Rodrigues AD, et al. Prevalence of metabolic syndrome and its components in the menopausal transition: a systematic review. *Cad Saude Publica.* 2012;28(8):1423-1437.

25. Wild RA, Manson JE. Insights from the Women's Health Initiative: individualizing risk assessment for hormone therapy decisions. *Semin Reprod Med.* 2014;32(6):433-437.

26. http://www.menopause.org/publications/clinical-care-recommendations/chapter-8-prescription-therapies. Accessed September 20, 2016.

Dyslipidemia in Chronic Kidney Disease

Aarthi Madhana Kumar, Madhan Nellaiyappan, and Indu G. Poornima

Key Points

- The incidence of chronic kidney disease (CKD) is increasing, and cardiovascular disease is the most significant cause of morbidity and mortality in this condition.
- Dyslipidemia is common in CKD and requires treatment.
- Although the lipid abnormalities are subtle, treatment with a statin to lower LDL cholesterol does improve cardiovascular outcomes.
- Measurement of LDL cholesterol does not impact decision for therapy in CKD unless over 190 mg/dL.
- Statins or statin and ezetimibe combinations are the drugs of choice for treatment of dyslipidemia in CKD.
- Doses of statin and mode of elimination of statin need to be considered in choosing appropriate regimen.
- Statins have not shown any benefit in patients on dialysis, and therefore, it is not recommended to start it at the time of initiation of dialysis.
- Patients undergoing renal transplantation benefit from statin treatment.

I.   Introduction

Chronic kidney disease (CKD) is associated with a higher risk of developing cardiovascular disease especially coronary artery disease, and in those with established cardiovascular disease, CKD is associated with progression of disease and recurrent cardiovascular events.[1] CKD is defined as kidney damage for ≥3 months as evidenced by structural or functional abnormalities of the kidneys with or without decreased glomerular filtration rate (GFR) and/or increased proteinuria as assessed by urine albumin to creatinine ratio with stages as shown in Table 15c.1.[2] Cardiovascular disease remains the largest cause of morbidity and mortality in this population,[3] and appropriate cardiovascular risk reduction in this group is imperative.[4] Kidney disease commonly coexists with other cardiovascular risk factors such as diabetes, hypertension, and dyslipidemia, and each of these risk factors carries independent and incremental risk. Thus, treatment of these additional risk factors is as critical as treatment of the underlying CKD to improve cardiovascular outcomes. In the Atherosclerosis Risk in Communities (ARIC) study, the risk that dyslipidemia carries for cardiovascular disease in

Table 15c.1.	Classification of CKD	
Stages	**GFR mL/min/1.73 m²ᵃ**	**Classification**
1	GFR ≥ 90	Mild CKD
2	GFR 60-89	Mild CKD
3A	GFR 45-59	Moderate CKD
3B	GFR 30-44	Moderate to severe CKD
4	GFR 15-29	Severe CKD
5	GFR < 15	Kidney failure

ᵃEach CKD stage can be further stratified based on degree of albuminuria ranging from <30 to >300 mg/g. For the treatment of dyslipidemia, the degree of albuminuria does not have any implications.

patients with CKD is similar to the risk seen in the general population.[5] Moreover, CKD is associated with distinct lipid abnormalities, and treatment has been shown to impact cardiovascular morbidity and mortality.

II.   Pathogenesis

The lipid profile in CKD is characterized by hypertriglyceridemia, low HDL, and, not uncommonly, normal total and LDL cholesterol levels.[6] Changes in key enzymes and receptors, presence of nephrotic range proteinuria, diabetes mellitus, concomitant hereditary disorders, and extrinsic factors such as type of renal replacement therapy and use of epoetin, steroids, and calcineurin inhibitors[7] contribute to these lipid abnormalities.

A. LDL in CKD

1. Total cholesterol and LDL-C levels are usually within the normal range or only slightly increased, but there are important qualitative changes in LDL particles that are acquired during prolonged residence in the circulation by the process of oxidation, glycation, and carbamylation.[6] These modified small dense LDL particles have decreased binding to their respective LDL receptors and hence are not cleared effectively by the liver but instead have high affinity for scavenger receptors on macrophages thereby contributing to atherogenesis.[8] Stable isotope kinetic studies have also shown that the plasma residence time of LDL particles is markedly prolonged in hemodialysis (HD) patients compared to controls further promoting atherosclerotic plaque formation.[9]

2. Elevated isoforms of lipoprotein(a) are described in CKD patients due to decreased elimination of this particle and may confer additional risk.[10]

3. Discordance between LDL levels and apolipoprotein B levels occurs in CKD due to the high levels of triglyceride-rich lipoprotein particles that exist in circulation, causing high apolipoprotein B levels in the setting of normal LDL levels.

4. The guidelines in management of dyslipidemia have therefore focused less on LDL levels and more on managing overall risk.

B. Hypertriglyceridemia of CKD

1. Mild to moderate hypertriglyceridemia (200-300 mg/dL) is seen in majority of the patients with CKD especially in patients with diabetes and specifically in patients undergoing continuous ambulatory peritoneal dialysis.[11] Several studies have shown that hypertriglyceridemia occurs in early stages of CKD even when serum creatinine levels are within normal limits.[12]

2. Hypertriglyceridemia is a consequence of increased production of endogenous triglycerides due to impaired carbohydrate tolerance and by the proteinuria and consequent hypoalbuminemia leading to compensatory stimulation of lipoprotein production by the liver, both of which can manifest as postprandial lipemia.[13] Reduced catabolism of triglycerides also occurs from decreased lipoprotein lipase and hepatic triglyceride lipase activity, the enzymes that are responsible for cleaving triglycerides into free fatty acids (FFA) for energy production and storage.[14] Studies have also shown that CKD patients have increased levels of lipase inhibitors in their plasma such as apolipoprotein C-III.[15]

3. In uremia, there is a disproportionate increase in apoC-III levels and decrease in the ratio of apoC-II/apoC-III. Accumulation of remnant particles that are rich in apolipoprotein E facilitates binding to the arterial wall for prolonged duration and predisposes to atherogenesis.[16]

C. **Low HDL-C**

1. Epidemiological studies have demonstrated that high HDL levels are associated with favorable cardiovascular outcomes, but at present, HDL is not a target for therapy in the general population or in CKD patients.[17]

2. Studies suggest that in CKD, the proteinuria leads to decreased apolipoprotein A-1, which in turn causes lower HDL levels.[18] However, the primary issue in CKD relates to the quality (functional properties) rather than the quantity of HDL with decreased maturation of cholesterol ester-poor HDL-3 to cholesterol ester-rich HDL-2 due to decreased lecithin-acetylcholine transferase (LCAT) activity. This decreased ability of the HDL particles to carry cholesterol leads to impairment of reverse cholesterol transport from peripheral cells to the liver, thereby burdening the vasculature with cholesterol and promoting atherosclerosis.[19]

III. Lipid Abnormalities With Renal Replacement Therapy

A. In patients with end-stage renal disease (ESRD) on dialysis, the abnormalities seen in the lipid profile are essentially the same as in predialysis patients. The choice of renal replacement therapy results in additional alterations in the lipid profile such as increased triglyceride levels.

B. In patients on hemodialysis (HD), the use of high-flux polysulfone or cellulose triacetate membranes instead of low flux membranes favors decreased triglyceride levels and increased apoA-I and HDL-C levels.[20] This could be partly explained by the increase in the ratio of apoC-II to apoC-III, which in turn increases lipoprotein lipase activity. Studies have also shown that using bicarbonate dialysate instead of acetate increases HDL-C levels.[21]

C. Although controversial, the use of heparin, which is known to release endothelial lipoprotein lipase leading to the depletion of the enzyme, can also adversely affect lipid levels, and low molecular weight heparin has shown more favorable effects, in comparison.[7,22]

D. Among patients on continuous ambulatory peritoneal dialysis (CAPD), increased atherogenic, small dense LDL and apolipoprotein B, higher Lp(a) levels, and decreased HDL-C levels have been reported.[23] The underlying mechanism seems to be the exaggerated proteinuria seen in CAPD patients resembling protein losses seen in patients with nephrotic syndrome, which may stimulate the liver to synthesize more albumin and cholesterol-enriched lipoproteins.[24] In addition, the glucose absorbed from the dialysate increases the insulin resistance and stimulates hepatic production of lipoproteins.[25] Recent studies show that the use of less absorbed icodextrin-containing dialysate for overnight dwell reduces the total cholesterol, triglycerides, and small dense LDL levels.[26]

IV. Dyslipidemia in Nephrotic Syndrome

A. Nephrotic syndrome (NS) is defined as the urinary total protein loss of ≥ 3.5 g/1.73 m^2 of body surface area per day[27] and may be the result of primary glomerular disease or associated with a systemic disease such as diabetes or lupus.

B. **Lipid profile in patients with NS**

1. A little over 50% of patients with NS have abnormal lipid profile, that is, elevated LDL or triglycerides. The dyslipidemia of NS has been associated with increased

cardiovascular risk, thrombotic risk, and also progression of glomerular disease to CKD. The duration of nephrotic hyperlipidemia appears to be critical to initiating vascular damage.[28] This is indirectly supported by analysis of data from an adult population with a history of childhood NS that did not progress to CKD or ESRD. In children where the NS resolved early with treatment, there was no increase in risk of coronary heart disease when compared to the general population, in the absence of treatment for the dyslipidemia.[29]

2. In about 75% of the cases, NS responds to steroids/immune suppressive therapy and goes into remission indicating that the duration of nephrotic hyperlipidemia may not be prolonged.

3. Lipoprotein(a) has characteristically been noted to be elevated in patients with nephrotic syndrome.

4. An increase in triglycerides (TGs) including VLDL remnants and chylomicron remnants is observed later in the course of the disease.[30]

C. Statin treatment for NS

1. Numerous trials in the 1990s evaluated the efficacy of a variety of statin agents showing reduction of LDL by 25%-50%, TC by 25%-37%, and TG by 13%-30% in treatment intervals ranging from 1 to 24 months in patients with nephrotic dyslipidemia.[30–35]

2. Based on current ACC/AHA guidelines, high-intensity statins may be warranted in most nephrotic syndrome patients as the average LDL cholesterol levels in this patient population is well above the 190 mg/dL placing patients in the statin benefit group.[36]

3. It is important to consider the age of the patient, the etiology of the NS, and the likely duration of the disease before initiation of statin therapy.

D. Current recommendations Current recommendations include assessing overall CVD risk using any of the risk scores in those with NS when LDL is <190 mg/dL, where the only manifestation of CKD is proteinuria and not a decline in GFR. The benefit from statins in NS is not limited to reduction in lipid numbers but also in decreasing anti-thrombotic effects and in decreasing disease proteinuria.[33,37,38]

V. Management of Dyslipidemia in Chronic Kidney Disease

A. CKD as a cardiovascular disease risk factor

1. CKD is a recognized risk factor for CVD, and the risk of coronary heart disease increases with age and worsening renal function as shown in Table 15c.2.[39] CKD has been evaluated as a CAD equivalent compared to diabetes.[40] While diabetes increases the incidence rate of MI 2.5 times, in those with CKD, the hazard ratio (HR) is 3.5 or even higher. When CKD and diabetes are present, the cumulative incidence of MI approaches 20% over 10 years.[41]

2. Guidelines
A summary of current guidelines is provided in Table 15c.3.
a. 2013 ACC/AHA Guidelines
The expert panel made "no recommendations regarding the initiation or discontinuation of statins in patients on maintenance hemodialysis" and does not include CKD in risk scoring.

Table 15c.2. Unadjusted Rates (95% CI) of Coronary Death or Nonfatal MI (per 1000 patient-years) From the Alberta Kidney Disease Cohort: Interaction Between Age and GFR

Age Groups GFR mL/min	Overall	Male	Female
Age >40 y GFR > 60 GFR ≤ 60	14.9 (14.6-15.3) 19.3 (18.8-19.8) 9.7 (9.3-10.0)	17.4 (16.9-17.9) 23.4 (22.6-24.2) 12.0 (11.4-12.6)	12.7 16.4 (15.8-17.0) 6.7 (6.3, 7.2)
Age 40-50 y GFR > 60 GFR ≤ 60	3.2 (2.9-3.6) 4.7 (3.7-6.0) 3.0 (2.6-3.3)	4.7 (4.2-5.4) 5.9 (4.3-8.1) 4.6 (4.0-5.3)	1.6 (1.2-2.0) 3.6 (2.5-5.3) 3.6 (2.5-5.3)
Age >50 y GFR > 60 GFR ≤ 60	17.3 (17.0-17.7) 19.9 (19.4-20.4) 12.9 (12.4-13.4)	20.2 (19.6-20.8) 24.3 (23.4-25.2) 15.2 (14.5-16.0)	14.8 (14.3-15.3) 16.9 (16.3-17.5) 6.7 (6.3, 7.2)

Table 15c.3. Comparison of Guidelines for Treatment of Dyslipidemia in Patients With CKD

CKD Stage	2013 ACC/AHA	NLA	KDIGO
Stage 1-3A	1. Moderate-intensity statin if clinical ASCVD/LDL >190 mg/dL 2. No clinical ASCVD but risk ≥7.5% moderate- to high-intensity statin in diabetic and nondiabetic	1. 1 ASCVD risk factor: treat if LDL > 160 mg/dL or non-HDL > 190 mg/dL 2. 2 ASCVD risk factors: treat if LDL > 130 mg/dL or non-HDL > 160 mg/dL 3. >3 ASCVD risk factors: treat if LDL > 100 mg/dL or non-HDL > 130 mg/dL 4. Clinical ASCVD or diabetes regardless of LDL	1. Age > 50 y: treat with moderate-intensity statin 2. Age 18-49 y: treat with moderate-intensity statin if the following present: • Known ASCVD • Diabetes • 10-y risk of MI or cardiac death >10%
Goal of treatment	None	1. For ASCVD and diabetes: LDL < 70 mg/dL Non-HDL < 100 mg/dL 2. For 1-3 or more RF LDL 100 mg/dL non-HDL 130-160 mg/dL	None
Stage 3B-4	1. Moderate-intensity statin if clinical ASCVD/LDL >190 mg/dL 2. No clinical ASCVD but risk ≥7.5% moderate- to high-intensity statin in diabetic and nondiabetic	All considered high risk and therefore would benefit from statin use	1. Age >50 y: treat with moderate-intensity statin + ezetimibe 2. Age 18-49 y: treat with moderate-intensity statin + ezetimibe if the following present: • Known ASCVD • Diabetes • 10-y risk of MI or cardiac death >10%
Goal of treatment	None	Treat to LDL < 100 mg/dL non-HDL to <130 mg/dL	None
Stage 5 (dialysis)	No recommendation	No recommendation	No treatment but continue statin if started previously
Post transplantation	No recommendation	No recommendation	Moderate-intensity statin

ACC/AHA, American College of Cardiology/American Heart Association; NLA, National Lipid Association; KDIGO, Kidney Disease-Improve Global Outcomes.

b. 2016 ACC Expert Consensus on Nonstatin therapy

The ACC publication on the use of nonstatin therapies in the management of dyslipidemia does include CKD, stages 1-4 (but excluding dialysis), as a comorbidity that entails higher risk that may benefit from greater LDL reduction especially if the LDL reduction is <50% with the maximally tolerated statin therapy.[42] It is however important to note that calculation of risk based on the ASCVD risk calculator would identify up to 92% of CKD patients as high risk and therefore would qualify for moderate- to high-intensity statin therapy.[43]

c. 2015 National Lipid Association Recommendations

The NLA identifies CKD ≥ stage 3B as a high or very high risk for ASCVD and isolated albuminuria (urine albumin/creatinine ratio ≥ 30 mg/g) as a risk indicator that might be considered for risk refinement. Stage 5 or on hemodialysis is noted to be a very high-risk condition but that "RCTs of lipid-altering therapies have not provided convincing evidence of reduced events in such patients." The NLA recommends addition of these variables to the standard ASCVD risk score to assess risk and define management strategies.

d. 2013 Kidney Disease-Improved Global Outcomes (KDIGO) Guidelines

These guidelines specifically address management of lipids in CKD. The KDIGO[44] guidelines only base treatment recommendations on age and GFR, and LDL is not required to estimate risk in this population. This arises from understanding of the pathophysiology of CVD in CKD that LDL levels may not be elevated in CKD but existing proatherogenic lipoprotein abnormalities promote the increased risk. The primary recommendations include the following:

   i. Initial screening with a fasting lipid panel in all patients with the initial diagnosis of CKD. Subsequent annual follow-up measurement is not recommended except in select circumstances.

   ii. In patients aged 18-49 years and CKD, treatment for hyperlipidemia with statin is recommended only if additional risk factors (known coronary artery disease, MI, or coronary revascularization; diabetes mellitus; prior ischemic stroke) are present or if calculated 10-year risk of coronary death or nonfatal MI is >10%.

   iii. In adults aged ≥50 years with eGFR < 60 mL/min/1.73 m^2 but not treated with chronic dialysis or kidney transplantation, treatment is recommended with a statin or statin/ezetimibe combination.

   iv. In adults aged ≥50 years with CKD and eGFR ≥ 60 mL/min/1.73 m^2, treatment with a statin is recommended. This includes adults with albuminuria or polycystic kidney disease that have preserved or increased GFR.

   v. In dialysis-dependent CKD patients, recommendations are to avoid initiating statin or statin/ezetimibe combination.

   vi. In patients already receiving statins or statin/ezetimibe combination at the time of dialysis initiation, recommendation is to continue the agents.

   vii. In adult kidney transplant recipients, recommendations favor treatment with statin.

VI.   Choice and Safety of Lipid-Lowering Agents in CKD

A. Lowering LDL with a statin continues to be the cornerstone of dyslipidemia treatment in CKD, similar to the general population.

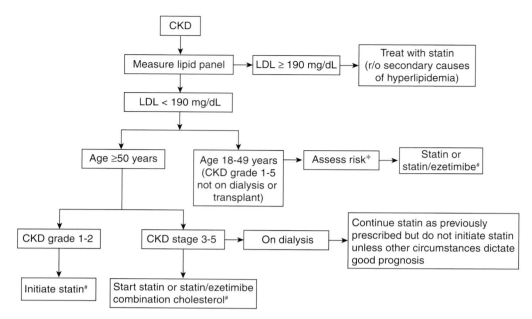

*High risk-prior coronary disease (MI or revascularization), diabetes, prior ischemic stroke, estimated 10 year incidence of coronary death or nonfatal MI > 10%.

Although KDIGO guidelines do not suggest a goal for LDL, the NLA guidelines suggest a goal of <100 mg/dL for LDL in those with Stage 3-5 CKD and the new ACC/AHA 2016 update suggest a 50% reduction in LDL in those with CKD.

FIGURE 15c.1: Algorithm for treatment of dyslipidemia in CKD in adults ages >18 years.

B. The treatment algorithm (Fig. 15c.1) should be based on GFR. Drugs eliminated mainly by the hepatic route should be preferred (fluvastatin, atorvastatin, pitavastatin, and ezetimibe). Statins metabolized via CYP3A4 may result in adverse effects due to drug-drug interactions, and dose adjustment becomes important in more advanced stages of CKD (stages 3-5), as adverse events are commonly dose related and due to increased blood concentration of the compound.[45] However, it is important to individualize statin dose based on underlying condition and patient tolerance such as the 55-year-old male with CKD, and a recent myocardial infarction would certainly benefit from a high-intensity statin as shown in the treating-to-target (TNT) trial[46] (See Table 15c.4).

Table 15c.4. Recommended Statin Doses for Patients With CKD and GFR < 60 mL/min/m^{2a}	
Lovastatin	**Not known**
Fluvastatin	80 mg
Atorvastatin	20 mg
Pravastatin	40 mg
Rosuvastatin	10 mg
Simvastatin	40 mg
Pitavastatin	2 mg
Simvastatin/Ezetimibe	20 mg/10 mg

^{a}These are the doses studied in the various trials reported under clinical trials.

C. In those with statin intolerance, ezetimibe can be used for LDL reduction although there is no evidence of reduced cardiac events with this drug when used alone.

D. Fibrates Fibrates are not first-line therapy in CKD and can be rarely used with some limitations listed below. Growing evidence indicates that fibrates increase serum creatinine without any effect on creatinine excretion into urine leading to erroneous estimation of GFR. Fenofibrate is also nondialyzable and should not be used in patients with GFR < 50 mL/min/1.73 m². The dose of gemfibrozil is recommended to be reduced to 600 mg/d if GFR is <60 mL/min/1.73 m² and avoided if GFR is <15 mL/min/1.73 m².

E. There is no concern for safety of niacin or fish oil, but there are also no data supporting its use in CKD.

F. Therapeutic lifestyle changes are recommended in all patients with CKD, especially those with persistent hypertriglyceridemia despite statin therapy.

G. The newer PCSK9 agents have not been studied in CKD, but it is interesting to note that PCSK9 levels in the blood are elevated in patients with CKD but decrease with initiation of HD.[45]

H. The 2016 update on use of nonstatin therapies supports the use of ezetimibe followed by bile acid resins or PCSK9 inhibitors as next line to statins in all patients including those with CKD not on dialysis.

I. No data or recommendations exist for use of mipomersen or lomitapide in patients with CKD.

VII. Clinical Trial Evidence Supporting Treatment Recommendations in Patients With CKD and ESRD on Dialysis

A. Initial evidence of dyslipidemia treatment in CKD came from post-hoc subgroup analyses of large secondary and primary prevention statin trials such as the Cholesterol and Recurrent Events (CARE) trial, Long-Term Intervention with Pravastatin in Ischemic Disease (LIPID) trial, and West of Scotland Coronary Prevention Study (WOSCOPS) and included patients with CKD who were not on dialysis with stage 1 and stage 2 disease.[47–49] These trials showed significant reductions in cardiovascular disease (CVD) events and total mortality in the CKD patients, which were comparable to the general population.

B. The Pravastatin Pooling Project (PPP)[50] showed that the benefit was most marked in subjects with both CKD and diabetes. In the Heart Protection Study (HPS), the absolute risk reduction was 11% in a subgroup of subjects with mild CKD as compared with 5.4% in the total cohort.[51] In early CKD identified only by proteinuria, CARE (Cholesterol and Recurrent Events) and CARDS (Collaborative Atorvastatin and Diabetes Study) trials found no significant interaction between presence of albuminuria and effect of statin on cardiovascular events[47,52] suggesting that the beneficial effect of statin is similar in patients with and without albuminuria. PREVEND IT (Prevention of Renal and Vascular End-stage Disease Intervention Trial) was a study of pravastatin/placebo in individuals with moderately increased albuminuria and preserved creatinine clearance[53] where pravastatin did not decrease the risk of cardiovascular events (HR, 0.87; 95% CI, 0.49-1.57). Hence, the evidence supporting statin use in those with isolated proteinuria and preserved GFR is low but nevertheless included in the KDIGO guidelines. It is important to recognize however that the majority of patients with this phenotype and age >50 years would typically qualify for a statin based on the ACC/AHA risk calculator since diabetes and hypertension are the most common causes of proteinuria in the United States.

C. Prospective randomized controlled trial evidence of lipid lowering in CKD primarily came from the SHARP (Study of Heart and Renal Protection) trial. This trial included 9270 participants older than 40 years with a serum creatinine level >1.7 mg/dL in men and >1.3 mg/dL in women and a mean estimated glomerular filtration of eGFR of 27 mL/min/1.73 m², who were randomized to receive simvastatin 20 mg plus ezetimibe 10 mg daily or placebo, and followed for 5 years. An average reduction of 0.85 mmol/L LDL resulted in a significant 17% reduction in major atherosclerotic events in patients on simvastatin and ezetimibe compared to placebo. Importantly, the benefits were proportionally equal among dialysis and nondialysis patients but not statistically significant in the dialysis subgroup.[54]

D. Dialysis patients

1. Trials that specifically examined treatment of lipids in dialysis patients have consistently been negative.

2. In a cohort of 1200 patients with diabetes on hemodialysis in the Die Deutsche Diabetes Dialyse Studie (4D) trial, atorvastatin had no positive effect on the primary composite end point of CVD.[55] The results from AURORA (A study to evaluate the Use of Rosuvastatin in subjects On Regular hemodialysis: an Assessment of survival and cardiovascular events) involving 2776 patients on hemodialysis showed that rosuvastatin lowered LDL-C as expected but had no significant effect on the composite CVD end point. The lack of efficacy was noted in all subgroup analyses including diabetics, LDL > 130, known CVD and high hs-CRP.[56]

3. Shorter duration of follow-up and causes of mortality not related to atherosclerotic disease, such as heart failure and arrhythmias, have all been proposed as plausible explanation for the lack of benefit of statin in this high-risk population.

4. Therefore, the KDIGO guidelines do not recommend initiation of a statin/statin and ezetimibe combination in patients being initiated on dialysis. Nevertheless, this practice can be embraced with a few caveats, namely, in those patients on dialysis, with recent MI or revascularization, the benefit of statin initiation outweighs the risk/lack of efficacy. Similarly younger individuals, such as those with diabetes who are commencing dialysis, should be initiated on a statin since the lifetime risk of CVD is very high and the longer duration of treatment may have benefits. Patients with CKD who have been on statin prior to commencing dialysis should be continued on the medication.

VIII. Dyslipidemia After Kidney Transplantation

A. Demographics

1. Hyperlipidemia is said to have an overall prevalence of 60% among transplant recipients.[57] The incidence of hypercholesterolemia peaks within 6 months of transplant, whereas hypertriglyceridemia peaks around 12 months after transplantation.[58] The prevalence of hypercholesterolemia is at least 2-3 times that of pretransplant at the end of 2 years.

2. In addition to traditional risk factors, pretransplant lipid profile, level of renal dysfunction, proteinuria, concomitant use of diuretics or beta-blockers, steroid use, and immunosuppressant use are implicated in the pathogenesis of dyslipidemia in this patient population.

3. Patients who develop postrenal transplantation coronary artery disease (CAD) tend to be older males, diabetics, higher cholesterol levels, smokers, and experienced greater number of acute renal allograft rejection episodes and, as a consequence, have received more cumulative dose of steroids.[59]

B. Recommendations

1. Hyperlipidemia not only increases cardiovascular risk but also increases the risk of chronic graft failure.[60] Assessment of hyperlipidemia should be initiated soon after transplantation and annually thereafter. KDIGO guidelines recommend that all adult kidney transplant recipients be treated with a statin.

2. The major study underpinning this recommendation was the ALERT (Assessment of Lescol in Renal Transplantation) trial. This randomized controlled trial noted that treatment with fluvastatin did not reduce major adverse cardiac events, the primary end point. However, cardiac deaths and nonfatal myocardial infarction, 2 of the 3 major adverse cardiac events (MACE) studied, were significantly reduced.[61] An unblinded extension study suggested that major adverse cardiac events—cardiac deaths, nonfatal MI, and coronary interventions—were attenuated in the long term.[62]

3. The KDIGO lipid guideline work group considered that the apparent benefits observed in ALERT are consistent with the effects of statins in the general population and suggests that statins offer benefit to kidney transplant recipients with a functioning transplant. The appropriate statin doses in this population are not well established but suffice to say that in the presence of immunosuppressants that may interfere with statin metabolism, dose adjustments must be considered.[63–65]

IX. Management of CKD and Dyslipidemia in Children and Young Adults

A. In children with CKD, progression is likely, and considering atherosclerosis as a long-term complication, it may be appropriate to visualize the lifetime trajectory of the particular child, teen, or young adult and assess cumulative risk exposures as they age. Half the children with eGFR < 75 mL/min/1.73 m^2 will reach ESRD in only 5 years and 70% in 10 years.[46] Likewise, most children with ESRD "progress" to transplantation: by 1 year after identification of ESRD, 50% of children receive a kidney transplant suggesting that long-term complications develop while moving through the stages of CKD and renal replacement therapies.

B. While there are data suggesting an association of lipids with increased carotid intima-media thickness in a subset of children in the CKiD (CKD in Children Cohort) study,[67] there have been no trials of lipid treatment with either clinical outcomes or surrogate outcomes in this population.[66] Therefore, there are no guidelines for initiation of statin or statin/ezetimibe combination therapy in children with CKD despite the understanding that CVD is the largest cause for decreased life expectancy in young adults with CKD.[68] It is however recommended to check a lipid panel at baseline and annual follow-up to identify inherited lipid abnormalities such as familial hypercholesterolemia, secondary causes of hyperlipidemia, and specifically hypertriglyceridemia that may occur in the setting of nephrotic syndrome.

X. Conclusions

Cardiovascular disease is the major cause of morbidity and mortality in CKD. There are data to support treatment of dyslipidemia in all stages of CKD both in the primary and in the secondary prevention settings. More research is warranted in this population to understand accurate assessment of risk while incorporating measures such as albuminuria and newer measures of lipoprotein assessment such as lipoprotein(a) and apolipoproteins.

References

1. Gansevoort RT, Correa-Rotter R, Hemmelgarn BR, et al. Chronic kidney disease and cardiovascular risk: epidemiology, mechanisms, and prevention. *Lancet.* 2013;382:339-352.
2. National Kidney Foundation. K/DOQI clinical practice guidelines for chronic kidney disease: evaluation, classification, and stratification. *Am J Kidney Dis.* 2002;39(2 suppl 1):S1-S266.
3. Keith DS, Nichols GA, Gullion CM, Brown JB, Smith DH. Longitudinal follow-up and outcomes among a population with chronic kidney disease in a large managed care organization. *Arch Intern Med.* 2004;164:659-663.
4. http://www.usrds.org. Accessed on March 31, 2016.
5. Muntner P, He J, Astor BC, Folsom AR, Coresh J. Traditional and nontraditional risk factors predict coronary heart disease in chronic kidney disease: results from the atherosclerosis risk in communities study. *J Am Soc Nephrol.* 2005;16(2):529-538.
6. Piecha G, Adamczak M, Ritz E. Dyslipidemia in chronic kidney disease: pathogenesis and intervention. *Pol Arch Med Wewn.* 2009;119(7-8):487-492.
7. Tsimihodimos V, Dounousi E, Siamopoulos KC. Dyslipidemia in chronic kidney disease: an approach to pathogenesis and treatment. *Am J Nephrol.* 2008;28(6):958-973.
8. Austin MA, King MC, Vranizan KM, Krauss RM. Atherogenic lipoprotein phenotype. A proposed genetic marker for coronary heart disease risk. *Circulation.* 1990;82:495-506.
9. Ikewaki K, Schaefer JR, Frischmann ME, et al. Delayed in vivo catabolism of intermediate-density lipoprotein and low-density lipoprotein in hemodialysis patients as potential cause of premature atherosclerosis. *Arterioscler Thromb Vasc Biol.* 2005;25(12):2615-2622.
10. Vaziri ND, Moradi H. Mechanisms of dyslipidemia of chronic renal failure. *Hemodial Int.* 2006;10(1):1-7.
11. Tsimihodimos V, Mitrogianni Z, Elisaf M. Dyslipidemia associated with chronic kidney disease. *Open Cardiovasc Med J.* 2011;5:41-48.
12. Sechi LA, Catena C, Zingaro L, Melis A, De Marchi S. Abnormalities of glucose metabolism in patients with early renal failure Diabetes *Diabetes.* 2002;51(4):1226-1232.
13. Charlesworth JA, Kriketos AD, Jones JE, Erlich JH, Campbell LV, Peake PW. Insulin resistance and postprandial triglyceride levels in primary renal disease. *Metabolism.* 2005;54:821–828.
14. Arnadóttir ML. Pathogenesis of dyslipoproteinemia in renal insufficiency: the role of lipoprotein lipase and hepatic lipase. *Scand J Clin Lab Invest.* 1997;57(1):1-11.
15. Moberly JB, Attman PO, Samuelsson O, Johansson AC, Knight-Gibson C, Alaupovic P. Apolipoprotein C-III hypertriglyceridemia and triglyceride-rich lipoproteins in uremia. *Miner Electrolyte Metab.* 1999;25:258-262.
16. Leary ET, Wang T, Baker DJ, et al. Evaluation of an immunoseparation method for quantitative measurement of remnant-like particle-cholesterol in serum and plasma. *Clin Chem.* 1998;44:2490-2498.
17. Kalil RS, Wang JH, de Boer IH, et al. Effect of extended-release niacin on cardiovascular events and kidney function in chronic kidney disease: a post hoc analysis of the AIM-HIGH trial. *Kidney Int.* 2015;87(6):1250-1257.
18. Cheung AK, Wu LL, Kablitz C, Leypoldt JK. Atherogenic lipids and lipoproteins in hemodialysis patients. *Am J Kidney Dis.* 1993;22(2):271-276.
19. Moradi H, Pahl MV, Elahimehr R, Vaziri ND. Impaired antioxidant activity of high-density lipoprotein in chronic kidney disease. *Transl Res.* 2009;153(2):77-85.
20. Blankestijn PJ, Vos PF, Rabelink TJ, van Rijn HJ, Jansen H, Koomans HA. High-flux dialysis membranes improve lipid profile in chronic hemodialysis patients. *J Am Soc Nephrol.* 1995;5(9):1703-1708.
21. Jung K, Scheifler A, Schulze BD, Scholz M. Lower serum high-density lipoprotein-cholesterol concentration in patients undergoing maintenance hemodialysis with acetate than with bicarbonate. *Am J Kidney Dis.* 1995;25(4):584-588.
22. Schrader J, Stibbe W, Armstrong VW, et al. Comparison of low molecular weight heparin to standard heparin in hemodialysis/hemofiltration. *Kidney Int.* 1988;33(4):890-896.
23. Kronenberg F, Lingenhel A, Neyer U, et al. Prevalence of dyslipidemic risk factors in hemodialysis and CAPD patients. *Kidney Int Suppl.* 2003;(84):S113-S116.
24. Heimburger O, Stenvinkel P, Berglund L, Tranoeus A, Lindholm B. Increased plasma lipoprotein(a) in continuous ambulatory peritoneal dialysis is related to peritoneal transport of proteins and glucose. *Nephron.* 1996;72:135-144.
25. Johansson AC, Samuelsson O, Attman PO, et al. Dyslipidemia in peritoneal dialysis—relation to dialytic variables. *Perit Dial Int.* 2000;20:306-314.
26. Bredie SJ, Bosch FH, Demacker PN, Stalenhoef AF, van Leusen R. Effects of peritoneal dialysis with an overnight icodextrin dwell on parameters of glucose and lipid metabolism. *Perit Dial Int.* 2001;21(3):275-281.
27. Stephan R, Orth MD, Eberhard Ritz MD. The nephrotic syndrome. *N Engl J Med.* 1998;338:1202-1211.
28. Park SJ, Shin JI. Complications of nephrotic syndrome. *Korean J Pediatr.* 2011;54(8):322-328.
29. Lechner BL, Bockenhauer D, Iragorri S, Kennedy TL, Siegel NJ. The risk of cardiovascular disease in adults who have had childhood nephrotic syndrome. *Pediatr Nephrol.* 2004;19(7):744-748.

30. Spitalewitz S, Porush JG, Cattran D, Wright N. Treatment of hyperlipidemia in the nephrotic syndrome: the effects of pravastatin therapy. *Am J Kidney Dis*. 1993;22(1):143-150.
31. Kasiske BL, Velosa JA, Halstenson CE, La Belle P, Langendörfer A, Keane WF. The effects of lovastatin in hyperlipidemic patients with the nephrotic syndrome. *Am J Kidney Dis*. 1990;15(1):8-15.
32. Prata MM, Nogueira AC, Pinto JR, et al. Long-term effect of lovastatin on lipoprotein profile in patients with primary nephrotic syndrome. *Clin Nephrol*. 1994;41(5):277-283.
33. Biesenbach G, Zazgornik J. Lovastatin in the treatment of hypercholesterolemia in nephrotic syndrome due to diabetic nephropathy stage IV-V. *Clin Nephrol*. 1992;37(6):274-279.
34. Warwick GL, Packard CJ, Murray L, et al. Effect of simvastatin on plasma lipid and lipoprotein concentrations and low-density lipoprotein metabolism in the nephrotic syndrome. *Clin Sci (Lond)*. 1992;82(6):701-708.
35. Valdivielso P, Moliz M, Valera A, et al. Atorvastatin in dyslipidaemia of the nephrotic syndrome. *Nephrology (Carlton)*. 2003;8(2):61-64.
36. Stone NJ, Robinson JG, Lichtenstein AH, et al.; American College of Cardiology/American Heart Association Task Force on Practice Guidelines. 2013 ACC/AHA guideline on the treatment of blood cholesterol to reduce atherosclerotic cardiovascular risk in adults: a report of the American College of Cardiology/American Heart Association Task Force on Practice Guidelines. *Circulation*. 2014;129(25 suppl 2):S1-S45.
37. Resh M, Mahmoodi BK, Navis GJ, Veeger NJ, Lijfering WM. Statin use in patients with nephrotic syndrome is associated with a lower risk of venous thromboembolism. *Thromb Res*. 2011;127(5):395-399.
38. Wei JL, Cui HM, Ma CY. Simvastatin inhibits tissue factor and plasminogen activator inhibitor-1 secretion by peripheral blood mononuclear cells in patients with primary nephrotic syndrome. *Eur J Med Res*. 2007;12(5):216-221.
39. Coresh J, Selvin E, Stevens LA, et al. Prevalence of chronic kidney disease in the United States. *JAMA*. 2007;298(17):2038-2047.
40. Debella YT, Giduma HD, Light RP, Agarwal R. Chronic kidney disease as a coronary disease equivalent—a comparison with diabetes over a decade. *Clin J Am Soc Nephrol*. 2011;6(6):1385-1392.
41. Debella YT, Giduma HD, Light RP, et al. Chronic Kidney Disease as a Coronary Disease Equivalent—A Comparison with Diabetes over a Decade. *Clin J Am Soc Nephrol*. 2011;6(6):1385-1392.
42. Lloyd-Jones DM, Morris PB, Ballantyne CM, et al. 2016 ACC Expert Consensus Decision Pathway on the Role of Non-Statin Therapies for LDL-Cholesterol Lowering in the Management of Atherosclerotic Cardiovascular Disease Risk. *J Am Coll Cardiol*. 2016;70(14):1785-1822.
43. Muntner P, Gutierrez OM, Zhao H, et al. Validation study of medicare claims to identify older US adults with CKD using the reasons for geographic and racial differences in stroke (REGARDS) study. *Am J Kidney Dis*. 2015;65(2):249-258.
44. Sarnak MJ, Bloom R, Muntner P, et al. KDOQI US commentary on the 2013 KDIGO Clinical Practice Guideline for Lipid Management in CKD. *Am J Kidney Dis*. 2015;65(3):354-366.
45. Konarzewski M, Szolkiewicz M, Sucajtys-Szulc E, et al. Elevated circulating PCSK-9 concentration in renal failure patients is corrected by renal replacement therapy. *Am J Nephrol*. 2014;40(2):157-163.
46. Shepherd J, Kastelein JJ, Bittner V, et al. Intensive lipid lowering with atorvastatin in patients with coronary heart disease and chronic kidney disease: the TNT (Treating to New Targets) Study. *J Am Coll Cardiol*. 2008;51(15):1448-1454.
47. Sacks FM, Pfeffer MA, Move LA, et al.; for the Cholesterol and Recurrent Events Trial Investigators. The effect of pravastatin on coronary events after myocardial infarction in patients with average cholesterol levels. *N Engl J Med*. 1996;335:1001-1009.
48. The Long Term Intervention with Pravastatin in Ischemic Disease (LIPID) Study group. Prevention of cardiovascular events and death with pravastatin in patients with coronary heart disease and a broad range of initial cholesterol levels. The Long-Term Intervention with Pravastatin in Ischaemic Disease (LIPID) Study Group. *N Engl J Med*. 1998;339(19):1349-1357.
49. Palmer SC, Navaneethan SD, Craig JC, et al. HMG CoA reductase inhibitors (statins) for people with chronic kidney disease not requiring dialysis. *Cochrane Database Syst Rev*. 2014;(5):CD007784.
50. Tonelli M, Keech A, Shepherd J, et al. Effect of pravastatin in people with diabetes and chronic kidney disease. *J Am Soc Nephrol*. 2005;16:3748–3754.
51. Collins R, Armitage J, Parish S, Sleigh P, Peto R; Heart Protection Study Collaborative Group. MRC/BHF Heart Protection Study of cholesterol-lowering with simvastatin in 5963 people with diabetes: a randomised placebo-controlled trial. *Lancet*. 2003;361:2005–2016.
52. Colhoun HM, Betteridge DJ, Durrington PN, et al. Effects of atorvastatin on kidney outcomes and cardiovascular disease in patients with diabetes: an analysis from the Collaborative Atorvastatin Diabetes Study (CARDS). *Am J Kidney Dis*. 2009;54(5):810-819.
53. Asselbergs FW, Diercks GF, Hillege HL, et al. Effects of fosinopril and pravastatin on cardiovascular events in subjects with microalbuminuria. *Circulation*. 2004;110(18):2809-2816.

54. Baigent C, Landray MJ, Reith C, et al.; SHARP Investigators. The effects of lowering LDL cholesterol with simvastatin plus ezetimibe in patients with chronic kidney disease (Study of Heart and Renal Protection): a randomised placebo-controlled trial. *Lancet.* 2011;377(9784):2181-2192.
55. Wanner C, Krane V, März W, et al.; German Diabetes and Dialysis Study Investigators. Atorvastatin in patients with type 2 diabetes mellitus undergoing hemodialysis. *N Engl J Med.* 2005;353:238–248.
56. Fellström BC, Jardine AG, Schmieder RE, et al.; AURORA Study Group. Rosuvastatin and cardiovascular events in patients undergoing hemodialysis. *N Engl J Med.* 2009;360:1395-1407.
57. Robertsen I, Asberg A, Granseth T, et al. More potent lipid-lowering effect by rosuvastatin compared with fluvastatin everolimus-treated renal transplant recipients. *Transplantation.* 2014;97(12):1266-1271.
58. Razeghi E, Shafipour M, Ashraf H, Pourmand G. Lipid disturbances before and after renal transplant. *Exp Clin Transplant.* 2011;9(4):230-235.
59. Diaz JM, Gich I, Bonfill X, et al. Prevalence evolution and impact of cardiovascular risk factors on allograft and renal transplant patient survival. *Transplant Proc.* 2009;41(6):2151-2155.
60. Raees-Jalali G, Eshraghian A, Faghihi A, et al. Hyperlipidemia after kidney transplantation: long-term graft outcome. *Iran J Kidney Dis.* 2012;6(1):49-55.
61. Holdaas H, Fellström B, Jardine AG, et al.; Assessment of LEscol in Renal Transplantation (ALERT) Study Investigators. Effect of fluvastatin on cardiac outcomes in renal transplant recipients: a multicentre, randomised, placebo-controlled trial. *Lancet.* 2003;361(9374):2024-2031.
62. Holdaas H, Fellström B, Cole E, et al.; Assessment of LEscol in Renal Transplantation (ALERT) Study Investigators. Long-term cardiac outcomes in renal transplant recipients receiving fluvastatin: the ALERT extension study. *Am J Transplant.* 2005;5(12):2929-2936.
63. Lemahieu WP, Hermann M, Asberg A, et al. Combined therapy with atorvastatin and calcineurin inhibitors: no interactions with tacrolimus. *Am J Transplant.* 2005;5(9):2236-2243.
64. Lemahieu WP, Maes BD, Verbeke K, Vanrenterghem Y. CYP3A4 and P-glycoprotein activity in healthy controls and transplant patients on cyclosporin vs. tacrolimus vs. sirolimus. *Am J Transplant.* 2004;4(9):1514-1522.
65. Shitara Y, Takeuchi K, Nagamatsu Y, Wada S, Sugiyama Y, Horie T. Long-lasting inhibitory effects of cyclosporin A, but not tacrolimus, on OATP1B1- and OATP1B3-mediated uptake. *Drug Metab Pharmacokinet.* 2012;27(4):368-378.
66. Jacobson TA, Ito MK, Maki KC, et al. National Lipid Association recommendations for patient-centered management of dyslipidemia: part 1—executive summary. *J Clin Lipidol.* 2014;8(5):473-488.
67. Brady TM, Schneider MF, Flynn JT, et al. Carotid intima-media thickness in children with CKD: results from the CKiD Study. *Clin J Am Soc Nephrol.* 2012;7(12):1930-1937.
68. Smith JM, Stablein DM, Munoz R, Hebert D, McDonald RA. Contributions of the Transplant Registry: the 2006 Annual Report of the North American Pediatric Renal Trials and Collaborative Studies (NAPRTCS). *Pediatr Transplant.* 2007;11(4):366-373.

Lipid Management in Older Patients

Joyce L. Ross

Key Points

- "Older" and "elderly" encompass ages from 65 to >100 years old and are very heterogeneous patient populations
- At present, there are no risk assessment tools or scoring systems specifically directed to older persons. Age is considered a risk factor
- Current guidelines and recommendations do not provide comprehensive information on diagnosis and management of older persons
- Statins as well as nonstatin medications should be considered safe and effective for older persons despite relative lack of information from observational studies and clinical trials

I.   Who Are Older Patients?

A. Definition

1. Most developed countries accept the chronological age of 65 as the definition of "elderly" per the World Health Organization.[1,2] The elderly or older patients are a complex and heterogeneous group of individuals encompassing a range of years from 65 to >100. No other chronological age classification is this expansive and is likely responsible for misinterpretation with regard to treatment in this population.

2. Chronological age varies culturally and historically; therefore, "elderly" is a social construct rather than a definitive biological score.[3] Forman et al.[4] recognize the diversity of old age by defining subgroups of the population into three areas, the young old, old, and the old-old, further demonstrating that all elderly are not comparable (Table 15d.1). Old age further comprises multiple dimensions, including chronological, biological, psychological, and social constructs.

3. Of note, an individual's chronological age may differ considerably from the functional age. Distinguishing markers of old age also occur in all five senses but at different times and at different rates. This diversity requires unique and often complex plans of care with regard to treatment of cardiovascular risk for both primary and secondary prevention.[1,2]

4. Cardiovascular disease represents a multifaceted and prevalent disease in the United States (US) and the world in general (Table 15d.2). Older patients are a population that requires careful consideration since they have been found to be underdiagnosed and therefore undertreated in primary care and cardiology.

Table 15d.1. Subgroups of Aging	
Chronological age	Subgroup
65-74	Young old
74-84	Old
85 plus	Old-old

Adapted from Forman DE, Berman AD, McCabe CH, Baim DS, Wei JY. PTCA in the elderly: the "young-old" versus the "old-old". *J Am Geriatr Soc.* 1992;40(1):19-22.

Table 15d.2.	The Elderly and Vascular Disease		
Age	**Cardiovascular Problem**	**Men**	**Women**
60-79 years of age	CVD, heart failure, stroke of hypertension, or some combination of all	69.1%	67.9%
≥80 years of age	CVD, stroke, or deaths attributable to CVD	84.7%	85%
	Age of first heart attack	65 years	71.8 years
	Stroke 70% in patients ≥65 years of age		

Data from Jacobson TA, et al. National Lipid Association Recommendations for Patient-Centered Management of Dyslipidemia: Part 2. *J Clin Lipidol*. 2015; 9(6 suppl):S1-S122.

B. Demographics

1. The proportion of people ≥65 years of age is expected to approach 19.6% worldwide by 2030. By 2050, the subgroup of persons ≥85 years of age in the United States is expected to triple.[5] While aging can vary substantially from one individual to another, ≥75 years of age is commonly used as the threshold for the beginning of old age. By 75, most adults have sustained sufficient aging changes to exhibit clinically relative differences in physiology and organ function and reserves.[2] In the United States, >80% and 85% of cardiovascular deaths and hospitalization, respectively, occur in persons >65 years of age.

   There are a number of reasons why older age predisposes to high cardiovascular mortality and morbidity,[2] which include a greater complexity of atherosclerotic lesions, delays in initiating therapy, multiple cardiovascular and noncardiovascular diseases occurring simultaneously, and compounding management challenges. These compounding liabilities relate to interactions of pathophysiologies such as anemia and coronary heart disease; interaction of medications, with a likelihood of polypharmacy; as well as the cumulative burden of care.[6]

II. Atherosclerotic Cardiovascular Risk (ASCVD Risk Assessment) in Older Adults

A. **Risk assessment** Improved cardiovascular management for the elderly must start with comprehensive assessment of the individual's health as well as a multifaceted health context, with therapy then personalized to the individual patient's situation. Both the 2013 ACC/AHA Guidelines[7] and the NLA Dyslipidemia Recommendations Parts 1 and 2[1,8] emphasize use of a patient-centered approach to care by delineating differences between treatment that are primarily oriented to prolonging life vs treatment that may be better suited to improving function, symptoms, and other aspects of quality of life. At present, we do not have a specific risk assessment tool or measures that apply to older patients to determine which patients will or will not be most likely to benefit from aggressive treatment.[8]

B. Scoring systems

1. Relationship to age current scoring systems that assess ASCVD risk in this population reflect the progressive increase in absolute risk that occurs with advancing age as evidenced by an age-related increase in atherosclerotic plaque burden. It is important, however, to note that population norms often do not apply to individual patients. Application of average risk scores applied to specific patients may lead to miscalculation of risk and inappropriate consideration of drug therapy.[2,8]

   A Rotterdam study of 4854 patients with a mean age of 65 years in which researchers applied the ACC/AHA Pooled Cohort Risk Equation, utilizing ≥7.5% 10 year as the threshold for consideration of initiation of moderate- or high-intensity statin therapy. Results identified 96.4% of men and 65.8% of women as potential candidates for such therapy. In this population, the average predicted vs observed cumulative incidence of ASCVD events was 21.5% vs 12.7% for men and 11.6% vs 7.9% in women, reflecting poor calibration of risk in this European sample.[2,8]

2. **Adjustments to risk scoring in older patients**
   a. In 1999, the AHA Scientific Statement on ASCVD Risk Assessment suggested that when risk scoring is used to adjust the intensity of risk factor management in elderly patients, relative risk reduction estimates, which eliminate the age factor and focuses on the major risk factors, might be more useful than absolute risk estimates. This approach allows providers to risk stratify and compare patients of the same age and select those at highest relative risk for the most aggressive treatment strategies. Other study results suggest that serum lipids partially lose their predictive power for relative ASCVD risk prediction in the elderly. A variety of reasons are identified for this phenomenon including the increased number of comorbidities among patients of advanced age.[2]
   b. It has been suggested that use of coronary artery calcification (CAC) may be of greater use in more fully assessing this population without known cardiovascular disease. Because calcification of the coronary arteries can be seen as a cumulative measure of lifetime exposure to cardiovascular risk factors, CAC may be especially important for assessment in the elderly. In a Rotterdam study evaluating 2028 patients using EBCT imaging of the epicardial arteries, CAC scores were reported utilizing Agatston's method of calculation. In a mean follow-up period of 9.2 years, there were 135 hard coronary events. Subjects were classified into low-, intermediate-, and high-risk categories using a Framingham refitted risk model.[9,10] The model was extended by coronary artery calcification, and reclassification percentages were calculated. Utilizing the results reclassification of a total of 52% of men and women were reclassified into either higher- or lower-risk categories. Of note, the need for reclassification was found primarily in those previously classified as intermediate risk.
   c. Although measurement of CAC appears to provide a more accurate means of risk assessment than traditional algorithms, certain caveats are noted including cost of the test, which is most often not covered by traditional insurance, lack of availability at health care institutions, and relative lack of studies linking results with outcomes. While these limiting factors are recognized in the general population and more so in the elderly population, nevertheless when such testing is available, it may be a valuable addition to CHD risk assessment.[2,4]

3. **Choice of risk calculator and scoring system** The National Lipid Association Recommendations suggest that risk calculation such as the ACC/AHA Pooled Cohort Risk Calculator or the ATP III Framingham Risk Calculator can be used in older individuals using the thresholds for high risk of ≥15% 10-year risk for a hard ASCVD event with the pooled cohort equations or ≥10% 10-year risk for a hard CHD event using the ATP III calculator. These risk calculators have several limitations for use in the older population since advanced age is often the predominate driver of increased ASCVD risk, which may result in overtreatment of lower-risk older individuals.[2]

C. Value of statin therapy in older patients

1. **Background** There appears to be a weaker correlation of cholesterol with ASCVD in older vs younger individuals since many patients with higher cholesterol and more susceptibility to CVD may have died before reaching old age, thereby reducing the number of patients with higher cholesterol among the population of older adults

and resulting in lower mean lipid levels among older survivors. Although lifelong dyslipidemia contributes to the development, promotion, and progression of atherosclerosis, clinical ASCVD events in older individuals may be more often related to nonlipid ASCVD risk factors.

2. **Statin therapy in primary prevention** Observational cohorts such as the Cardiovascular Health Study sponsored by NHLBI have provided information on dyslipidemia and primary prevention of coronary heart disease; however, relatively few randomized clinical trials have been designed to investigate interventions in this age group.

    The 2013 ACC/AHA Guideline did not include specific recommendations for either primary or secondary prevention in people >75 years old as it was felt that fewer people in the age group were included in the statin randomized clinical trials that were reviewed.

3. **Secondary prevention studies in older adults treated with statin therapy** Lipid-lowering therapy in older patients is a valuable adjunct to secondary prevention of ASCVD. Few studies have specifically addressed use of lipid-lowering therapy in older patients, although many statin studies have included subjects between the ages of 65 and 75 and have demonstrated similar relative risk reduction (RRR) and safety in older and younger individuals.[11,12] (see Table 15d.3.)

4. **Statin safety in older adults**
    a. Biases

        There are recognized biases in reporting side effects of statin therapy in older adults. Randomized controlled trials (RCTs) often suggest a higher incidence of side effects in older vs younger populations treated with statins; however, this concept has certain limitations. Observational studies often report a higher incidence of side effects than do RCTs in elderly patients. Patients entering RCTs and experiencing side effects during run-in periods or exhibiting conditions that predispose to side effects are often excluded. Validated injury instruments that assess for harm may not be employed. Other issues including definition of adverse events, selective reporting of outcomes, and publication bias may affect the reported incidence of side effects as well.[2,13]

    b. Muscle symptoms

        It is generally reported that older individuals have a higher incidence of statin-associated muscle symptoms than do younger patients. It is unclear whether these effects are related to a decrease in muscle mass that occurs with normal aging or polypharmacy, also common among older patients, increasing the potential for drug-drug interactions, and a loss in the function of enzymes necessary for drug metabolism are responsible for these muscle symptoms. Either independently or

Table 15d.3. Meta-analysis of Patients 65-82 for Risk Reduction from 9 Secondary Statin Trials of 19 569 Subjects	Absolute Risk Reduction	Relative Risk Reduction
All cause mortality	22%	3.1%
CHD mortality	30%	2.6%
Nonfatal MIs	26%	2.3%
Need for revascularizations	30%	Not reported

Adapted from Afilalo J, Duque G, Steele R, Jukema JW, de Craen AJ, Eisenberg MJ. Statins for secondary prevention in elderly patients: a hierarchical Bayesian meta-analysis. *J Am Coll Cardiol.* 2008;51:3.

in combination, these factors need to be considered with statin therapy in the elderly population. Results from a study based on the Understanding Statin Use in America and Gaps in Education (USAGE) Internet survey[14] revealed more muscle side effects in older patients and that older patients were more likely to discontinue a statin due to muscle side effects.[2]

 c. Diabetes

   Another issue for consideration in the elderly population is diabetes, which has high known prevalence in this population. In JUPITER, patients with a median age of 66.0 years and at least 1 major diabetes risk factor were at higher risk for developing diabetes than were patients without a major diabetes risk factor.[14] This is consistent with the finding from the 2014 NLA Task Force on Statin Safety Update, clinical trial data, including meta-analyses, which suggest a modest, but statistically significant increase in the incidence of new-onset type 2 diabetes with statin vs no statin use or higher- and lower-intensity statin use. However, since cardiovascular events and mortality benefits of statins have exceeded the diabetes hazard in all patients, it is recommended that periodic glucose monitoring, and when appropriate glycated hemoglobin measurement, be performed when administering statin therapy in this population.[2,13]

 d. Cognitive function

   i. Cognitive dysfunction with statin use has also been an area of concern in the elderly population. The NLA Task Force on Statin Safety—2014 Update[13] defined cognitive dysfunction as impairment in any of four domains, including executive function, memory, language, and visuospatial ability. Mild cognitive impairment was defined as a state of cognitive dysfunction between normal cognition and dementia involving 2 domains and is sufficiently severe to interfere with activities of daily living associated with progressive loss of independence. Clinically, it is especially important to differentiate a potential medication side effect causing cognitive impairment from other causes of dementia in older patients, including Alzheimer disease, frontoparietal dementia, Parkinson disease, Lewy body dementia, infectious processes, inflammatory vascular or metabolic disorders, and depression.[1,2,8]

   ii. The NLA Task Force on Statin Safety put forth the following perspectives on statins and cognitive dysfunction. They specify that statins as a class are not associated with adverse effects on cognition and therefore suggest that a baseline cognitive assessment does not need to be performed prior to initiation of therapy. In patients who report cognitive symptoms after beginning a statin, cognitive testing should be performed, other potential contributors ruled out, and the risk of stopping a statin assessed. Other considerations indicate that the provider may consider stopping the statin to assess the reversibility of symptoms, lowering the dose, or switching to an alternative statin. Consideration for selection of other statins should include starting a statin that is less likely to penetrate the brain including pravastatin or rosuvastatin.[1,2,8]

D. Nonstatin therapy in older patients The 2016 ACC Expert Consensus document on use of nonstatins follows the 2013 ACC/AHA Guidelines and does not specifically address nonstatin drug use in patients >75 years old. Use of nonstatin drugs for older patients should be based on information for the general population. See discussion in Chapter 10 of this text.

E. Polypharmacy and drug-drug interactions

 1. Polypharmacy, defined as the concurrent use of five or more medications, is common in older patients and is likely contributed to by normal changes in aging such as absorption, bioavailability, and volume of distribution. Multiple pathways of altered metabolism have been described in statin drug-drug interactions; the CYP3A4 and CYP2C9 pathways are most commonly implicated.[17]

2. In addition, single-nucleotide polymorphisms in organic anion transporter 1B1 may be an additional cause of statin-related drug interactions. Greater than 50% of medications prescribed to the elderly are metabolized by this pathway thereby increasing the risk for drug-to-drug interaction to occur. It has been suggested that older patients on polypharmacy regimens be regularly evaluated for drug-to-drug interactions with medication reconciliation carefully performed at each clinic visit.[1,2]

III. Conclusion

The elderly, who are becoming an increasing proportion of our population, represent a diverse group of the population who are often underdiagnosed and undertreated for the prevention of cardiovascular disease. Specific and directed assessment techniques will be necessary for a thorough evaluation including the use of risk calculators. Until we have more dedicated guidelines and recommendations, those for the general population should be used for older patients. The National Lipid Association Recommendations for Patient-Centered Management of Dyslipidemia: Part 2 synthesize current literature and best practices to provide a hands-on tool for the provider who treats the elderly patient (see Tables 15d.4 and 15d.5).

Table 15d.4.	**Guideline Recommendations for Lipid Management in Older Patients**		
Organizations	**Treatment in Those >65 Years of Age**	**Patients >75 Years of Age**	**Patients >80 Years of Age**
2013 ACC/AHA Guidelines for Treatment of Blood Cholesterol	• **LDL-C is the target of treatment for cardiovascular risk reduction.** • **Primary prevention**—use of Pooled Cohort Risk Equation to inform statin treatment • Use of provider-patient discussion with regard to treat or not • **Secondary prevention**—high-intensity statin therapy recommended • Triglyceride reduction/goals are not addressed within these guidelines.	• **Primary prevention** in those >75 to <80 y • The Pooled Cohort Risk Equation can be used to provide information on expected 10-y ASCVD risk as well as for those 76-79 y of age that may inform the treatment decision. • Use of provider-patient discussion with regard to decision to use statin therapy is necessary. • **Secondary prevention** in those >75 to >80 y of age may be treated similar to those >65 to <75 y of age. • Moderate-intensity statin therapy recommended vs high-intensity therapy after a consideration of the risk-benefit ratio of such therapy	• Recommendations for patients >80 y of age were not clearly delineated within these guidelines. • Few data are available to indicate an ASCVD risk reduction in primary care in those >75 y. • RCT evidence supports the continuation of statins beyond 75 y in persons who are already taking and tolerating them. • Few data were available to indicate an ASCVD event reduction benefit in primary prevention among individuals >75 y who do not have clinical ASCVD; therefore, initiation of statins for primary prevention of ASCVD in that population requires consideration of additional factors including increasing comorbidities, safety consideration, and priorities of care. • A larger amount of data support the use of moderate-intensity statin therapy for secondary prevention in individuals with ASCVD > 75 y old. Available data did not clearly support initiation of high-intensity statin therapy in individual >75 y. • Initiation of high-intensity statin

(Continued)

Table 15d.4. Guideline Recommendations for Lipid Management in Older Patients (*Continued*)			
Organizations	**Treatment in Those >65 Years of Age**	**Patients >75 Years of Age**	**Patients >80 Years of Age**
2015 NLA Recommendations for the Patient-Centered Management of Dyslipidemia: Parts 1 and 2	• **Primary prevention**—primary prevention strategies in those 65-79 y of age should first focus on exclusion and correction of secondary causes of dyslipidemia. • Strategies in those 65 to <80 y lifestyle management should be used for 3-6 mo. If unable to achieve goal, should discuss pros and cons of therapy. If feasible, moderate-intensity statin therapy, particularly for those with 1 or more ASCVD risk factors aside from age using the Pooled Risk Equation or ATP III Framingham Risk Calculator. CAC scoring may be useful in this population to inform decisions. • **Secondary prevention** • In patients >65 to <80 y of age, moderate- or high-intensity statin therapy should be considered after a careful consideration of the risk-benefit ratio. • Those with serum triglycerides 150-499 mg/dL should receive dietary counseling focusing on the following: • Initial goal of 5%-10% body weight loss in those who are overweight or obese • Reduction in simple carbohydrate intake • Increased consumption of dietary fiber • Elimination of dietary trans-fatty acids • Reduction in consumption of fructose and saturated fat • Intake and increased consumption of marine-based long-chain omega-3 fatty acids • A minimum of 150 min/wk of moderate-intensity cardiorespiratory exercise is advised. • The initial objective is to reduce serum triglycerides to <500 mg/dL, at which point the therapeutic target then becomes achievement of non–HDL-C and LDL-C goals as suggested by the NLA Recommendations: Part 1. • For those with fasting triglycerides 500-999 mg/dL • The concomitant use of triglyceride-lowering pharmacotherapy, often with statins as the first step in those with no history of pancreatitis, should be considered although the FDA recently pulled the approval of use with statins and fibrates and niacin. • For those with serum triglycerides ≥1000 mg/dL • Nonstatin triglyceride-lowering drug therapy with fibrates, long-chain marine omega-3 fatty acids, and/or niacin is a reasonable therapeutic option.	• **Secondary prevention**—moderate-intensity statin therapy should be considered based upon a provider-patient discussion of the risk and benefits of therapy. • Aggressive treatment with lifestyle management and medication to reduce non–HDL-C when necessary in this age group	• **Secondary prevention**—in those >80 with atherogenic lipoproteins above stated goals and ASCVD. Moderate-intensity statin therapy should be considered based upon a provider-patient discussion of risks and benefits of such therapy. • Drug-to-drug interactions, polypharmacy, and concomitant medical conditions including frailty need to be considered as well as cost considerations and patient preferences.

Adapted from Stone NJ, et al. 2013 ACC/AHA Blood Cholesterol Guidelines. *J Am Coll Cardiol.* 2014;63:2889-2934; Jacobson TA, et al. NLA dyslipidemia recommendations: part 2. *J Clin Lipidol.* 2015;9(6 suppl):S1-S122.

Table 15d.5.   Recommendations for Older Patients From the NLA Dyslipidemia Recommendations: Part 2

Recommendation	Strength	Quality
Primary prevention strategies in patients 65-79 y of age should be managed in accordance with the NLA Recommendations for the Patient-Centered Management of Dyslipidemia: Part 1.1	A	High
For patients aged ≥65 to <80 y of age with ASCVD or diabetes mellitus, moderate- or high-intensity statin therapy should be considered after a careful consideration of the risk-benefit ratio.	A	High
For secondary prevention in patients ≥80 y of age, moderate-intensity statin therapy should be considered based upon a provider-patient discussion of the risks and benefits of such therapy, consideration of drug-drug interactions, polypharmacy, concomitant medical conditions including frailty, cost considerations, and patient preference.	B	Moderate
Risk calculators such as the ACC/AHA Pooled Cohort Risk Calculator or the ATP III Framingham Risk Calculator can be used in select older individuals with one additional risk factor to further assess risk, using the thresholds for high risk of ≥15% 10-year risk for a hard ASCVD event (MI, stroke, or death from CHD or stroke) with the Pooled Cohort Equations and ≥10% 10-year risk for a hard CHD event (MI or CHD death) using the ATP III Framingham Risk Calculator. However, these risk calculators have several limitations for use in older patients, since advanced age is often the predominate driver of increased ASCVD risk, and this may result in overtreatment of lower-risk older individuals.	E	Low
Older, primary prevention patients who are statin eligible should undergo a patient-centered discussion with their provider about the risks and benefits of statin therapy so that they can make a more informed decision about taking statins over the long term.	E	Low
If the older primary prevention patient is unable to achieve atherogenic cholesterol goals after a minimum 3-6 mo trial on lifestyle modification, the provider should discuss the pros and cons of drug therapy and, if feasible, prescribe moderate-intensity statin therapy, particularly for patients with one or more ASCVD risk factor aside from age, with risk exceeding the high-risk threshold using the Pooled Risk Equation or ATP III Framingham Risk Calculator.	E	Moderate
CAC scoring may be useful to further assess risk in older patients for whom questions remain about whether to prescribe drug therapy.	E	Low
If statin intolerance is an issue, consideration should be given to the use of alternate statin regimens such as low-intensity statin therapy or nondaily moderate-intensity statin therapy; low-dose statin combination therapy with ezetimibe, bile acid sequestrants, or niacin; or non-statin monotherapy (ie, ezetimibe or bile acid sequestrant) or their combination, with a goal of at least a 30% reduction in LDL-C.	B	Moderate

Adapted from Jacobson TA, et al. NLA dyslipidemia recommendations: part 2. *J Clin Lipidol.* 2015;9(6 suppl):S1-S122.

References

1. Mozaffarian D, Benjamin EJ, et al. American Heart Association Statistics Committee and Stroke Statistics 2015 Update. *Circulation.* 2015;131:e29-e322.
2. Forman DE, Rich MW, Alexander KP, et al. Cardiac care for older adults. Time for a new paradigm. *J Am Coll Cardiol.* 2011;57:1801-1810.
3. Jacobson TA, et al. NLA dyslipidemia recommendations: part 2. *J Clin Lipidol.* 2015;9(6 suppl):S1-S122.
4. Stone NJ, Robinson JG, Lichtenstein AH, et al. 2013 ACC/AHA guidelines on the treatment of blood cholesterol to reduce atherosclerotic cardiovascular risk in adults: a report of the American College of Cardiology/American Heart Association Task Force on Practice Guidelines. *J Am Coll Cardiol.* 2014;63(25 Pt B):2889-2934.
5. Jacobson TA, Ito MK, Mak KC, et al. National lipid association recommendations for patient-centered management of dyslipidemia: part 1—full report. *J Clin Lipidol.* 2015;9:129-169.
6. Baigent C, Keech A, Kearney PM, et al.; Cholesterol Treatment Trialists' (CTT) Collaborators. Efficacy and safety of cholesterol-lowering treatment: prospective meta-analysis of data from 90,056 participants in 14 randomized trials of statins. *Lancet.* 2005;366:1267-1278.
7. Orringer C, Grundy S, Ross J, CRNP in Jacobson et al. NLA dyslipidemia recommendations: part 2. *J Clin Lipidol.* 2015;9(6 suppl):S1-S122.
8. Vliegenthart R, Oudkerk M, Holman A, et al. Coronary calcification improves cardiovascular risk prediction in the elderly. *Circulation.* 2005;112:572-577.
9. Afilalo J, Duque G, Steele R, Jukema JW, de Craen AJ, Eisenberg MJ. Statins for secondary prevention in elderly patients: a hierarchical Bayesian meta-analysis. *J Am Coll Cardiol.* 2008;51:37-45.

10. Fleg JL, Forman DE, Berra K, et al.; American Heart Association Committees on Older Populations and Exercise Cardiac Rehabilitation and Prevention of Council on Clinical Cardiology, Council on Cardiovascular and Stroke Nursing, Council on Lifestyle and Cardiometabolic Health. Secondary prevention of atherosclerotic cardiovascular disease in older adults: a scientific statement from the American Heart Association. *Circulation.* 2013;128:2422-2446.

11. Cohen JD, Brinton EA, Ito MK, Jacobson TA. Understanding Statin Use in America and Gaps in Patient Education (USAGE): an internet-based survey of 10,138 current and former statin users. *J Clin Lipidol.* 2012;6:208-215.

12. Ridker P. The JUPITER trial. *Circ Cardiovasc Qual Outcomes.* 2009;2:279-285.

13. Rojas-Fernandez CH, et al. *J Clin Lipidol.* 2014;8-8:S5-S16.

14. Kellick KA, et al. *J Clin Lipidol.* 2014;8:S30-S46.

15. Rosenson RS, Baker SK, Jacobson TA, Kopecky SL, Parker BA; The National Lipid Association's Muscle Safety Expert Panel. An assessment by the Statin Muscle Safety Task Force: 2014 update. *J Clin Lipidol.* 2014;8(3 suppl): S58-S71. doi:10.1016/j.jacl.2014.03.004.

16. Forman D, Wenger NK. What do the recent ACC/AHA Foundation Clinical Practice Guidelines tell us about the evolving management of coronary heart disease in older adults? *J Geriatr Cardiol.* 2013;10:123-128.

Index

Note: Page numbers in *italics* denote figures; those followed by "b" and "t" denote boxes and tables.